Male Fertility and Lipid Metabolism

Editors

Stephanie R. De Vriese
Scientific Institute of Public Health
Brussels, Belgium

Armand B. Christophe
Ghent University Hospital
Ghent, Belgium

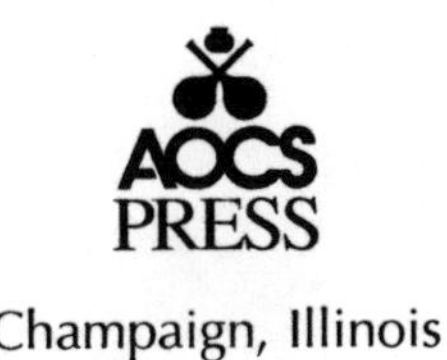

AOCS
PRESS

Champaign, Illinois

Library of Congress Cataloging-in-Publication Data
Male fertility and lipid metabolism / editors, Stephanie R. De Vriese, Armand B. Christophe.
    p. cm.
  ISBN 1-893997-39-1
1. Spermatozoa. 2. Fertility. 3. Unsaturated fatty
acids—Metabolism. 4. Lipids—Metabolism. I. Vriese, Stephanie R. De.
II. Christophe, Armand B.

  QP255.M2123 2003
  612.6'1--dc21

                                                                    2003006193

Printed in the United States of America with vegetable oil-based inks.

5 4 3 2 1

Preface

The interest in lipid metabolism and, more specifically, in polyunsaturated fatty acids in relation to sperm production has increased during the last decade. The motivation for the research described in this book originates from the discovery that sperm lipids contain extremely high proportions of long-chain polyunsaturated fatty acids, thus establishing a link between lipid biochemistry and male fertility. Moreover, the fact that polyunsaturated fatty acids must, in some form, be supplied in the diet suggests a relationship between fertility and nutrition and raises the possibility of improving male fertility by dietary means.

Reactive oxygen species play a pivotal role in male fertility. Increased generation of reactive oxygen species has been documented in subfertile men with varicocele, immunological infertility, and idiopathic oligozoospermia. Excessive reactive oxygen species can cause oxidative damage to the sperm DNA and the sperm membrane. The long-chain polyunsaturated fatty acids in the sperm membrane are highly susceptible to peroxidation. However, the high content of these long-chain polyunsaturated fatty acids is necessary for the optimal membrane fluidity required for the acrosome reaction and membrane fusion. Furthermore, sperm motility plays an important role in male fertility, as spermatozoa with decreased motility have reduced fertilizing capacity. It has been suggested that the fluidity of the membranes of the spermatozoa, which among others depends on the fatty acid composition of the phospholipids in the membrane, is related to sperm motility.

These new insights have contributed to the development of supplementation therapies with fatty acid mixtures and antioxidants.

This book intends to give the reader an up-to-date view of several aspects of male fertility in relation to lipid and fatty acid metabolism.

An overview of the different factors related to male fertility is given in chapter 1. Chapter 2 discusses the synthesis of long-chain polyunsaturated fatty acids by Sertoli cells in the testis. Chapters 3 to 5 deal with the phospholipid and fatty acid composition of human testicular cells and human sperm. The effect of supplementation of docosahexaenoic acid on male fertility is also described. Chapter 6 discusses the manipulation of the lipid composition of boar spermatozoa and its effect on reproductive efficiency in pigs. Chapters 7 and 8 address the lipid and fatty acid composition of avian semen. The regulation of mammalian and avian sperm production by dietary fatty acids is summarized in chapter 9. The role of sterols in the epididymis is discussed in chapter 10, whereas the physiological and biophysical properties of sulfogalactosylglycerolipid in male germ cells are handled in chapter 11. Chapter 12 discusses the regulation of oxytocinase activity in the testis by dietary lipids. Finally, chapters 13 to 16 deal with oxidative stress and oxidative damage of polyunsaturated fatty acids in spermatozoa and antioxidant protection of sperm.

The book should be useful for: researchers in the domain of male fertility, fatty acid metabolism, and antioxidants; medical personnel involved in the treatment of male infertility; fat technologists; students in nutrition, dietetics, biochemistry, pharmacy, and medicine; and everybody interested in the field.

Finally, we would like to express our thanks to all of the authors for their valuable discussions, suggestions, and contributions. The assistance provided by the AOCS Press staff in Champaign is gratefully acknowledged.

February 2003
Stephanie R. De Vriese
Armand B. Christophe
Editors

Contents

Chapter 1

Factors Affecting Male Fertility

F. Comhaire[a], A. Mahmoud[a], A. Zalata[b], and W. Dhooge[a]

[a]Ghent University Hospital, Department of Internal Medicine, Center for Medical and Urological Andrology, 6K12 IE, De Pintelaan 185, B-9000, Ghent, Belgium
[b]Biochemistry Department, Faculty of Medicine, Mansoura University, Egypt

Abstract

Male infertility is a multifactorial disease resulting from the interaction between genetic, lifestyle, and environmental factors and urogenital pathologies. In particular, endogenous and exogenous estrogenic substances and oxidative overload have been implicated in synergistic damage to male fertility. The deleterious effects are mediated through changes in the phospholipid composition of the sperm membrane, oxidative changes to DNA, and the suppression of the neuroendocrine regulation of spermatogenesis. The treatment of specific pathologies, *e.g.*, varicocele or accessory gland infection, even though it has significantly increased the effective rate of conception resulting in live birth of healthy children, has limited effectiveness. Complementary treatment with a pure antiestrogen and with antioxidants appears to enhance the reversal of pathogenic processes, resulting in improvement of the fertility status of infertile men.

Introduction

Spermatogenesis takes place in the seminiferous tubules of the testes. Male fertility requires adequate testicular stimulation (Fig. 1.1) and optimal function of the accessory sex glands. In developed countries, between 8 and 10% of all men are infertile and unable to attain conception in their partner within a time period of 12 months (1). The mechanisms through which impairment of male fertility occur are progressively being unravelled, and an efficient approach to the standardized investigation and diagnosis, as well as the clinical management, of the infertile male has been developed (1).

Regulation of Spermatogenesis

Pulsatile secretion of luteinizing hormone releasing hormone (LHRH) by the hypothalamus induces pulsatile release of luteinizing hormone (LH) by the pituitary, which causes pulsatile secretion of testosterone by the cells of Leydig in the interstitial space of the testes. Testosterone is released into the interstitial fluid surrounding the seminiferous tubules, which are themselves exposed to extremely high concentrations of

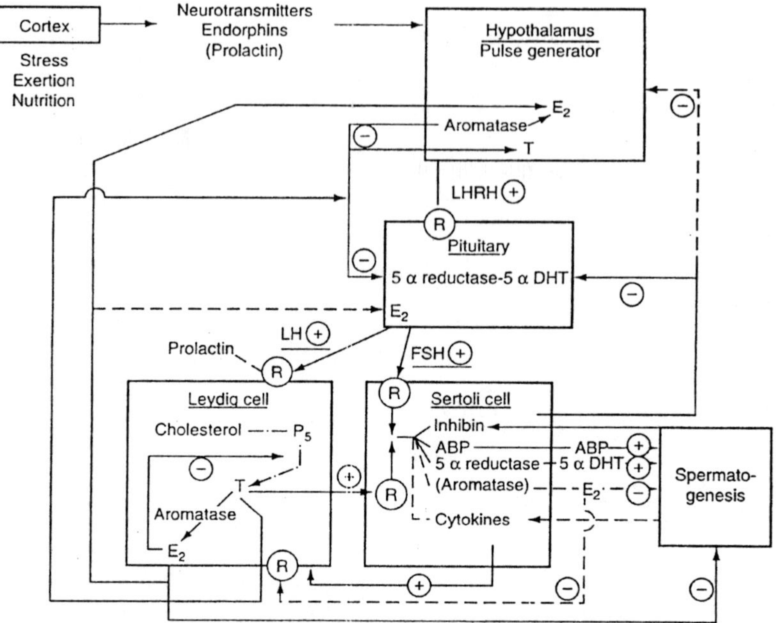

Fig. 1.1. Hormonal regulation of spermatogenesis.

this steroid (2). It is not known whether constant exposure of the seminiferous tubules to a high testosterone concentration has the same effect as pulsatile exposure, which may pace the tightly timed sequence of spermatogenesis. On the other hand, stimulation of the intratubular nutritive cells of Sertoli by follicle stimulating hormone (FSH) is required for optimal spermatogenesis, though some degree of sperm production can be maintained by the effect of testosterone alone (3).

The stimulatory system is controlled by neurotransmitters affecting the LHRH pulse generator and by feedback regulation (Fig. 1.1). The hypothalamo-pituitary unit is inhibited by testosterone that is aromatized to estradiol by the neuroendocrine cells of the hypothalamus and to 5-alfa-dihydrotestosterone in the pituitary. FSH secretion by the pituitary is under the feedback control of Inhibin B, a secretory product of the cells of Sertoli (4). There is some evidence that Inhibin B also exerts a direct inhibitory effect on spermatogenesis (5,6).

Male Infertility: A Multifactorial Disease

Four groups of factors act in synergy to reduce male fertility (Fig. 1.2). *Genetic causes* include, among others, translocations of autosomal chromosomes, numeric and structural abnormalities of the sex chromosomes (such as Klinefelter's syndrome), mutations of the cystic fibrosis gene, and microdeletions of the long arm of the Y chromo-

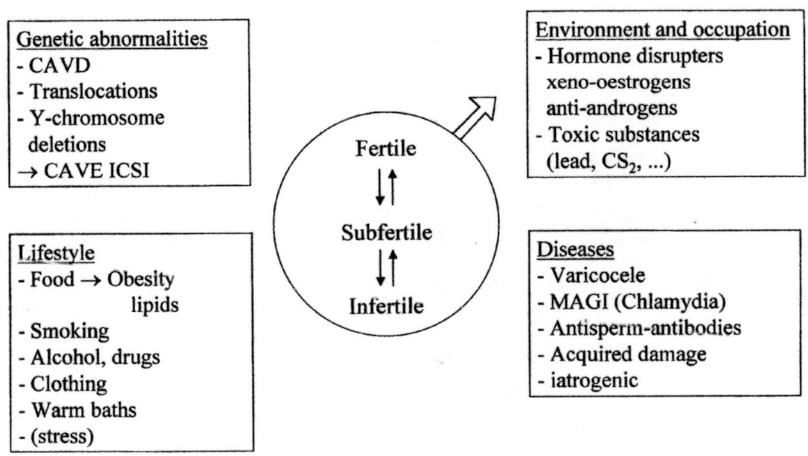

Fig. 1.2. Sub/infertility: A multifactorial disease.

some (Yq11.23). *Life style factors* include the excessive use of tobacco, alcohol, or recreational drugs; certain nutritional habits and obesity; regular exposure to high temperatures, such as during hot baths; tight clothing; and perhaps stress. There is strong evidence that *exposure to professional and environmental toxic agents* exerts major deleterious influence on sperm quality. In particular, substances with a hormone disrupting effect have been blamed because of their pseudo-estrogenic and/or antiandrogenic effects (7). Hormone disrupters include pesticides such as DDT and DDE, alkyl-phenols, polychlorinated biphenyls, dioxines, and also pharmaceutical products such as ethinylestradiol and, possibly, testosterone itself. The fourth group of factors refers to the more specific *andrological diseases of the urogenital tract* including varicocele, male accessory gland infection, immunological causes from anti-sperm-antibodies, and hormonal diseases such as hypogonadotropic hypogonadism. It has become increasingly evident that factors in different groups act in synergy. For instance, men with varicocele that do not smoke have a better sperm quality than those who smoke (8), and the number of white blood cells required to cause deterioration of sperm quality and production is lower in cases with than without coincidental genital pathology (Fig. 1.3a and b, A.M. Mahmoud *et al.*, unpublished data). The presence of certain gene mutations in men with varicocele might render them more susceptible to sperm DNA oxidative damage (9). Also, patients with varicocele are more susceptible to the known toxic effects of cadmium on spermatogenesis due to selective accumulation of this element in their testes (10).

Mechanisms of Sperm Deterioration

Whereas some infertile men present a single causal factor amendable to treatment (*e.g.,* hypogonadotropic hypogonadism), many others present a combination of fac-

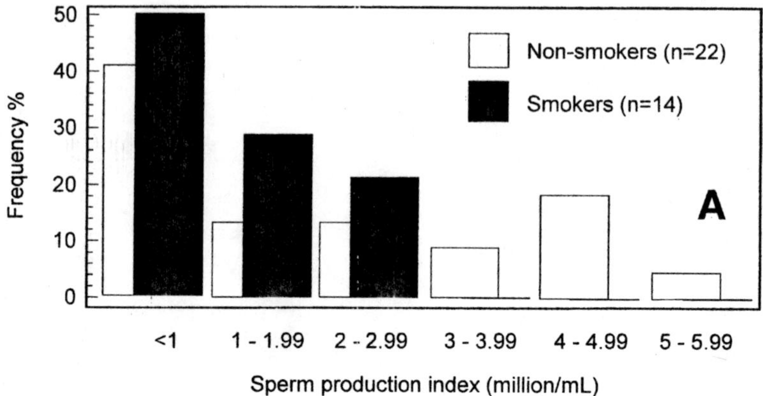

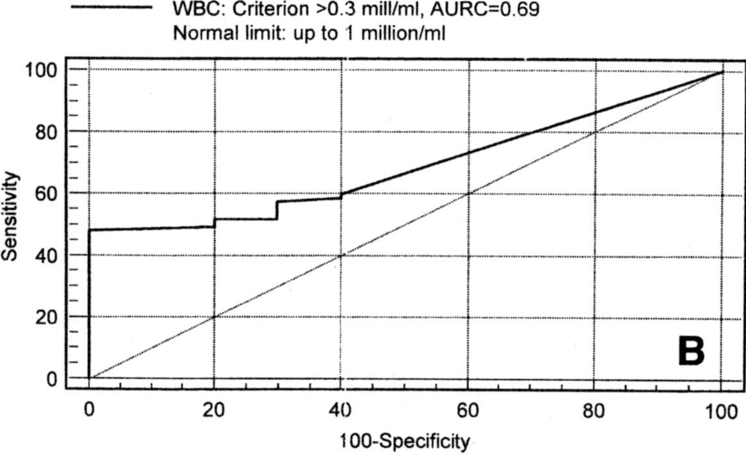

Fig. 1.3. A. Sperm production index: Total number of spermatozoa in the ejaculate (in million) divided by the total testicular volume in mL, normal value > 4.9 million/mL testis. B. White blood cells (WBC) (Receiver Operating Characteristic (ROC) curve) differentiate between varicocele patients with abnormal ($n = 75$) or normal ($n = 10$) sperm production index. Criterion = criterion value; AURC = area under ROC curve

tors. In the latter cases common mechanisms may be involved in disrupting spermatogenesis. We suggest that reactive oxygen species and hormonal imbalance are instrumental in this process (Fig. 1.4). Hormonal imbalance results from increased exposure of both the testes and the hypothalamo-pituitary unit to endogenous and/or exogenous estrogens. These decrease the mass of LHRH secreted during the pulses, reducing the secretion of LH and of testosterone. Also, the physiological increase of FSH fails to occur in response to low sperm concentration (oligozoospermia). In fact, estrogens have been documented to increase the Inhibin B secretion by cells of Sertoli cultured

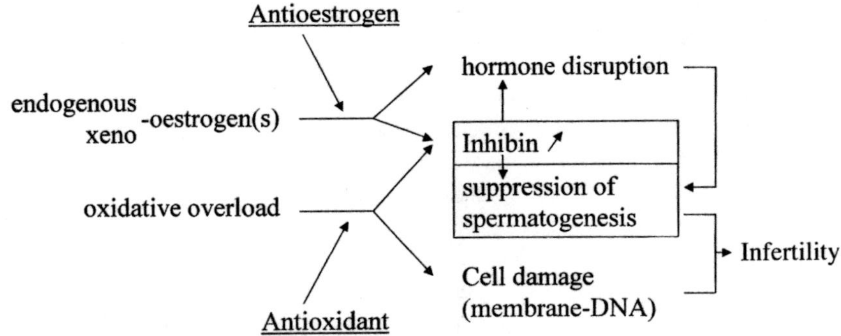

Fig. 1.4. Mechanisms of sperm deterioration.

in vitro (11). Also, oligozoospermic patients with normal concentrations of FSH and Inhibin B in serum were found to present increased serum concentrations of estradiol and probably of dehydroepiandrosterone (12). Since the concentration of testosterone (a major estrogen precursor) was not increased in these cases, it is suggested that estrogen precursors originating from the adrenal gland, increased aromatase activity, and/or decreased sulfotransferase-catalyzed estradiol inactivation are involved in the relative hyper-estrogenism (7,12,13). On the other hand, persons exposed to lead were found to present a lower mean sperm concentration and higher serum Inhibin B concentration than unexposed controls (14). This suggests a direct effect of lead on the cells of Sertoli, similar to that seen in patients with (endogenous) hyper-estrogenisms. Today the level of exposure to exogenous pseudo- or xeno-estrogens is very high in certain geographic regions (7). It is hypothesized that this causes excessive Inhibin B secretion by the cells of Sertoli, contributing to the development of "idiopathic" oligozoospermia.

Men suffering from idiopathic oligozoospermia who do not present elevated serum gonadotropin levels benefit from treatment with the specific antiestrogen Tamoxifen (Nolvadex®) that increases sperm concentration (15) and significantly enhances the probability of conception (16).

The pathologic factors of lifestyle, environment, and genitourethral origin all generate increased production of reactive oxygen species (ROS) and imbalance the oxidative status while also reducing the antioxidant capacity of seminal plasma (*e.g.,* in cases with male accessory gland infection) (17). The resulting oxidative overload exerts deleterious effects on both the membrane and the DNA content of spermatozoa that possess little antioxidant potential. Oxidative damage has been shown to change the phospholipid composition of the sperm membrane, with decreased content of polyunsaturated fatty acids (22:6n-3 in particular) reducing membrane fluidity (18). These changes diminish the fusogenic capacity of spermatozoa evidenced by a decrease of the induced acrosome reaction and by an impaired capacity of spermatozoa to fuse with the oocyte membrane. Oxidative DNA damage results in excessive amounts of 8-hydroxy-2-deoxyguanosin that may induce transition mutagenesis (19).

Also, the high concentration of oxidized DNA may overwhelm the natural capacity to repair DNA damage, allowing minor genetic DNA deletions or errors to come to expression.

Oxidative damage of the sperm membrane reduces the probability of spontaneous conception and the success rate of intrauterine insemination (20) and conventional *in vitro* fertilization (21). Since fertilization fails to occur, there is no increased risk of the oxidized DNA causing mutagenesis of the (pre)embryo(s). When intracytoplasmic injection (ICSI) of spermatozoa is performed, bypassing membrane fusion, damaged DNA can be introduced into the oocytes. This may result in an increased risk of embryonic abnormalities with both a higher rate of spontaneous (and induced) abortions and an increased prevalence of major congenital abnormalities in the offspring (22–25).

The Value of Antioxidants, Nutritional Supplementation, and Antiestrogens in the Treatment of the Infertile Male

Since hormone disruption as well as oxidative overload seems to play a pivotal role in the pathogenesis of male infertility, treatment should aim at eliminating possible causes of these factors. This includes lifestyle adaptations, such as smoking habits, exposure to excessive heat, changes in clothing, and adjustment of nutrition (26). Specific treatment of andrological diseases includes transcatheter embolization of the internal spermatic vein(s) in varicocele (27), antibiotic treatment in male accessory gland infection (28), injections of gonadotropins in men with hypogonadotropic hypogonadism, etc. Whenever possible, professional and environmental exposure to hormone disrupting or toxic agents should be avoided or reduced.

Although this approach significantly increases the effective rate of conception resulting in live birth of healthy children, its effectiveness is limited. In our patient population the effective cumulative pregnancy rate increases from approximately 1% per month in untreated controls to 3.5–4% per month in couples treated according to this approach (29,30).

Antiestrogen treatment of men with idiopathic oligozoospermia has a similar success rate and the majority of pregnancies occur within 6 to 9 months of treatment (31). These "conventional" treatment modalities produce better results in terms of pregnancy rates if the initial sperm concentration is low (less than approximately 10 million/mL), and they seem to be less effective in patients with moderate or borderline sperm deficiency. In the latter it is assumed that mainly sperm function is defective, requiring complementary management.

Infertile men were found to present oxidative imbalance in their serum; the lag time before oxidation of LDL cholesterol was shorter than that in fertile controls (32). In a double-blind trial we demonstrated that stability of LDL cholesterol against oxidative stress can be increased and that the lag time can be prolonged through the intake of a combination of vitamin A, vitamin E (d-α-tocopherol), vitamin C, selenium, and zinc (Quatral®, Nycomed) (33).

In an open label trial we studied the effects of 6 months of food supplementation with fish oil and natural vitamin E or acetylcysteine on semen quality and fertility of infertile men. This treatment significantly reduced the amount of reactive oxygen species in spite of unchanged concentrations of peroxidase positive white blood cells in semen. The phospholipid composition of the sperm membrane was shifted toward highly polyunsaturated fatty acids, increasing membrane fluidity. The induced, but not the spontaneous, acrosome reaction was increased, sustaining the beneficial effect of treatment on the function of the sperm membrane. There was a highly significant decrease in the concentration of oxidized DNA (8-hydroxy-2-deoxyguanosin), which reached normal values in all treated cases. The per-month rate of spontaneous conception was 9% in couples where the man was a (ex)smoker (34).

Finally, we performed a double-blind study in which infertile men were given 3 months of either natural Astaxanthin (AstaCarox®, Astacarotene, Sweden) or placebo. All patients received conventional treatment as recommended by WHO (1). Among patients receiving the complementary treatment with Astaxanthin, there was a significant decrease of ROS and an increase of linear progressive motility of the spermatozoa. Also, the attachment of spermatozoa to the zona-free hamster oocytes increased in the treated cases as compared to the controls, as well as the percentage of oocyte penetration (Fig. 1.5). A significant decrease of serum Inhibin B concentration was observed, in spite of unchanged sperm concentration. This suggests that ROS may stimulate the secretion of Inhibin B by the cells of Sertoli and that antioxidant supplementation can counteract this phenomenon.

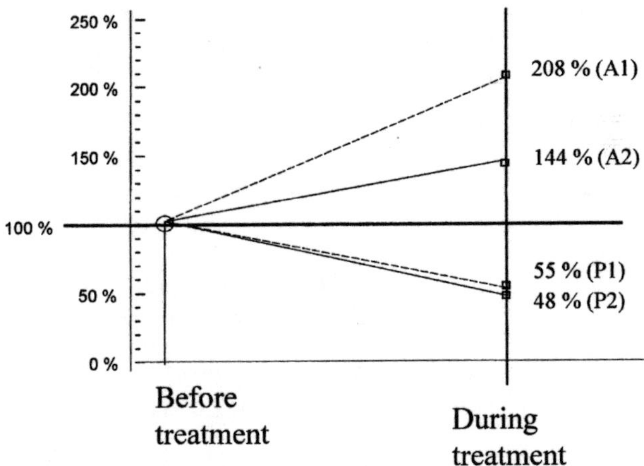

Fig. 1.5. Effects of Astaxantin (A1 & A2) compared to placebo (P1 & P2) on the average number of spermatozoa that have penetrated and are decondensed in the zona free hamster oocytes (A1 & P1), and the average number of spermatozoa that are firmly attached to the zona free hamster oocytes (A2 & P2). The average rate of penetration or attachment before treatment is set at 100 %.

In the 3 months follow-up period the per-month pregnancy rate was 23% in the treated group as compared to 3.6% in the controls. Post hoc analysis revealed that men with moderate sperm deficiency were more likely to benefit from the Astaxantin treatment.

Conclusion

The facts listed in the present paper support the concept of synergistic damage to male fertility resulting from estrogenic agents and oxidative overload. Deleterious effects are mediated through changes in the phospholipid composition of the sperm membrane, oxidative changes to DNA, and the suppression of the neuroendocrine regulation of spermatogenesis. Complementary treatment with a pure antiestrogen and with appropriate antioxidants can counteract these pathogenic processes, resulting in remarkable improvement of the fertility status of infertile men.

References

1. Rowe, P.J., Comhaire, F.H., Hargreave, T.B., and Mahmoud, A.M.A. (2000) *WHO Manual for the Standardized Investigation, Diagnosis and Management of the Infertile Male,* First Edition, Cambridge University Press, Cambridge.
2. de Kretser, D.M., Loveland, K.L., Meinhardt, A., Simorangkir, D., and Wreford, N. (1998) Spermatogenesis, *Hum. Reprod. 13 (Suppl. 1),* 1–8.
3. Kerr, J.B., Maddocks, S., and Sharpe, R.M. (1992) Testosterone and FSH Have Independent, Synergistic and Stage-Dependent Effects Upon Spermatogenesis in the Rat Testis, *Cell. Tissue. Res. 268,* 179–189.
4. Anderson, R.A., and Sharpe, R.M. (2000) Regulation of Inhibin Production in the Human Male and Its Clinical Applications, *Int. J. Androl. 23,* 136–144.
5. Weinbauer, G.F., and Wessels, J. (1999) 'Paracrine' Control of Spermatogenesis, *Andrologia. 31,* 249–262.
6. Bame, J.H., Dalton, J.C., Degelos, S.D., Good, T.E., Ireland, J.L., Jimenez-Krassel, F., Sweeney, T., Saacke, R.G., and Ireland, J.J. (1999) Effect of Long-Term Immunization Against Inhibin on Sperm Output in Bulls, *Biol. Reprod. 60,* 1360–1366.
7. Oliva, A., Spira, A., and Multigner, L. (2001) Contribution of Environmental Factors to the Risk of Male Infertility, *Hum. Reprod. 16,* 1768–1776.
8. Klaiber, E.L., Broverman, D.M., Pokoly, T.B., Albert, A.J., Howard, P.J.J., and Sherer, J.F.J. (1987) Interrelationships of Cigarette Smoking, Testicular Varicoceles, and Seminal Fluid Indexes, *Fertil. Steril. 47,* 481–486.
9. Chen, S.S., Chang, L.S., Chen, H.W., and Wei, Y.H. (2002) Polymorphisms of Glutathione S-Transferase M1 and Male Infertility in Taiwanese Patients With Varicocele, *Hum. Reprod. 17,* 718–725.
10. Benoff, S., Jacob, A., and Hurley, I.R. (2000) Male Infertility and Environmental Exposure to Lead and Cadmium, *Hum. Reprod. Update 6,* 107–121.
11. Depuydt, C.E., Mahmoud, A.M., Dhooge, W.S., Schoonjans, F.A., and Comhaire, F.H. (1999) Hormonal Regulation of Inhibin B Secretion by Immature Rat Sertoli Cells *in Vitro*: Possible Use As a Bioassay for Estrogen Detection, *J. Androl. 20,* 54–62.
12. Mahmoud, A.M., Comhaire, F.H., and Depuydt, C.E. (1998) The Clinical and Biologic Significance of Serum Inhibins in Subfertile Men, *Reprod. Toxicol. 12,* 591–599.

13. Kester, M.H.A., Bulduk, S., van Toor, H., Tibboel, D., Meinl, W., Glatt, H., Falany, C.N., Coughtrie, M.W.H., Schuur, A.G., Brouwer, A., and Visser, T.J. (2002) Potent Inhibition of Estrogen Sulfotransferase by Hydroxylated Metabolites of Polyhalogenated Aromatic Hydrocarbons Reveals Alternative Mechanism for Estrogenic Activity of Endocrine Disrupters, *J. Clin. Endocrinol. Metab. 87*, 1142–1150.

14. Mahmoud, A., Kiss, P., Kaufman, J.M., Comhaire, F., and Asclepios (2000) The Influence of Age and Lead Exposure on Inhibin B Serum Levels in Men, *Int. J. Androl. 23 (Suppl. 1)*, PO94.

15. Adamopoulos, D.A., Nicopoulou, S., Kapolla, N., Karamertzanis, M., and Andreou, E. (1997) The Combination of Testosterone Undecanoate With Tamoxifen Citrate Enhances the Effects of Each Agent Given Independently on Seminal Parameters in Men With Idiopathic Oligozoospermia, *Fertil. Steril. 67*, 756–762.

16. Comhaire, F. (1976) Treatment of Oligospermia with Tamoxifen, *Int. J. Fertil. 21*, 232–238.

17. Comhaire, F.H., Mahmoud, A.M., Depuydt, C.E., Zalata, A.A., and Christophe, A.B. (1999) Mechanisms and Effects of Male Genital Tract Infection on Sperm Quality and Fertilizing Potential: The Andrologist's Viewpoint, *Hum. Reprod. Update. 5*, 393–398.

18. Zalata, A.A., Christophe, A.B., Depuydt, C.E., Schoonjans, F., and Comhaire, F.H. (1998) The Fatty Acid Composition of Phospholipids of Spermatozoa from Infertile Patients, *Mol. Hum. Reprod. 4*, 111–118.

19. Loft, S., and Poulsen, H.E. (1996) Cancer Risk and Oxidative DNA Damage in Man, *J. Mol. Med. 74*, 297–312.

20. D'Agata, R., Vicari, E., Moncada, M.L., Sidoti, G., Calogero, A.E., Fornito, M.C., Minacapilli, G., Mongioi, A., and Polosa, P. (1990) Generation of Reactive Oxygen Species in Subgroups of Infertile Men, *Int. J. Androl. 13*, 344–351.

21. Geva, E., Bartoov, B., Zabludovsky, N., Lessing, J.B., Lerner-Geva, L., and Amit, A. (1996) The Effect of Antioxidant Treatment on Human Spermatozoa and Fertilization Rate in an *in Vitro* Fertilization Program, *Fertil. Steril. 66*, 430–434.

22. Kurinczuk, J.J., and Bower, C. (1997) Birth Defects in Infants Conceived by Intracytoplasmic Sperm Injection: An Alternative Interpretation, *Br. Med. J. 315*, 1260–1265.

23. Simpson, J.L., and Lamb, D.J. (2001) Genetic Effects of Intracytoplasmic Sperm Injection, *Semin. Reprod. Med. 19*, 239–249.

24. Rubio, C., Gil-Salom, M., Simon, C., Vidal, F., Rodrigo, L., Minguez, Y., Remohi, J., and Pellicer, A. (2001) Incidence of Sperm Chromosomal Abnormalities in a Risk Population: Relationship with Sperm Quality and ICSI Outcome, *Hum. Reprod. 16*, 2084–2092.

25. Hansen, M., Kurinczuk, J.J., Bower, C., and Webb, S. (2002) The Risk of Major Birth Defects After Intracytoplasmic Sperm Injection and *in Vitro* Fertilization, *N. Engl. J. Med. 346*, 725–730.

26. De Vriese, S.R., Christophe, A.B., and Comhaire, F.H. (2002) *Relation Between the Fatty Acid Composition of Phospholipids of Spermatozoa and Plasma and the Effect of Dietary Intake of PUFA*, 93rd AOCS Annual Meeting and Expo, Palais des Congrés de Montréal, Montréal, Québec, Canada.

27. Comhaire, F.H., and Kunnen, M. (1985) Factors Affecting the Probability of Conception After Treatment of Subfertile Men with Varicocele by Transcatheter Embolization with Bucrylate, *Fertil. Steril. 43*, 781–786.

28. Comhaire, F.H. (1987) Concentration of Pefloxacine in Split Ejaculates of Patients with Chronic Male Accessory Gland Infection, *J. Urol. 138*, 828–830.

29. Comhaire, F., Zalata, A., and Mahmoud, A. (1996) Critical Evaluation of the Effectiveness of Different Modes of Treatment of Male Infertility, *Andrologia. 28 (Suppl 1)*, 31–35.

30. Mahmoud, A.M., Tuyttens, C.L., and Comhaire, F.H. (1996) Clinical and Biological Aspects of Male Immune Infertility: A Case-Controlled Study of 86 Cases, *Andrologia. 28*, 191–196.

31. Comhaire, F. (2000) Clinical Andrology: From Evidence-Base to Ethics. The 'E' Quintet in Clinical Andrology, *Hum. Reprod. 15*, 2067–2071.

32. Christophe, A., Zalata, A., Mahmoud, A., and Comhaire, F. (1998) Fatty Acid Composition of Sperm Phospholipids and Its Nutritional Implications, *Middle East Fertility Society Journal 3*, 46–53.

33. Bernard, D., Christophe, A., Delanghe, J., Langlois, M., De Buyzere, M., and Comhaire, F. (2003) The Effect of Supplementation with an Antioxidant Preparation on LDL-oxidation is Determined by Haptoglobin Polymorphism, *Redox. Rep.,* in press.

34. Comhaire, F.H., Christophe, A.B., Zalata, A.A., Dhooge, W.S., Mahmoud, A.M., and Depuydt, C.E. (2000) The Effects of Combined Conventional Treatment, Oral Antioxidants, and Essential Fatty Acids on Sperm Biology in Subfertile Men, *Prostaglandins Leukot. Essent. Fatty. Acids. 63*, 159–165.

Chapter 2

Metabolism of Long-Chain Polyunsaturated Fatty Acids in Testicular Cells

Thien N. Tran[a], Kjetil Retterstøl[b], and Bjørn O. Christophersen[a]

[a]Institute of Clinical Biochemistry, The Lipid Clinic, Department of Internal Medicine, and [b]National Hospital, University of Oslo, N-0027 Oslo, Norway

Abstract

Testicular cells and spermatozoa contain high amounts of 20- and 22-carbon n-3 and n-6 polyunsaturated fatty acids (PUFA). It is well established that testicular cells are able to convert dietary 18:2n-6 and 18:3n-3 to more highly unsaturated fatty acids via a sequence of alternate desaturations and elongations. Also, 18:1n-9 is converted to 20- and 22-carbon n-9 PUFA in the testis. The capacities for elongation of unsaturated fatty acids in the testis are high. Human and rat testicular cells are more active in the conversion of 18- and 20-carbon n-3 PUFA to 22-carbon n-3 PUFA than in the conversion of the corresponding 18- and 20-carbon n-6 to 22-carbon n-6 PUFA. However, rat testicular cells contain high amounts of 22:5n-6, whereas human testicular cells contain high amounts of 22:6n-3. These findings suggest that high capacities for the metabolism of unsaturated fatty acids and the specificity for incorporation of PUFA into testicular lipids might regulate the patterns of fatty acid composition in the testis. The cDNA encoding enzymes involved in the conversion of 18:2n-6 and 18:3n-3 to 20- and 22-carbon n-3 and n-6 fatty acids, i.e. desaturases and elongase, have recently been cloned. High levels of $\Delta 5$ and $\Delta 6$-desaturase mRNA were found in rat and mouse testes. Also mRNA levels of an enzyme involved in the elongation of 18 and 20-carbon PUFA in human testes were high. The presence of high mRNA levels of these enzymes is consistent with the high activities of the testis in the biosynthesis of highly unsaturated fatty acids.

Introduction

Testicular lipids contain high levels of unsaturated fatty acids. The compositions of testicular unsaturated fatty acids vary from species to species. The testes of rat, hamster, rabbit, and dog (1) have high contents of docosapentaenoic acid (22:5n-6), whereas human (2,3) and monkey (4) testes have high contents of docosahexaenoic acid (22:6n-3) (5,6). High amounts of polyunsaturated fatty acids (PUFA) in the membrane phospholipids of germ cells are known to contribute to membrane fluidity and flexibility (7).

Previous studies have shown a positive correlation between sperm motility and sperm phospholipid 22:6n-3 content (8–10). Recent studies have shown that the 22:6n-3 content was significantly lower in sperm of asthenozoospermic men compared with those of normozoospermic men (5,8,10). This suggested a reduction in the synthesis of 22:6n-3 or a metabolic difference in asthenozoospermic men (10).

The 22:6n-3 levels were much higher in sperm than in blood serum of both asthenozoospermic and normozoospermic men (10). Furthermore, dietary DHA supplementation in asthenozoospermic men increased serum and possibly seminal plasma phospholipid 22:6n-3 levels without affecting the incorporation of 22:6n-3 into the spermatozoa phospholipid and sperm motility (11). These findings are consistent with the view that the accumulation of high 22:6n-3 levels in human testicular cells is the result of an active biosynthesis of unsaturated fatty acids in the testis.

Studies in rat (12) and monkey (4) have shown that the content of PUFA is higher in germ cells than in Sertoli cells. Further studies have shown that Sertoli cells are more active than germ cells in the metabolism of 18:2n-6 to 22:5n-6 (13) and that more 20- and 22-carbon PUFA were elongated by Sertoli cells than germ cells (14). These findings suggest that Sertoli cells synthesize PUFA to supply germ cells. However, there was no direct experimental evidence for such a transport of PUFA from Sertoli cells to germ cells.

This chapter focuses on the metabolism of 18-, 20-, and 22-carbon PUFA by testicular cells. In addition, a brief review of the incorporation of PUFA in the testicular lipids and the effects of pituitary gonadotrophins and testosterone on enzymes involved in the metabolism of unsaturated fatty acids, *i.e.*, desaturases and elongase, is also included.

Biosynthesis of 22-Carbon PUFA

The biosynthesis of 22-carbon PUFA from 18-carbon unsaturated fatty acids proceeds via a sequence of alternate desaturations and elongations (Fig. 2.1) (15,16). Studies in rats have shown that various cell types of testicular cells are able to metabolize 18-carbon PUFA to more highly unsaturated fatty acids. The capacities for the biosynthesis of 20- and 22-carbon PUFA differ in each cell type of the testicular cells. It appears that interactions between different cell types and the selective incorporation of fatty acids into testicular lipids may regulate the content of PUFA composition in the testis.

Elongation and Desaturation of 18-Carbon Unsaturated Fatty Acids

Desaturation of 18-carbon fatty acids. The predominant pathway in the biosynthesis of highly n-6 unsaturated fatty acids from 18:2n-6 is initiated by Δ6-desaturation of 18:2n-6 to 18:3n-6. The amounts of 20- and 22-carbon n-6 PUFA were increased when 18:2n-6 was added to primary cultures of Sertoli cells (17–19). Only a small amount of 18:3n-6 was detected. A low level of 18:3n-6 suggested that Δ6-desaturation product, 18:3n-6, was rapidly elongated to 20:3n-6 (19). When 18:3n-3 was incubated with cultured Sertoli cells, only a small amount of 18:4n-3 was detected (19).

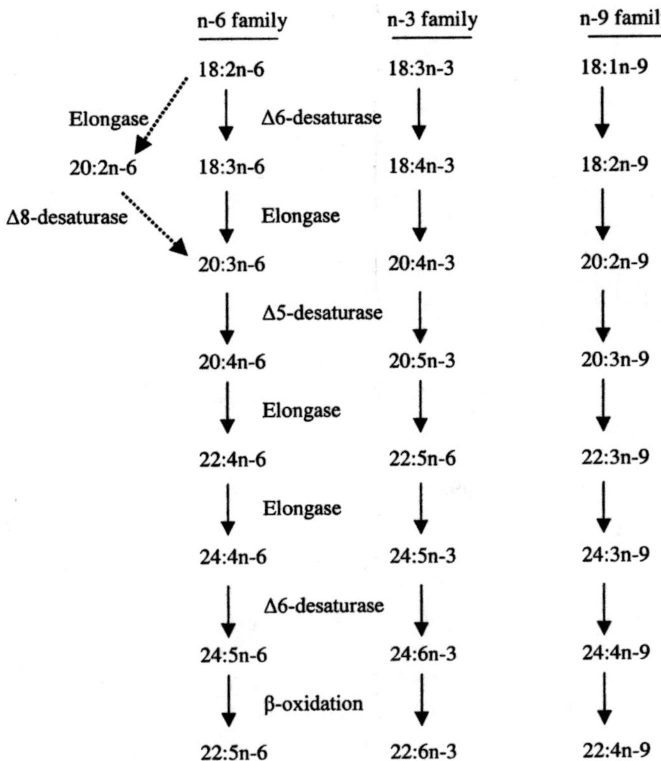

Fig. 2.1. The metabolism pathways of 18-carbon unsaturated fatty acids to more highly unsaturated fatty acids.

As observed with 18:2n-6, the levels of 20- and 22-carbon n-3 were increased by addition of 18:3n-3 to the incubation (19). Furthermore, studies on the metabolism of ^{14}C-labeled 18:2n-6 and 18:3n-3 in cell cultures enriched in Sertoli cells from 19-day-old rats have also shown that the amounts of Δ6-desaturation products, ^{14}C-labeled 18:3n-6 or 18:4n-3, respectively, were reduced with long incubation time (20). These results were consistent with the suggestion that Δ6-desaturation products, *i.e.,* 18:3n-6 and 18:4n-3, were rapidly metabolized to 20- and 22-carbon PUFA.

18:3n-3 was preferentially metabolized to 22-carbon n-3 PUFA, particularly 22:6n-3, and 24-carbon n-3 PUFA, whereas a large amount of 18:2n-6 was metabolized to 20:3n-6 and 20:4n-6 (20). Small amounts of 18:2n-6 was converted to 24:4n-6, 24:5n-6, and 22:5n-6 (20). The total amount of 18:3n-3 metabolized to longer and more highly n-3 PUFA was higher than that of 18:2n-6 to longer and more highly unsaturated n-6 PUFA (20).

In contrast to 18:2n-6 and 18:3n-3, only a small amount of ^{14}C-labeled 18:1n-9 was Δ6-desaturated to 18:2n-9, which was further converted to 20:2n-9 and 22:3n-9 by cultured Sertoli cells from rats raised on standard pellets (20). It has been suggested that Δ6-desaturation of 18-carbon PUFA may be a rate-limiting step in the metabolism of 18-carbon to 20- and 22-carbon PUFA by cultured Sertoli cells (19).

The cDNA encoding Δ6-desaturase from rat (21), mouse (22), and human (23,24) have recently been cloned. High mRNA levels of Δ6-desaturase have been found in mouse testes (22). The high expression of Δ6-desaturase mRNA in the testis was consistent with the findings that in the testis high amounts of 18-carbon unsaturated fatty acids were converted to more highly unsaturated fatty acids.

Elongation of 18-carbon unsaturated fatty acids. When ^{14}C-labeled 18:2n-6 was injected into rat testes, high amounts of ^{14}C-labeled 20:3n-6, 20:4n-6, 22:4n-6, and 22:5n-6 were formed (13). Further analysis on the fatty acid patterns in germ cells and Sertoli cells has shown that the proportions of ^{14}C-labeled 20:3n-6 and 20:4n-6 found in germ cells and Sertoli cells were similar (13). This finding indicates that both germ cells and Sertoli cells were able to metabolize 18-carbon PUFA to 20-carbon PUFA.

In vitro studies with cell preparations enriched in different germ cell types of mouse testes, *i.e.*, spermatids and spermatocytes, have shown that various germ cell types were able to incorporate ^{14}C-labeled acetate in the incubation medium into different PUFA with chain lengths of 20- and 22-carbon in cultures (25). The formation of ^{14}C-labeled 20- and 22-carbon PUFA in various germ cell types indicates that germ cells were able to elongate cellular 18- and 20-carbon PUFA. As in the liver, the acetyl-CoA carboxylase in the testis converts acetate to malonyl-CoA, which is used as the substrate for the elongation of cellular fatty acids (26). Consistent with this report, human testicular cells have also been shown to utilize ^{14}C-labeled acetate in the elongation of cellular 18-carbon (and possibly 20-carbon) n-6 fatty acids to 20- and 22-carbon n-6 fatty acids (27). In primary cultures of rat Sertoli cells high amounts of ^{14}C-labeled 18:2n-6 were also elongated to 20-carbon PUFA (18).

Incubation of cultured Sertoli cells with 18:2n-6 resulted in increased levels of 20:2n-6 in the membrane lipids (19). This finding was consistent with a previous study in cultured rat Sertoli cells, which has reported that high amounts of ^{14}C-labeled 18:2n-6 was elongated to ^{14}C-labeled 20:2n-6 (18). Furthermore, incubation of cultured Sertoli cells with 18:3n-3 resulted in increased levels of 20:3n-3 in the membrane lipids (19). This result indicated that high amounts of incubated 18:3n-3 were elongated to 20:3n-3 (19).

Elongation and Desaturation of 20-Carbon Unsaturated Fatty Acids

Elongation of 20-carbon unsaturated fatty acids. The *in vivo* metabolism of 20:4n-6 to other PUFA have been studied by intratesticular injection of ^{14}C-labeled 20:4n-6 into rat testes (13). The ^{14}C-labeled 22:4n-6 was detected in both Sertoli cells and germ cells 1.5 hr after intratesticular injection of ^{14}C-labeled 20:4n-6. This finding suggested that both Sertoli cells and germ cells were able to elongate 20:4n-6 to 22:4n-6. However, a higher amount of ^{14}C-labeled 22:5n-6 was found in Sertoli cells than in germ cells a short time after intratesticular injection, suggesting that Sertoli cells were more active than germ cells in the biosynthesis of 22:5n-6 from 20:4n-6 (13).

In vitro studies have shown that when ^{14}C-labeled acetate was added to the incubation medium of cultured Sertoli cells, ^{14}C-labeled 22:4n-6 was formed. The presence of ^{14}C-labeled 22:4n-6 was suggested to be a result of an elongation reaction where ^{14}C-labeled acetate was utilized to elongate cellular 20:4n-6 (28). Furthermore, it has also been reported that mouse spermatids and spermatocytes in cultures were able to metabolize 20:4n-6 to 24:5n-6 and 26:5n-6 (25,29).

The metabolism of 20:5n-3 to 22:6n-3 was more efficient than the metabolism of 20:4n-6 to 22:5n-6 in primary cultures enriched in rat Sertoli cells (20,30). Isolated human testicular cells also elongated more 20:5n-3 than 20:4n-6 to 22- and 24-carbon PUFA (31). In the cell cultures, the metabolism of 20:5n-3 to 22- and 24-carbon PUFA might be dependent on the concentration of the substrate in the incubation medium. Cultured Sertoli cells from rats raised on a standard diet also elongated considerable amounts of 20:3n-9 to 22:3n-9 (20).

Studies in cell cultures have suggested that there might be a competition between n-6 and n-3 fatty acids for elongations and desaturations of 20- and 22-carbon n-3 and n-6 PUFA. The metabolism of ^{14}C-labeled 20:4n-6 to 22:5n-6 was suppressed by the addition of 20:5n-3 to the incubation medium of cultures enriched in Sertoli cells (30). Conversely, addition of 20:4n-6 to the incubation medium of cultures enriched in rat Sertoli cells did not affect the conversion of 20:5n-3 to 22:6n-3 (30). Furthermore, a recent study in humans has shown that dietary 22:6n-3 supplementation in asthenozoospermic men was associated with decreases in the 22:4n-6 content of the sperm phospholipid but did not result in any other sperm phospholipid fatty acid composition modification (11). These findings suggest that 22:6n-3 decreased the elongation of 20:4n-6 to 22:4n-6 *in vivo* (11).

Human testicular cells (cell suspension consisting of a mixture of the cells in seminiferous tubules) elongated more 20:4n-6 and 20:5n-3 to 22-carbon PUFA than did fractions enriched in germ cells, *i.e.,* spermatocytes and round spermatids (31). The data suggest that human germ cells have a low capacity for fatty acid elongation (31). In support of this finding, rat germ cells were also found to have low capacities for elongation of unsaturated fatty acids (14). It appears that the difference in the elongation of 20-carbon n-3 and n-6 PUFA may play regulatory roles in the biosynthesis of 22:6n-3 and 22:5n-6 in the rat testis.

Recently, cDNA encoding for an enzyme involved in elongation of PUFA was cloned (32). This elongation enzyme was shown to have high capacities for elongation of 18- and 20-carbon PUFA, but not 22-carbon PUFA (32). Highest mRNA levels of this elongation enzyme were found in the human testis. These findings were consistent with previous studies based on the measurement of fatty acid metabolites showing that testicular cells have high activities in elongating 18- and 20-carbon PUFA.

Desaturation of 20-carbon unsaturated fatty acids. An alternative pathway for the biosynthesis of 20:4n-6 from 18:2n-6 in the testis has been suggested to be initiated by an elongation of 18:2n-6 to 20:2n-6 and then followed by Δ8-desaturation to 20:3n-6 and Δ5-desaturation to 20:4n-6, thus bypassing the requirement of Δ6-desaturation (Fig. 2.1). However, this synthesis pathway remains controversial. It has been reported that Δ8-desaturation of 20:2n-6 was not observed in the rat brain (33) and liver (34). Furthermore, kinetic studies on the metabolism of n-3 and n-6 PUFA in cultured rat Sertoli cells have suggested that no Δ8-desaturation was detected (19). A recent study on the metabolism of unsaturated fatty acids by testicular cells from rats raised on a fat-free diet has also suggested that only a small amount, if any, of 20:2n-6 might be metabolized to 20:4n-6 via Δ8-desaturation pathway (35). In contrast to these studies, previous studies have reported an active Δ8-desaturation of 20:2n-6 to 20:3n-6 in rat (36) and human testes (37).

In primary cultures enriched in rat Sertoli cells high amounts of incubated ^{14}C-labeled 20:3n-6 was converted to ^{14}C-labeled 20:4n-6, indicating a high activity of Δ5-desaturase (17,38). Also Leydig cells from testes of mature rats were able to take up ^{14}C-labeled 20:3n-6 from incubation medium and convert it to ^{14}C-labeled arachidonic acid (38). A low Δ5-desaturase activity has been suggested to suppress the conversion of 20:3n-6 to 20:4n-6 in cultured rat Sertoli cells (17,19).

At the molecular levels, it has been reported that high mRNA levels of Δ5-desaturase have been found in mouse (22) and rat testes (21). This finding was consistent with the observation that the rat testis was able to synthesize high amounts of 20- and 22-carbon n-3 and n-6 PUFA from 18:3n-3 and 18:2n-6, respectively (13).

Metabolism of 22-Carbon Unsaturated Fatty Acids

In primary cultures enriched in Sertoli cells 22:5n-3 was metabolized to 24-carbon PUFA and 22:6n-3 to a larger extent than the corresponding conversion of 22:4n-6 to 24-carbon n-6 PUFA and 22:5n-6 at a low (4 μM) substrate concentration (30). The metabolism of 22:4n-6 and 22:5n-3 fatty acids did not, however, differ much at a high (40 μM) substrate concentration (3). The percentage of the added substrates elongated was lower at high substrate concentrations as compared with low substrate concentrations (30).

As observed with 20:4n-6 and 20:5n-3, there might also be a competition between elongation of 22:4n-6 and 22:5n-3 to 24:4n-6 and 24:5n-3, respectively. In cultures enriched in Sertoli cells 22:5n-3 suppressed the elongation of 22:4n-6 (30). Conversely, 22:4n-6 did not affect the elongation of 22:5n-3 (30). These findings indicate that n-3 fatty acids were preferentially metabolized in the primary cultures enriched in rat Sertoli cells (30). Thus, it appears that the formation of 22:6n-3 was given priority over the formation of 22:5n-6 when little n-3 fatty acid precursor was available. However, in the presence of higher n-3 fatty acid concentrations, the formation of 22:6n-3 was suppressed. In this respect, it was demonstrated that the two elongation reactions (from C20 to C22 and from C22 to C24) are important for the regulation of the synthesis of 22:6n-3 and 22:5n-6.

Considerable amounts of 22:3n-9 and 22:4n-9 were formed in the testes of rats fed a fat-free diet for 10 to 15 weeks, but these 22-carbon PUFA were not detected in the testes of rats fed fat supplemented diets (26). Consistent with this finding, a previous study in cell cultures enriched in Sertoli cells isolated from rats fed standard pellets has shown that 22:3n-9 was not elongated to 24:3n-9 (20).

There was no significant difference in Δ6-desaturation of 24:4n-6 *versus* 24:5n-3 or retroconversion of 24:5n-6 *versus* 24:6n-3 to 22:5n-6 *versus* 22:6n-3 by primary cultures enriched in rat Sertoli cells (30). In contrast to the elongation of 22-carbon n-3 and n-6 PUFA, it appears that Δ6-desaturation of 24:4n-6 and 24:5n-3 was not dependent on the concentration of these fatty acids (30). Recent studies have suggested that a single Δ6-desaturase catalyzed the desaturation of 18- and 24-carbon n-3 and n-6 PUFA (39,40). At present, there is no kinetic study to compare the Δ6-desaturation of 18-carbon n-3 and n-6 PUFA versus 24-carbon n-3 and n-6 PUFA.

In vivo studies on the metabolism of 24:4n-6 and 24:5n-3 by injection of 14C-labeled 24:4n-6 and 24:5n-3 into rat testes have shown that more ^{14}C-labeled 22:6n-3 than ^{14}C-labeled 22:5n-6 were formed (41). More ^{14}C-labeled 22:6n-3 than ^{14}C-labeled 22:5n-6 was also formed after intratesticular injection with ^{14}C-labeled 22:5n-3 versus 22:4n-6 (41). These findings indicated that the low level of 22:6n-3 versus the abundance of 22:5n-6 does not appear to be due to differences in the ability of testes to metabolize n-3 and n-6 PUFA (41). Thus, the data in the literature raise the possibility that the accumulation of high amounts of 20- and 22-carbon n-6 PUFA in rat testicular cells may be due to the selective uptake or incorporation of n-6 fatty acids into the rat testis.

The daily sperm production per gram testis is 5 to 6 times higher in rat than in man (42). The testis is an organ that loses 22-carbon PUFA by the transport of sperm to vesiculae seminalis. The rat testis seems to have a very high capacity for producing both 22:6n-3 and 22:5n-6. Since more n-6 than n-3 precursor fatty acids are available, this may be important for the formation of high levels of 22:5n-6 in rat testis.

Oxidation of Unsaturated Fatty Acids

When [1-^{14}C]18:2n-6 was injected into rat testes approximately 16 to 20% of the recovered radioactivity was in the palmitic acid (16:0), and small amounts of ^{14}C-label were present in 18:0 and 18:1n-9 after 3 to 48 hr (13). These *de novo* synthesized fatty acids were derived from ^{14}C-acetyl-CoA produced by β-oxidation of [1-^{14}C]18:2n-6. When [1-^{14}C]20:4n-6 was injected into rat testes, less ^{14}C-label was incorporated into palmitic acid and 18-carbon fatty acids (approximately 3 to 4% of the recovered radioactivity) than occurred following an intratesticular injection of [1-^{14}C]18:2n-6 (13). These results indicated that more 18:2n-6 than 20:4n-6 was oxidized. The data were also consistent with studies in primary cultures of rat Sertoli cells, which have shown that the ^{14}C-label incorporated into *de novo* synthesized 16- and 18-carbon fatty acids was approximately 16% of ^{14}C-label in total fatty acids after 48 hr incubation with [1-^{14}C]18:2n-6 (18). Another study in primary cultures of rat Sertoli cells has suggested that the amounts of radioactive oxidation products from oxidation of ^{14}C-labeled 20:5n-3 was higher than those found with 20:4n-6, 22:4n-6, and 22:5n-3 (30).

Incorporation of PUFA into Testicular Lipids

The testis consists of many different cell types with different phospholipid classes and fatty acid compositions. Rat germ cells contained mostly phosphatidylcholine (PC) and phosphatidylethanolamine (PE), whereas Sertoli cells had a more evenly distributed phospholipid pattern (43). A greater proportion of the phospholipid of rat Sertoli cells than of germ cells was composed of phosphatidylserine (PS), phosphatidylinositol (PI), and sphingomyelin and lysophosphatides (43).

The fatty acid profiles of phospholipids of rat Sertoli cells contained less 16:0 and 22:5n-6 and more 18:1, 20:4n-6, and 22:4n-6 than did the corresponding phospholipids of the germ cells (43). These findings were also consistent with data from studies of the lipid composition of separated rat testicular germ cell types, which showed that PE and PS contained a high concentration of 22:5n-6 (12). Also, the fatty acid patterns of the total lipids of separated cell fractions enriched in rat Sertoli cells or germ cells have previously been studied (43). The fractions enriched in rat Sertoli cells contained less 22:5n-6 and 22:6n-3 than did the germ cell fractions (43). 24-carbon PUFA were only detected in the triacylglycerols, but not in the phospholipids (12,43), and were present in higher concentrations in triacylglycerols in germ cells than in Sertoli cells (43).

In vitro studies have shown that after incubation of ^{14}C-labeled 22:4n-6 or 22:5n-3 with isolated human testicular cells, higher amounts of these fatty acids were esterified into triacylglycerols than in phospholipids (31). With 20-carbon n-3 and n-6 as the substrates more 20:5n-3 and 20:4n-6 were esterified into phospholipids than in triacylglycerols (31). In the phospholipid fraction more fatty acid substrates were esterified into PC than in PE, PS or PI (31).

In cultures of cell preparations enriched in rat Sertoli cells most of the incubated 18:2n-6, 18:3n-3, 20:3n-9, 20:4n-6, and 20:5n-3 were incorporated into PC and PE (20). The metabolites, 22:5n-6 and 22:6n-3, were esterified in triacylglycerols, cholesterol esters, and phospholipid classes PC and PE (20). After incubation of Sertoli cells with 20- and 22-carbon n-3 and n-6 PUFA, more n-6 than n-3 fatty acids were esterified into phospholipids, and fewer n-6 PUFA than n-3 PUFA were esterified into triacylglycerols (30). With high substrate concentrations, high amounts of 20- and 22-carbon n-3 and n-6 PUFA were esterified into PC, and small amounts of these PUFA were esterified into PE, PI, or PS (30).

Hormonal Regulation of Metabolism of PUFA in the Rat Testis

Studies of the fatty acid composition of testes from hypophysectomized rats have shown that the levels of 22:5n-6, 24:4n-6, and 24:5n-6 were increased, whereas the levels of 18:2n-6 and 20:4n-6 were greatly decreased (44). Testicular phospholipids of hypophysectomized rats had more 20:3n-6 and 22:5n-6 and less 18:0, 18:2n-6, and 22:4n-6 than did those of control rats (45). When ^{14}C-labeled 18:2n-6 was injected intratesticularly, there was an accumulation of ^{14}C-labeled 20:3n-6 and a decreased amount of ^{14}C-labeled 20:4n-6 in the testis of hypophysectomized compared to control rats (45). Furthermore, following intratesticular injection of ^{14}C-labeled 20:3n-6, there was less ^{14}C-labeled 20:4n-6 and 22:4n-6 of both phospholipids and triacylglycerols of hypophysectomized compared to control rats (45). This finding indicates that the Δ5-desaturation of 20:3n-6 to 20:4n-6 was suppressed in hypophysectomized rats. Administration of adrenocorticotropin (ACTH) to the mature normal rats decreased the Δ5-desaturase activity in the testicular cells (38). Similar results were obtained when ACTH was added to the incubation medium of cultured cells isolated from non-hormone treated rats (38). The total fatty acid composition of the Sertoli cells isolated from ACTH-treated rats showed a significant increase in the relative percentage of 18:2n-6 and a decrease in 20- and 22-carbon PUFA biosynthesis (38). The data suggested that ACTH exerts an inhibitory effect on Δ5- and Δ6-desaturase (38).

The effects of luteinizing hormone (LH), follicle-stimulating hormone (FSH), and testosterone on the metabolism of 18:2n-6 to highly unsaturated fatty acids have also been studied in hypophysectomized rats. Analysis of the testicular phospholipids in the immature hypophysectomized rats has shown a significant increase in the concentration of 24:5n-6 after both LH and testosterone treatment (46). However, in the immature hypophysectomized rats these hormonal treatments have only small effects on the metabolism of 18:2n-6 into more highly unsaturated fatty acids (46).

In hypophysectomized mature rats the metabolism of ^{14}C-labeled 18:2n-6 to longer PUFA was lower than that in any of the hormone-treated, *i.e.,* FSH, LH, and testosterone (46). LH treatment caused a pronounced increase in the incorporation of ^{14}C-label into 20:4n-6 and 22:5n-6 (46). The effect of testosterone was similar to that of LH (46). LH and testosterone treatments resulted in significant increases in the concentrations of ^{14}C-label 20:4n-6 and 22:5n-6 fatty acids, whereas FSH had a less marked effect (46).

Summary

In vivo and *in vitro* studies have shown that testicular cells have high capacities for metabolism of dietary 18:2n-6 and 18:3n-3 to more highly unsaturated fatty acids. There is a preference for the synthesis of 22:6n-3 *versus* 22:5n-6 from n-3 *versus* n-6 fatty acid precursors, respectively, by testicular cells. Studies in humans and rats have suggested that Sertoli cells are more active than germ cells in the metabolism of 18-carbon to 22-carbon PUFA. However, higher levels of 22-carbon PUFA have been found in germ cells than in Sertoli cells. These findings suggested, but did not prove, that Sertoli cells produce PUFA for germ cells.

The activities of Δ5, Δ6-desaturase and elongase measured by metabolisms of fatty acid substrates in the testis were high. These results were also consistent with high mRNA levels of these genes in the testis. It has been suggested that Δ5- and Δ6-desaturase might play regulatory roles in the metabolism of 18:2n-6 and 18:3n-3 to

22:5n-6 and 22:6n-3, respectively. Several hormones, *e.g.*, ACTH and LH, have been suggested to change unsaturated fatty acid composition in the testis by changing activities of enzymes involved in the metabolism of unsaturated fatty acids, *e.g.*, $\Delta 5$- and $\Delta 6$-desaturase.

Acknowledgments

This work was supported by the Medinnova fund. We thank Trine B. Haugen and Thomas Sæther at the Department of Gynecology and Obstetrics, Andrology Laboratory, Rikshospitalet University Hospital for collaboration in working out several of the papers making this review possible.

References

1. Bieri, J.G., and Prival, E.L. (1965) Lipid Composition of Testes from Various Species, *Comp. Biochem. Physiol. 15*, 275–282.
2. Coniglio, J.G., Grogan, W.M., Jr., and Rhamy, R.K. (1974) Lipids of Human Testes Removed at Orchidectomy, *J. Reprod. Fertil. 41*, 67–73.
3. Coniglio, J.G., Grogan, W.M., Jr., and Rhamy, R.K. (1975) Lipid and Fatty Acid Composition of Human Testes Removed at Autopsy, *Biol. Reprod. 12*, 255–259.
4. Connor, W.E., Lin, D.S., and Neuringer, M. (1997) Biochemical Markers for Puberty in the Monkey Testis: Desmosterol and Docosahexaenoic Acid, *J. Clin. Endocrinol. Metab. 82*, 1911–1916.
5. Zalata, A.A., Christophe, A.B., Depuydt, C.E., Schoonjans, F., and Comhaire, F.H. (1998) The Fatty Acid Composition of Phospholipids of Spermatozoa from Infertile Patients, *Mol. Hum. Reprod. 4*, 111–118.
6. Alvarez, J.G., and Storey, B.T. (1995) Differential Incorporation of Fatty Acids into and Peroxidative Loss of Fatty Acids from Phospholipids of Human Spermatozoa, *Mol. Reprod. Dev. 42*, 334–346.
7. Lenzi, A., Gandini, L., Lombardo, F., Picardo, M., Maresca, V., Panfili, E., Tramer, F., Boitani, C., and Dondero, F., (2002) Polyunsaturated Fatty Acids of Germ Cell Membranes, Glutathione, and Blutathione-Dependent Enzyme-Phgpx: from Basic to Clinic, *Contraception 65*, 301–304.
8. Gulaya, N.M., Margitich, V.M., Govseeva, N.M., Klimashevsky, V.M., Gorpynchenko, I.I., and Boyko, M.I. (2001) Phospholipid Composition of Human Sperm and Seminal Plasma in Relation to Sperm Fertility, *Arch. Androl. 46*, 169–175.
9. Nissen, H.P., and Kreysel, H.W. (1983) Polyunsaturated Fatty Acids in Relation to Sperm Motility, *Andrologia 15*, 264–269.
10. Conquer, J.A., Martin, J.B., Tummon, I., Watson, L., and Tekpetey, F. (1999) Fatty Acid Analysis of Blood Serum, Seminal Plasma, and Spermatozoa of Normozoospermic *vs.* Asthenozoospermic Males, *Lipids 34*, 793–799.
11. Conquer, J.A., Martin, J.B., Tummon, I., Watson, L., and Tekpetey, F. (2000) Effect of DHA Supplementation on DHA Status and Sperm Motility In Asthenozoospermic Males, *Lipids 35*, 149–154.
12. Beckman, J.K., Gray, M.E., and Coniglio, J.G. (1978) The Lipid Composition of Isolated Rat Spermatids and Spermatocytes, *Biochim. Biophys. Acta. 530*, 367–374.
13. Beckman, J.K., and Coniglio, J.G. (1980) The Metabolism of Polyunsaturated Fatty Acids in Rat Sertoli and Germinal Cells, *Lipids 15*, 389–394.

14. Retterstol, K., Tran, T.N., Haugen, T.B., and Christophersen, B.O. (2001) Metabolism of Very Long Chain Polyunsaturated Fatty Acids in Isolated Rat Germ Cells, *Lipids 36*, 601–606.

15. Voss, A., Reinhart, M., Sankarappa, S., and Sprecher, H. (1991) The Metabolism of 7,10,13,16,19-Docosapentaenoic Acid To 4,7,10,13,16,19-Docosahexaenoic Acid in Rat Liver Is Independent of A 4-Desaturase, *J. Biol. Chem. 266*, 19995–20000.

16. Mohammed, B.S., Sankarappa, S., Geiger, M., and Sprecher, H. (1995) Reevaluation of the Pathway for the Metabolism of 7,10,13,16-Docosatetraenoic Acid To 4,7,10,13,16-Docosapentaenoic Acid in Rat Liver, *Arch. Biochem. Biophys. 317*, 179–184.

17. Hurtado De Catalfo, G.E., and De Gomez Dumm, I.N. (2002) Polyunsaturated Fatty Acid Biosynthesis from 1-^{14}C 20:3 N-6 Acid in Rat Cultured Sertoli Cells Linoleic Acid Effect, *Int. J. Biochem. Cell Biol. 34*, 525–532.

18. Coniglio, J.G., and Sharp, J. (1989) Biosynthesis of [^{14}C]Arachidonic Acid from [14C]Linoleate in Primary Cultures of Rat Sertoli Cells, *Lipids 24*, 84–85.

19. Oulhaj, H., Huynh, S., and Nouvelot, A. (1992) The Biosynthesis of Polyunsaturated Fatty Acids By Rat Sertoli Cells, *Comp. Biochem. Physiol. B 102*, 897–904.

20. Retterstol, K., Haugen, T.B., Woldseth, B., and Christophersen, B.O. (1998) A Comparative Study of the Metabolism of N-9, N-6, and N-3 Fatty Acids in Testicular Cells from Immature Rat, *Biochim. Biophys. Acta. 1392*, 59–72.

21. Zolfaghari, R., Cifelli, C.J., Banta, M.D., and Ross, A.C. (2001) Fatty Acid Δ(5)-Desaturase Mrna Is Regulated by Dietary Vitamin A and Exogenous Retinoic Acid in Liver of Adult Rats, *Arch. Biochem. Biophys. 391*, 8–15.

22. Matsuzaka, T., Shimano, H., Yahagi, N., Amemiya-Kudo, M., Yoshikawa, T., Hasty, A.H., Tamura, Y., Osuga, J., Okazaki, H., Iizuka, Y., Takahashi, A., Sone, H., Gotoda, T., Ishibashi, S., and Yamada, N. (2002) Dual Regulation of Mouse Δ(5)- and Δ(6)-Desaturase Gene Expression By SREBP-1 and PPARalpha, *J. Lipid Res. 43*, 107–114.

23. Cho, H.P., Nakamura, M.T., and Clarke, S.D. (1999) Cloning, Expression, and Nutritional Regulation of the Mammalian Δ-6 Desaturase, *J. Biol. Chem. 274*, 471–477.

24. Cho, H.P., Nakamura, M., and Clarke, S.D. (1999) Cloning, Expression, and Fatty Acid Regulation of the Human Δ-5 Desaturase, *J. Biol. Chem. 274*, 37335–37339.

25. Grogan, W.M., and Lam, J.W., (1982) Fatty Acid Synthesis in Isolated Spermatocytes and Spermatids of Mouse Testis, *Lipids 17*, 604–611.

26. Whorton, A.R., and Coniglio, J.G. (1977) Fatty Acid Synthesis in Testes of Fat-Deficient and Fat-Supplemented Rats, *J. Nutr. 107*, 79–86.

27. Coniglio, J.G., Grogan, W.M., Jr., and Rhamy, R.K. (1977) Fatty Acid Synthesis in Human Testis Incubated with 1-^{14}C Acetate, *J. Reprod. Fertil. 51*, 463–465.

28. Fisher, D.M., and Coniglio, J.G. (1983) Composition of, and [^{14}C]Acetate Incorporation into, Lipids of Rat Sertoli Cells in Culture, *Biochim. Biophys. Acta 751*, 27–32.

29. Grogan, W.M., and Huth, E.G. (1983) Biosynthesis of Long-Chain Polyenoic Acids from Arachidonic Acid in Cultures of Enriched Spermatocytes and Spermatids from Mouse Testis, *Lipids 18*, 275–284.

30. Retterstol, K., Haugen, T.B., and Christophersen, B.O. (2000) The Pathway from Arachidonic to Docosapentaenoic Acid (20:4n-6 To 22:5n-6) and from Eicosapentaenoic to Docosahexaenoic Acid (20:5n-3 To 22:6n-3) Studied in Testicular Cells from Immature Rats, *Biochim. Biophys. Acta. 1483*, 119–131.

31. Retterstol, K., Haugen, T.B., Tran, T.N., and Christophersen, B.O. (2001) Studies on the Metabolism of Essential Fatty Acids in Isolated Human Testicular Cells, *Reproduction 121*, 881–887.

32. Leonard, A.E., Bobik, E.G., Dorado, J., Kroeger, P.E., Chuang, L.T., Thurmond, J.M., Parker-Barnes, J.M., Das, T., Huang, Y.S., and Mukerji, P. (2000) Cloning of a Human cDNA Encoding a Novel Enzyme Involved in the Elongation of Long-Chain Polyunsaturated Fatty Acids, *Biochem. J. 350*, 765–770.

33. Dhopeshwarkar, G.A., and Subramanian, C. (1976) Intracranial Conversion of Linoleic Acid to Arachidonic Acid: Evidence for Lack of Δ8 Desaturase in the Brain, *J. Neurochem. 26*, 1175–1179.

34. Ullman, D., and Sprecher, H. (1971) An *in Vitro* and *in Vivo* Study of the Conversion of Eicosa-11,14-Dienoic Acid to Eicosa-5,11,14-Trienoic Acid and of the Conversion of Eicosa-11-Enoic Acid to Eicosa-5,11-Dienoic Acid in the Rat, *Biochim. Biophys. Acta. 248*, 186–197.

35. Chen, Q., Yin, F.Q., and Sprecher, H. (2000) The Questionable Role of a Microsomal Δ8 Acyl-CoA-Dependent Desaturase in the Biosynthesis of Polyunsaturated Fatty Acids, *Lipids 35*, 871–879.

36. Albert, D.H., and Coniglio, J.G. (1977) Metabolism of Eicosa-11,14-Dienoic Acid in Rat Testes. Evidence for Δ8-Desaturase Activity, *Biochim. Biophys. Acta. 489*, 390–396.

37. Albert, D.H., Rhamy, R.K., and Coniglio, J.G. (1979) Desaturation of Eicosa-11,14-Dienoic Acid in Human Testes, *Lipids 14*, 498–500.

38. Hurtado De Catalfo, G.E., Mandon, E.C., and De Gomez Dumm, I.N. (1992) Arachidonic Acid Biosynthesis in Non-Stimulated and Adrenocorticotropin-Stimulated Sertoli and Leydig Cells, *Lipids 27*, 593–598.

39. De Antueno, R.J., Knickle, L.C., Smith, H., Elliot, M.L., Allen, S.J., Nwaka, S., and Winther, M.D. (2001) Activity of Human Δ5 and Δ6 Desaturases on Multiple N-3 and N-6 Polyunsaturated Fatty Acids, *FEBS Lett. 509*, 77–80.

40. D'andrea, S., Guillou, H., Jan, S., Catheline, D., Thibault, J.N., Bouriel, M., Rioux, V., and Legrand, P. (2002) The Same Rat Δ6-Desaturase not only Acts on 18- but also on 24-Carbon Fatty Acids in Very-Long-Chain Polyunsaturated Fatty Acid Biosynthesis, *Biochem. J. 364*, 49–55.

41. Yin, F.Q., Chen, Q., and Sprecher, H. (1999) A Comparison of the Metabolism of [3-^{14}C]-Labeled 22- and 24-Carbon (N-3) and (N-6) Unsaturated Fatty Acids By Rat Testes and Liver, *Biochim. Biophys. Acta. 1438*, 63–72.

42. Sharp, R.M., (1994) *In the Physiology of Reproduction*, Knobil, E., and Nistal, M. (Eds.), Raven Press, New York, pp. 1363–1419.

43. Beckman, J.K., and Coniglio, J.G. (1979) A Comparative Study of the Lipid Composition of Isolated Rat Sertoli and Germinal Cells, *Lipids 14*, 262–267.

44. Nakamura, M., Jensen, B., and Privett, O.S. (1968) Effect of Hypophysectomy on the Fatty Acids and Lipid Classes of Rat Testes, *Endocrinology 82*, 137–142.

45. Marzouki, Z.M., and Coniglio, J.G. (1984) The Effects of Hypophysectomy and Testosterone Treatment on the Composition and Metabolism of Testicular Lipids, *Lipids 19*, 609–616.

46. Goswami, A., and Williams, W.L. (1967) Effect of Hypophysectomy and Replacement Therapy on Fatty Acid Metabolism in the Rat Testis, *Biochem. J. 105*, 537–543.

Chapter 3

Fatty Acid Remodeling during Sperm Maturation: Variation of Docosahexaenoic Acid Content

Mario Ollero[a,b,c] and Juan G. Alvarez[c,d]

Departments of [a]Obstetrics, Gynecology, and Reproductive Biology, and [b]Medicine, Beth Israel Deaconess Medical Center, [c]Harvard Medical School, Boston, MA, and [d]Instituto de Infertilidad Masculina, USP-Hospital Santa Teresa, La Coruña, Spain

Abstract

Sperm maturation involves a broad range of events that occur during sperm migration through the seminiferous tubules and the epididymis, including the remodeling of sperm membrane components. The oxidation of membrane phospholipid bound docosahexaenoic acid (DHA) has been shown to be one of the major factors that limit the motile lifespan of sperm *in vitro*. Sperm samples show high cell-to-cell variability in lifespan and, consequently, in susceptibility toward lipid peroxidation. Therefore, it is postulated that there is also cell-to-cell variability in DHA content in human spermatozoa and that the content of the main substrate of lipid peroxidation (DHA) is critical and highly regulated during the sperm maturation process. Several studies have been performed to analyze the fatty acid content of germ cells and sperm at different stages of maturation, including *in vivo* studies in animal models, and *in vitro* approaches in human spermatozoa. The latter have been carried out in spermatozoa isolated from semen by techniques based on density gradients. In a recent work, we determined DHA content in subsets of human spermatozoa at different stages of maturation isolated by a discontinuous Percoll density gradient. The results of this study indicated that (i) there is significant cell-to-cell variability in DHA content in human sperm; and (ii) there is a net decrease in DHA content in sperm during the process of sperm maturation. These results suggest that DHA content may be critical in determining the fertilizing ability of mature spermatozoa and at the same time the susceptibility to lipid peroxidative damage leading to loss of membrane integrity, decreased lifespan, and increased DNA damage.

Overview of Sperm Maturation

In order to fertilize the oocyte *in vivo* and *in vitro*, spermatozoa must undergo a complex process of maturation in the seminiferous epithelium and the epididymis (1,2). This process involves a broad range of events, including the remodeling of membrane components (2) leading to the acquisition of motility (3,4) and the ability to undergo the acrosome reaction, (5–7) that require an overall increase in membrane fluidity

(8,9). Therefore, polyunsaturated fatty acids, and especially docosahexaenoic acid (DHA), are thought to play a key role in regulating membrane fluidity and sperm function.

Testicular Maturation: Spermatogenesis and Spermiogenesis

The process of spermatogenesis takes place in the seminiferous epithelium of the testis and is closely regulated and coordinated by the Sertoli cell (10–14). This paracrine process is synergistically regulated by testosterone and follicle stimulating hormone (FSH) (15–17). Regulation of spermatogenesis involves genetically programmed changes in chromatin structure and gene expression in the developing germ cells (18–20). The disruption of this double regulation system could lead to alterations in the development of sperm cell function.

Spermatogenesis in the seminiferous epithelium is conventionally divided into stages and steps (21). Each stage contains a specific set of cell types (e.g., spermatogonia, primary and secondary spermatocytes and round spermatids). The number of these stages varies significantly in a species-specific manner. For example, spermatogenesis in the rat involves 14 stages (22), whereas 6 stages are involved in the human (23).

The process of differentiation of a round spermatid into a differentiated spermatozoon, known as spermiogenesis, involves 19 steps in the rat, whereas the same process is completed in the human in only 8 steps. In the mouse and Rhesus monkey, spermiogenesis spans a total of 16 steps, whereas in dog, stallion, and bovine sperm it spans 12 steps (23).

Epididymal Maturation

The remodeling of the sperm plasma membrane, which occurs during sperm passage through the epididymis, is believed to be crucial in the acquisition of motility and the ability to penetrate and fertilize the egg (3,24). This remodeling process includes the uptake of secreted epididymal glycoproteins, removal or utilization of specific phospholipids from the inner leaflet of the bilayer, processing of existing or acquired glycoproteins by endoproteolysis, and repositioning of both protein and lipid molecules to different membranes (24,25). These modifications are carefully coordinated at different zones of the epididymis and indirectly affect intracellular membranes, organelles and even nuclear components (24). Lipid composition of the plasma membrane may be key in the interaction of spermatozoa with the epididymal environment. Secretion by epididymal cells of lipid-binding proteins may mediate changes in sterol content of particular membrane domains. The contact of sperm cells with membranous vesicles and merocrine secretions may be crucial in the development of physiological changes (26,27).

The Human Paradigm: A Deficiency in Quality Control?

A measure of spermatogenesis efficiency is the estimated number of spermatozoa produced per gram of testicular parenchyma (28). This depends on the proportional abundance of germ cells, their lifespan, the amount of germ cell degeneration, pubertal development, season, and aging (28,29).

In the plain rat (*Pseudomys australis*) the mean duration of the cycle of the seminiferous epithelium has been reported to be 11.2 days, the duration of spermatogenesis 45 days, and an epididymal transit time of approximately 9 days (caput 0.8 days; corpus 1.5 days; cauda 6.5 days) (30). In the human, the duration of each cycle is approximately 16 days with a total of 74 days required for a spermatogonia to become a differentiated spermatozoon. However, daily sperm production is only 25 to 35% of that of most species, including rats and nonhuman primates (31).

In the rat, a total of 19 steps are required for a round spermatid to become differentiated sperm. Of these 19 steps, eight (12 to 19) involve significant remodeling of the nucleus and cytoplasm. (21). The prevalence of morphological abnormalities (*e.g.,* abnormal head morphology and cytoplasmic retention) in species with a relatively complex process of spermiogenesis, such as the rat, mouse, *Rhesus* monkey, and stallion, is relatively low. In contrast, in man, a species in which there is a relatively high prevalence of immature sperm with head abnormalities and proximal cytoplasmic retention in the ejaculate, spermiogenesis spans 8 steps of which only two involve remodeling of the nucleus and cytoplasm. Therefore, it is conceivable that human sperm, because of a less rigorous quality control in the testis, are more prone to alterations in normal spermiogenesis and membrane remodeling.

Lipid Peroxidation

One of the consequences of defective sperm maturation in the seminiferous epithelium is the retention of residual cytoplasm. This residual cytoplasm, which is attached to the midpiece and retronuclear area of the sperm head, has been shown to produce high levels of reactive oxygen species (ROS) (32–35). In addition, the membranes enclosing the residual cytoplasm are enriched in polyunsaturated fatty acids such as DHA (35,36). The combination of high polyunsaturated fatty acid content and high ROS production in these immature sperm has been shown to lead to increased lipid peroxidation and subsequent loss of sperm function (32,33). ROS-mediated damage to human spermatozoa was characterized in the early 1980s (5,37–41) and has been shown by many authors to be an important factor in the pathogenesis of male infertility (32,42–44).

To a first approximation, the process of lipid peroxidation involves the initial abstraction of a hydrogen atom from the bis-allylic methylene groups of polyunsaturated fatty acids, mainly DHA, by molecular oxygen. This leads to molecular rearrangement to a conjugated diene and addition of oxygen, resulting in the production of a lipid peroxide radical. This peroxyradical can now abstract a new hydrogen atom from an adjacent DHA molecule leading to a chain reaction that ultimately results in lipid fragmentation and the production of malonaldehyde and toxic short-chain alkanes (*e.g.,* propane). These propagation reactions are mediated by oxygen radicals (Figure 3.1A).

DHA (Fig. 3.1B) is the major polyunsaturated fatty acid in sperm from a number of mammalian species, including the human (5,45,46), accounting in this species for up to 30% of phospholipid-bound fatty acid and 73% of polyunsaturated fatty acids (5). At the same time, DHA is the main substrate of lipid peroxidation, accounting for 90% of the overall rate of lipid peroxidation in human spermatozoa (5). Lipid peroxidation has profound consequences in biological membranes. The generation of the polar lipid peroxides ultimately results in the disruption of the membrane hydrophobic packing, inactivation of glycolytic enzymes, damage of axonemal proteins (loss of motility), acrosomal membrane damage, and DNA alterations (47–49). Oxidation of phospholipid-bound DHA has been shown to be the major factor that determines the motile lifespan of sperm *in vitro* (5,50,51).

Three basic factors determine the overall rate of lipid peroxidation of sperm *in vitro*: oxygen concentration and temperature in the medium (OXIDANT), the presence of antioxidant defenses (ANTIOXIDANT), and the content of membrane-bound DHA (SUBSTRATE) (Fig. 3.2). Thus, the higher the temperature and the concentration of oxygen in solution, the higher the rate of lipid peroxidation as measured by malonaldehyde production (41). Conversely, the higher the activity of antioxidant enzymes, the lower the rate of lipid peroxidation (41). The balance between these key factors determines the overall rate of peroxidation *in vitro*.

In this system, the substrate seems to play a key role. The main substrates for lipid peroxidation are polyunsaturated fatty acids, especially docosahexaenoic acid (Fig. 3.3). Since DHA is essential in maintaining membrane fluidity leading to the acquisition of motility and the zona-induced acrosome reaction, mammalian sperm have been forced during evolution to develop a powerful enzymatic antioxidant defense system, involving superoxide dismutase, glutathione peroxidase, and phospholipase A_2 (41,52).

The Cell-to-Cell Variability Theory and the Substrate Hypothesis

Since the motile lifespan of sperm *in vitro* and *in vivo* displays a cell-to-cell variability and is determined by the rate of lipid peroxidation, it would appear reasonable to hypothesize that there is a cell-to-cell variability in the rate of lipid peroxidation in sperm. As shown in Fig. 3.3, if all the sperm cells in a sample underwent lipid peroxidation at the same rate (as in A), they would be expected to lose motility at the same time. However, this is not what is observed *in vitro* and *in vivo*: as shown in B, a sperm sample is comprised of discrete subsets of spermatozoa that undergo motility loss in a stepwise fashion with some cells losing motility faster than others, thus suggesting that not all sperm cells in a given sample undergo lipid peroxidation at the same rate.

Since all sperm cells in a homogeneous suspension are assumed to be exposed to the same temperature and oxygen concentration, a potential strategy to minimize lipid peroxidation in sperm may be to maximize the activity and/or expression of antioxidant enzymes. However, the activity and cell-to-cell distribution of superoxide dismu-

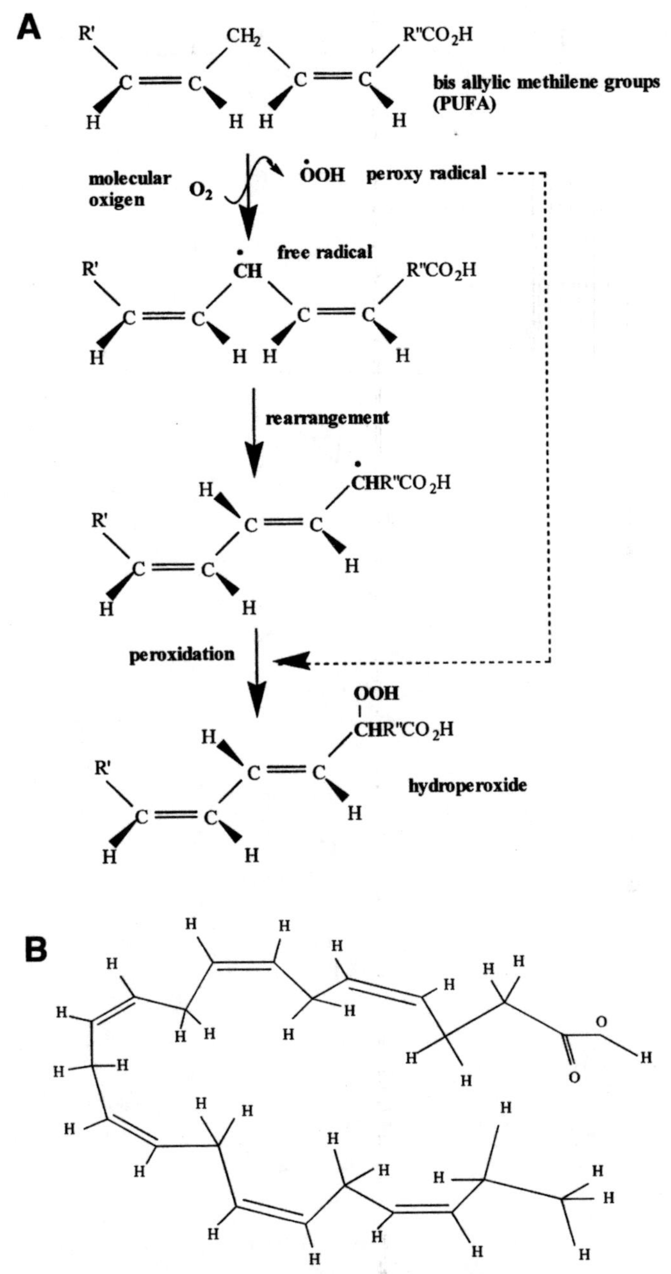

Fig. 3.1. (A) Schematic representation of the initial steps of fatty acid peroxidation. (B) Molecule of docosahexaenoic acid (DHA), the major substrate of lipid peroxidation.

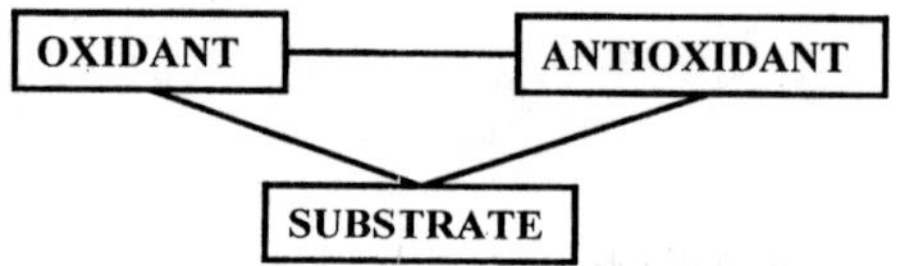

Fig. 3.2. The triad of lipid peroxidation.

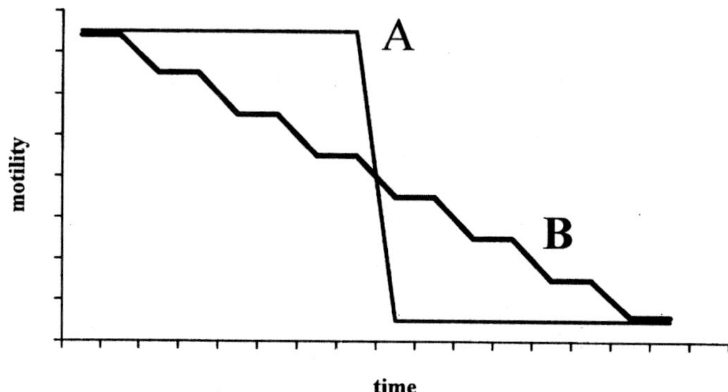

Fig. 3.3. The cell-to-cell variability theory. *A* corresponds to an ideal situation in which all spermatozoa in a given sample lose motility at the same time. *B* corresponds to an ideal situation in which cell subpopulations of a given sample undergo motility loss at different times.

tase and glutathione peroxidase, the main antioxidant defenses in human sperm, has been reported to be remarkably constant (52,53). Therefore, the only strategy left for sperm to minimize the risk of oxygen-induced damage would be to reduce the content of the SUBSTRATE during the process of membrane remodeling that takes place during sperm maturation in the seminiferous epithelium. However, as it was indicated previously, the efficiency of this process in the human testis is relatively low, leading to the release into the seminiferous tubules of relatively high numbers of sperm at different stages of maturation and membrane remodeling. It has been previously reported that the rate of lipid peroxidation and the production of ROS is significantly higher in immature sperm compared to mature sperm (33,34,35,42,54). According to the "substrate hypothesis" this observation can be related, at least in part, to the relatively high DHA content in the membranes of these immature sperm.

Fatty Acid Composition of Sperm at Different Stages of Maturation: The *in Vivo* Model

Most of the studies dealing with the analysis of fatty acid content in sperm and germ cells have been performed on experimental models, especially in rodents. It is worth noting that there are interspecific differences in the relative importance of polyunsaturated fatty acids, and the identity of the most abundant polyunsaturates. DHA, or 22:6n-3, is the predominant polyunsaturated fatty acid in sperm from humans and ruminants, whereas rodent and rabbit sperm contain mostly the n-6 docosapentaenoic acid (DPA, 22:5n-6) (45).

In an early study performed in the mouse, Grogan *et al.* isolated different populations of germ cells by light scattering sorting and assessed their lipid content (55). They found that 22:5n-6 (the most abundant polyunsaturate) increased progressively from 2 to 20% of total fatty acid in the progression of germinal cell differentiation from preleptotene spermatocyte to condensing spermatid but decreased in mature sperm. Its precursor, arachidonic acid (20:4n-6), showed a roughly reciprocal relationship, whereas 22:6n-3 showed no significant correlation with cell type. 22:5n-6 was found highest in triglycerides at later stages of differentiation, whereas 20:4n-6 and 22:6n-3 were found primarily in phospholipids from all cell fractions (55).

The same authors showed that the n-6 polyunsaturated fatty acids of the germinal cells labeled with radioactive acetate contained levels of radioactivity in each lipid class that were consistent with the importance of long-chain polyenoic fatty acid metabolism in germ cell function. Cells at later stages of maturation incorporated much higher levels of radioactivity into fatty acids derived from 20:4n-6 by elongation-desaturation pathways than did less mature cells or whole testis *in vitro* (56). Therefore, germ cells reach the epididymis containing the biochemical tools necessary for polyunsaturated fatty acid biosynthesis.

However, the changes that sperm undergo in their membrane components during epididymal transit seem to be mostly due to redistribution rather than to acquisition of new components. Thus, immature spermatozoa of the caput epididimys show higher ability to incorporate labeled fatty acids compared with mature spermatozoa from the cauda (57). Nevertheless, a change of the typical asymmetric pattern of membrane phospholipids has been attributed to postgonadal maturation of sperm. A marked decrease in the phosphatidylethanolamine/phosphatidylcholine ratio in the inner membrane has been reported (58), as well as profound changes in the distribution of saturated and unsaturated phospholipid-bound fatty acids.

Also, depletion of components has been reported. Aveldano *et al.* described a decrease in phosphatidylcholine and phosphatidylethanolamine in rat epididymis, leading to a relative increase in plasmenylcholine, which becomes the main phospholipid. Oleate and linoleate are decreased, whereas the proportion of longer chain and more unsaturated fatty acids is increased. The most relevant change corresponds to the relative increase in n-9 polyenes, accounting for more than half of the acyl chains present in plasmenylcholine of cauda spermatozoa (59,60).

In an early study, Adams *et al.* showed how spermatozoa from the caput epididymis had a significantly greater content of phospholipid, cholesterol, cholesterol ester, and free fatty acid than those from the cauda epididymis (61). Spermatozoa from the corpus epididymis had a significantly greater content of monoglyceride than those from the caput epididymis and a greater content of phospholipid, cholesterol, free fatty acids, and monoglyceride than those from the cauda epididymis (61).

In the ram and in the boar, the species containing the highest proportion of polyunsaturated fatty acids in mature spermatozoa (45), a net loss in phospholipid content and phospholipid-bound fatty acids has been described (62,63). This decrease in phospholipid content seems to be due to phosphatidylethanolamine, resulting in an increase in the phosphatidylcholine/phosphatidylethanolamine ratio, as well as in the cholesterol/phospholipid ratio, whereas desmosterol becomes negligible after maturation. The relative predominant fatty acids switch from palmitic in the less mature to DHA on the more mature spermatozoa (64).

In a more recent study performed in the epididymal sperm of human patients of prostate carcinoma, Haidl and Opper found that the ratio between phosphatidylcholine and phosphatidylserine plus phosphatidylethanolamine plus sphingomyelin was significantly higher in spermatozoa from the cauda compared to those from the caput and corpus. This was attributed to both an increase of phosphatidylcholine and a decrease of other phospholipids. With regard to fatty acids, those with saturated chains predominated in caput spermatozoa, whereas the highest concentration of unsaturated long-chain fatty acids was found in cauda spermatozoa (65).

In another study using rat epididymal sperm, 56% of the phospholipid consisted of choline and ethanolamine phosphoglycerides; the remainder consisted of sphingomyelin, phosphatidylserine, and diphosphatidylglycerol. The mole percent of phosphatidylethanolamine increased in sperm proceeding from the caput to the corpus epididymis and then declined from the corpus to the cauda epididymis. The phospholipid-bound fatty acids consisted primarily of palmitate and stearate (saturated), with a significant increase in the mole percent 22:5n-6 in cauda sperm (66).

More recently we analyzed the fatty acid content of cells isolated from the seminiferous tubules and the epididymis of adult mice, and we found that the content in both 22:5n-6 and 22:6n-3 is higher in cells from seminiferous tubules than from epididymis. The total fatty acid content was found to be 6-fold higher in cells from the seminiferous tubules. Since the decrease in fatty acid content per cell in epididymal sperm, compared to cells from the seminiferous tubules, was much more pronounced than the decrease in 22:6n-3 content, when DHA was expressed as the percent of total fatty acid, there appeared to be an apparent increase in DHA in epididymal sperm (36).

The *in Vitro* Model: Isolation of Sperm Subsets by Density Gradient Centrifugation

In a recent study, we analyzed the content of phospholipid-bound DHA in subsets of human spermatozoa isolated by a discontinuous Percoll density gradient (36). Since most human ejaculated sperm samples contain a relative high proportion of immature cells, the use of these gradients allows the study *in vitro* of sperm at different stages of maturation.

The four panels of Fig. 3.4 show the morphology of the cells found in the different fractions obtained by a discontinuous density gradient of Percoll. Fraction 1 (panel A) is enriched in immature germ cells and immature sperm with abnormal head morphology and cytoplasmic retention. These immature forms and germ cells look closer to the cells that can be found in the seminiferous epithelium. Fraction 2 (panel B) con-

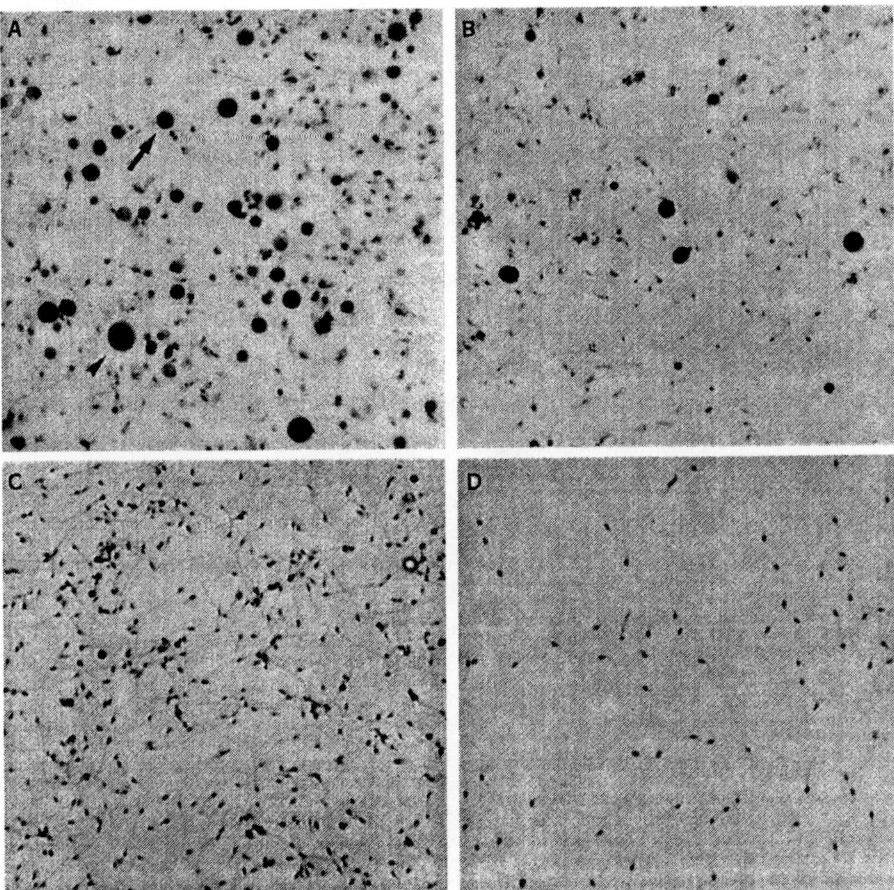

Fig. 3.4. The *in vitro* density gradient model for sperm maturation. Light micrography of hematoxylin-eosin-stained human spermatozoa. In order to obtain subpopulations of sperm at different stage of maturation, samples are processed through a 50, 70, and 95% discontinuous Percoll gradient. After 20 minutes of centrifugation at 800 g, four fractions are recovered: Fraction 1 (A), from the interphase between seminal plasma and 50% Percoll; Fraction 2 (B), from the 50%/70% interphase; Fraction 3 (C), from the 70%/95% interphase; and Fraction 4 (D), corresponding to the pellet. Arrowhead: primary spermatocyte. Arrow: round spermatid (from Ollero *et al.* [36]).

tains, mostly, immature sperm with cytoplasmic retention, looking closer to those that could be found in the seminiferous tubules. Fraction 3 (panel C) contains a mixture of morphologically normal and abnormal sperm. The proportion of cells with normal morphology is higher than in the previous panels, and the most frequent morphological abnormality is the presence of the cytoplasmic droplet. This is similar to the cells that can be found in the caput/corpus epididymis. Finally, fraction 4 (panel D) contained, for the most part, morphologically normal sperm, looking closer to mature cells found in the cauda epididymis or vas deferens (36).

In this study as in many others using similar gradients (67–69), percent sperm motility was significantly lower in fractions 1, 2, and 3 compared to fraction 4. The opposite happens with percent abnormal forms (35,67–80). DHA content (Table 3.1 and Fig. 3.5) in the most immature fraction is 2.5 times higher than in the most mature, whereas total fatty acid content is 2.7-fold higher in the former. However, no significant differences in phospholipid-bound DHA were found when expressed as the percent of total fatty acid. Although there is a slight increase from fraction 1 to 3, differences were not statistically significant (36).

Using fairly similar Percoll gradients, Lenzi *et al.* compared the fatty acid profile, expressed as the relative amount of each fatty acid, of human immature germ cells and mature spermatozoa. A higher proportion of saturated fatty acid and essential fatty acid was present in immature cells, as well as a lower percentage of DHA, showing a direct linear correlation between percent DHA and percent Percoll in the gradient layer (81).

Gradients of Percoll or similar products separate cells as a function of cell density or lipid/protein ratio. In general, we would expect that samples with a higher content in lipids would be in fraction 1, at the top of the gradient. This is consistent with the presence of cytoplasm in immature cells. These cells have more volume, more surface, and are expected to have more lipids and display lower density.

Table 3.1

Fatty Acid and Sterol Composition of the Different Percoll Fractions of Human Sperm Samples. Values Are Expressed in nmoles per Million Cells (from Ollero *et al.* [36]).

	Fraction 1	Fraction 2	Fraction 3	Fraction 4
16:0	9.49 ± 1.06	5.46 ± 0.50	3.61 ± 0.25	3.46 ± 0.36
16:1	0.35 ± 0.06	0.33 ± 0.08	0.15 ± 0.03	0.12 ± 0.04
18:0	0.79 ± 0.10	0.51 ± 0.08	0.38 ± 0.04	0.53 ± 0.10
18:1	0.80 ± 0.09	0.44 ± 0.05	0.23 ± 0.02	0.23 ± 0.04
18:2n-6	0.70 ± 0.09	0.31 ± 0.03	0.17 ± 0.01	0.14 ± 0.01
20:3n-6	0.24 ± 0.03	0.11 ± 0.01	0.07 ± 0.01	0.05 ± 0.00
20:4n-6	0.18 ± 0.02	0.09 ± 0.01	0.07 ± 0.01	0.07 ± 0.01
22:6n-3 (DHA)	2.17 ± 0.30	1.46 ± 0.19	1.07 ± 0.14	0.86 ± 0.12
Cholesterol	0.86 ± 0.07	0.62 ± 0.04	0.38 ± 0.02	0.39 ± 0.04
Desmosterol	0.18 ± 0.02	0.12 ± 0.01	0.10 ± 0.01	0.11 ± 0.02
Cholesterol/Desmosterol	7.50 ± 1.33	7.17 ± 1.04	5.32 ± 0.87	5.58 ± 0.98
DHA/cholesterol	2.95 ± 0.57	2.83 ± 0.49	3.24 ± 0.59	3.19 ± 0.58

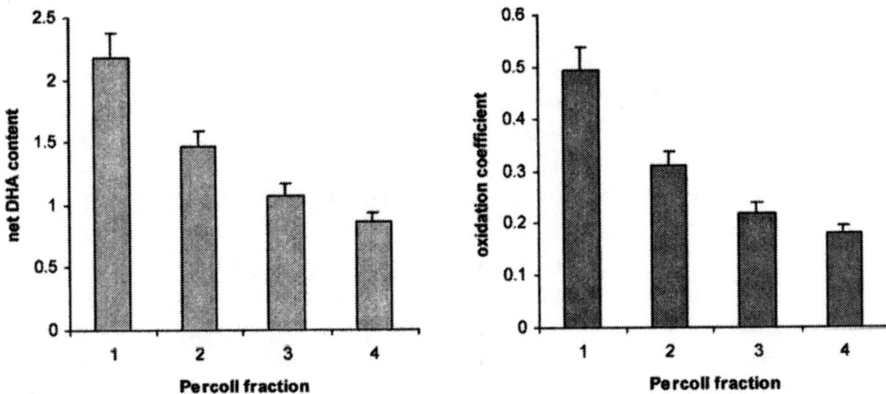

Fig. 3.5. DHA content (left) and oxidation coefficients (right) in human sperm from the different Percoll fractions. DHA values are expressed in nmoles per million (from Ollero *et al.* [36]). Oxidation coefficients were calculated from the exponential curves of time course of loss of fatty acids from the phospholipid components of human sperm cells described by Alvarez and Storey (5).

Swim-up is another commonly used method for the isolation of sperm subsets, in this case, as a function of motility through layers of different density. In a recent study, the cholesterol and total phospholipid content was found to be significantly lower in swim-up selected sperm compared to total sperm (82). The authors estimated membrane fluidity by fluorescence polarization and found this parameter comparable between the swim-up sperm fraction (more mature) and total sperm. The sperm membrane fluidity obtained in normospermic patients was compared with abnormospermic ones (oligoasthenoteratospermia), and in the latter it was found to be decreased in migrated spermatozoa compared with total sperm. The authors suggest that the swim-up selects a subpopulation of mature spermatozoa characterized by a low content of cholesterol and phospholipid, likely related to a reduced membrane area. The fact that the cholesterol/phospholipid and phophatidylcholine/(phophatidylcholine+phophatidylethanolamine) molar ratios were unchanged suggests that membrane quality is somehow maintained. This was confirmed by the measurement of fluorescence anisotropy, showing no difference in plasma membrane fluidity between swim-up selected sperm and total sperm (82).

Putting Things Together: DHA Up or Down?

The results of the *in vitro* approach for the isolation of subsets of human spermatozoa at different stages of maturation demonstrate the presence of cell-to-cell differences in DHA content, and, by extension, in content of polyunsaturates, as well as marked changes in lipid composition in spermatozoa during the process of maturation.

When lipid data are expressed as moles/cell, it can be concluded that there is a net decrease in total fatty acid and DHA content as sperm migrate from the seminiferous tubules to the epididymis (36,82). These results are in agreement with the *in vivo* model approach in which data are expressed in the same fashion (83,84). Interestingly, when the lipid data are expressed as the relative concentration of the different fatty acids, there are either no significant differences or an "apparent" increase in polyunsaturated fatty acid concentration during the process of sperm maturation (36,64–66). However, based on the *in vivo* and *in vitro* studies, we can conclude that there is a net decrease in DHA content in sperm membranes during the process of sperm maturation and a "relative increase" or a "lower decrease" in DHA concentration compared to other fatty acids.

A selective loss of phospholipids, probably associated with the extrusion of the residual cytoplasm occurs during sperm maturation. As a consequence, there is a higher decrease in total fatty acid mass compared to plasmalogens (64), which could explain this apparent increase in DHA. The fact that the net decrease in DHA is concomitant with a net decrease in saturated fatty acid and sterol content (36,82) (Table 1) would explain why the overall sperm membrane fluidity may not significantly change or even increase. On the other hand, removal of DHA (substrate) during sperm maturation will decrease the susceptibility of sperm toward lipid peroxidation. Figure 3.5 shows the calculated oxidation coefficients of sperm in mature and immature sperm isolated by density gradient centrifugation.

This is consistent with the notion that loss of DHA during sperm maturation may be part of the genomically regulated cellular maturational steps that take place within the adluminal compartment. By the time sperm arrive to the epididymis, these events are completed (85). If these events do not occur, immature sperm in the ejaculate would exhibit cytoplasmic retention, a high rate of lipid peroxidation (42,54), and ROS production (33), and presumably these sperm also show higher levels of DHA and shortened cell viability (33,86). It is possible that the same spermiogenic remodeling described for membrane bound galactosyl transferase, cytoplasmic droplet extrusion, and creatine phosphokinase-M expression also applies to loss of DHA (87). It is likely that the decline in DHA content, similar to the reported decline in galactosyl transferase, reflects this developmental membrane remodeling.

DHA has been shown to induce apoptosis in somatic cells (88) and to regulate the cell cycle (89,90). Therefore, since DHA content is relatively high in immature germ cells, and given that these cells are capable of synthesizing polyunsaturated fatty acids, it is possible that DHA may also play a role in the regulation of spermatogenesis through diverse mechanisms, including programmed death of spermatogenic cells.

It can be concluded that during the process of sperm maturation a critical level of DHA may be retained, resulting in optimal membrane fluidity required for sperm motility and the induction of the acrosome reaction and, at the same time, minimizing peroxidative damage to sperm.

Acknowledgments

We express our gratitude to the Andrology Laboratory at Boston IVF for their help in the processing and collection of samples; John Zeind, director of the Core Laboratory at Beth Israel Deaconess Medical Center, for technical support; and Dr. Bayard T. Storey for his intellectual contribution to the thoughts and hypotheses expressed in this chapter.

References

1. Amann, R.P., Hammerstedt, R.H., and Veeramachaneni, D.N. (1993) The Epididymis and Sperm Maturation: A Perspective, *Reprod. Fertil. Dev. 5*, 361–381

2. Jones, R. (1989) Membrane Remodeling during Sperm Maturation in the Epididymis, *Oxf. Rev. Reprod. Biol. 11*, 285–337

3. Esponda, P. (1991) Spermatozoon Maturation in Vertebrates with Internal Fertilization, *Microsc. Electron Biol. Cell. 15*, 1–23.

4. Hegde, U.C. (1996) Epididymal Sperm Maturation Proteins, *Indian J. Biochem. Biophys. 33*, 103–110.

5. Alvarez, J.G., and Storey, B.T. (1995) Differential Incorporation of Fatty Acids Into and Peroxidative Loss of Fatty Acids from Phospholipids of Human Spermatozoa, *Mol. Reprod. Dev. 42*, 334–346.

6. Toshimori, K. (1998) Maturation of Mammalian Spermatozoa: Modifications of the Acrosome and Plasma Membrane Leading to Fertilization, *Cell Tissue Res. 293*, 177–187.

7. Yeung, C.H., Cooper, T.G., and Weinbauer, G.F. (1996) Maturation of Monkey Spermatozoa in the Epididymis with Respect to Their Ability to Undergo the Acrosome Reaction, *J. Androl. 17*, 427–432.

8. Flechon, J.E. (1985) Sperm Surface Changes during the Acrosome Reaction as Observed by Freeze-Fracture, *Am. J. Anat. 174*, 239–248.

9. Myles, D.G., Hyatt, H., and Primakoff, P. (1987) Binding of Both Acrosome-Intact and Acrosome-Reacted Guinea Pig Sperm to the Zona Pellucida during *in Vitro* Fertilization, *Dev. Biol. 121*, 559–567.

10. De Kretser, D.M., Loveland, K.L., Meinhardt, A., Simorangkir, D., and Wreford, N. (1998) Spermatogenesis, *Hum. Reprod. 13 (Suppl. 1)*, 1–8.

11. Griswold, M.D. (1995) Interactions Between Germ Cells and Sertoli Cells in the Testis, *Biol. Reprod. 52*, 211–216.

12. Griswold, M.D. (1998) The Central Role of Sertoli Cells in Spermatogenesis, *Semin. Cell Dev. Biol. 9*, 411–416.

13. Griswold, M.D., Morales, C., and Sylvester, S.R. (1988) Molecular Biology of the Sertoli Cell, *Oxf. Rev. Reprod. Biol. 10*, 124–161.

14. Kerr, J.B. (1995) Macro, Micro, and Molecular Research on Spermatogenesis: The Quest to Understand Its Control, *Microsc. Res. Tech. 32*, 364–384.

15. Mclachlan, R.I., O'Donnell, L., Meachem, S.J., Stanton, P.G., De Kretser, D.M., Pratis, K., and Robertson, D.M. (2002) Identification of Specific Sites of Hormonal Regulation in Spermatogenesis in Rats, Monkeys, and Man, *Recent Prog. Horm. Res. 57*, 149–179.

16. Tesarik, J., Guido, M., Mendoza, C., and Greco, E. (1998) Human Spermatogenesis *in Vitro*: Respective Effects of Follicle-Stimulating Hormone and Testosterone on Meiosis, Spermiogenesis, and Sertoli Cell Apoptosis, *J. Clin. Endocrinol. Metab. 83*, 4467–4473.

17. Weinbauer, G.F., and Nieschlag, E. (1997) Endocrine Control of Germ Cell Proliferation in the Primate Testis. What Do We Really Know? *Adv. Exp. Med. Biol. 424*, 51–58

18. Escalier, D. (2001) Impact of Genetic Engineering on the Understanding of Spermatogenesis, *Hum. Reprod. Update 7*, 191–210.

19. Grootegoed, J.A., Baarends, W.M., Hendriksen, P.J., Hoogerbrugge, J.W., Slegtenhorst-Eegdeman, K.E., and Themmen, A.P. (1995) Molecular and Cellular Events in Spermatogenesis, *Hum. Reprod. 10 (Suppl. 1)*, 10–14.

20. Grootegoed, J.A., Siep, M., and Baarends, W.M. (2000) Molecular and Cellular Mechanisms in Spermatogenesis, *Baillieres Best Pract. Res. Clin. Endocrinol. Metab. 14*, 331–343.

21. Russell, L.D., Ettlin, R.A., Sinha-Hikim, A.P., and Clegg, E.D. (1990) *Histological and Histopathological Evaluation of the Testis*, pp. 286, Cache River Press, Vienna, IL.

22. Clermont, Y., and Leblond, C.P. (1953) Renewal of Spermatogonia in the Rat, *Am. J. Anat. 93*, 475–501.

23. Clermont, Y. (1963) The Cycle of the Seminiferous Epithelium in Man, *Am. J. Anat. 112*, 35–51.

24. Jones, R. (1998) Plasma Membrane Structure and Remodeling during Sperm Maturation in the Epididymis, *J. Reprod. Fertil. Suppl. 53*, 73–84.

25. James, P.S., Wolfe, C.A., Ladha, S., and Jones, R. (1999) Lipid Diffusion in the Plasma Membrane of Ram and Boar Spermatozoa during Maturation in the Epididymis Measured by Fluorescence Recovery after Photobleaching, *Mol. Reprod. Dev. 52*, 207–215.

26. Cooper, T.G. (1998) Interactions Between Epididymal Secretions and Spermatozoa, *J. Reprod. Fertil. Suppl. 53*, 119–136

27. Kirchhoff, C., Pera, I., Derr, P., Yeung, C.H., and Cooper, T. (1997) The Molecular Biology of the Sperm Surface. Post-Testicular Membrane Remodeling, *Adv. Exp. Med. Biol. 424*, 221–232

28. Johnson, L. (1995) Efficiency of Spermatogenesis, *Microsc. Res. Tech. 32*, 385–422.

29. Johnson, L., Varner, D.D., Roberts, M.E., Smith, T.L., Keillor, G.E., and Scrutchfield, W.L. (2000) Efficiency of Spermatogenesis: A Comparative Approach, *Anim. Reprod. Sci. 60–61*, 471–480.

30. Peirce, E.J., and Breed, W.G. (2001) A Comparative Study of Sperm Production in Two Species of Australian Arid Zone Rodents (*Pseudomys Australis, Notomys Alexis*) with Marked Differences in Testis Size, *Reproduction 121*, 239–247.

31. Johnson, L., Chaturvedi, P.K., and Williams, J.D. (1992) Missing Generations of Spermatocytes and Spermatids in Seminiferous Epithelium Contribute to Low Efficiency of Spermatogenesis in Humans, *Biol. Reprod. 47*, 1091–1098.

32. Aitken, J., Krausz, C., and Buckingham, D. (1994) Relationships Between Biochemical Markers for Residual Sperm Cytoplasm, Reactive Oxygen Species Generation, and the Presence of Leukocytes and Precursor Germ Cells in Human Sperm Suspensions, *Mol. Reprod. Dev. 39*, 268–279.

33. Gil-Guzman, E., Ollero, M., Lopez, M.C., Sharma, R.K., Alvarez, J.G., Thomas, A.J., Jr., and Agarwal, A. (2001) Differential Production of Reactive Oxygen Species by Subsets of Human Spermatozoa at Different Stages of Maturation, *Hum. Reprod. 16*, 1922–1930.

34. Gomez, E., Buckingham, D.W., Brindle, J., Lanzafame, F., Irvine, D.S., and Aitken, R.J. (1996) Development of an Image Analysis System to Monitor the Retention of Residual Cytoplasm by Human Spermatozoa: Correlation with Biochemical Markers of the Cytoplasmic Space, Oxidative Stress, and Sperm Function, *J. Androl. 17*, 276–287.

35. Huszar, G., and Vigue, L. (1993) Incomplete Development of Human Spermatozoa Is Associated with Increased Creatine Phosphokinase Concentration and Abnormal Head Morphology, *Mol. Reprod. Dev. 34*, 292–298.

36. Ollero, M., Powers, R.D., and Alvarez, J.G. (2000) Variation of Docosahexaenoic Acid Content in Subsets of Human Spermatozoa at Different Stages of Maturation: Implications for Sperm Lipoperoxidative Damage, *Mol. Reprod. Dev. 55*, 326–334.

37. Alvarez, J.G., Holland, M.K., and Storey, B.T. (1984) Spontaneous Lipid Peroxidation in Rabbit Spermatozoa: A Useful Model for the Reaction of O_2 Metabolites with Single Cells, *Adv. Exp. Med. Biol. 169*, 433–443

38. Alvarez, J.G., and Storey, B.T. (1982) Spontaneous Lipid Peroxidation in Rabbit Epididymal Spermatozoa: Its Effect on Sperm Motility, *Biol. Reprod. 27*, 1102–1108.

39. Alvarez, J.G., and Storey, B.T. (1984) Assessment of Cell Damage Caused by Spontaneous Lipid Peroxidation in Rabbit Spermatozoa, *Biol. Reprod. 30*, 323–331.

40. Alvarez, J.G., and Storey, B.T. (1984) Lipid Peroxidation and the Reactions of Superoxide and Hydrogen Peroxide in Mouse Spermatozoa, *Biol. Reprod. 30*, 833–841.

41. Alvarez, J.G., Touchstone, J.C., Blasco, L., and Storey, B.T. (1987) Spontaneous Lipid Peroxidation and Production of Hydrogen Peroxide and Superoxide in Human Spermatozoa. Superoxide Dismutase as Major Enzyme Protectant Against Oxygen Toxicity, *J. Androl. 8*, 338–348.

42. Aitken, J., and Fisher, H. (1994) Reactive Oxygen Species Generation and Human Spermatozoa: The Balance of Benefit and Risk, *Bioessays 16*, 259–267.

43. De Lamirande, E., and Gagnon, C. (1994) Reactive Oxygen Species (Ros) and Reproduction, *Adv. Exp. Med. Biol. 366*, 185–197

44. Sharma, R.K., and Agarwal, A. (1996) Role of Reactive Oxygen Species in Male Infertility, *Urology 48*, 835–850.

45. Poulos, A., Darin-Bennett, A., and White, I.G. (1973) The Phospholipid-Bound Fatty Acids and Aldehydes of Mammalian Spermatozoa, *Comp. Biochem. Physiol. B 46*, 541–549.

46. Zalata, A.A., Christophe, A.B., Depuydt, C.E., Schoonjans, F., and Comhaire, F.H. (1998) The Fatty Acid Composition of Phospholipids of Spermatozoa from Infertile Patients, *Mol. Hum. Reprod. 4*, 111–118.

47. Alvarez, J.G., Sharma, R.K., Ollero, M., Saleh, R.A., Lopez, M.C., Thomas, A.J., Evenson, D.P., and Agarwal, A. (2002) Increased DNA Damage in Sperm from Leukocytospermic Semen Samples as Determined by the Sperm Chromatin Structure Assay, *Fertil. Steril. 78*, 319–329.

48. Fraga, C.G., Motchnik, P.A., Shigenaga, M.K., Helbock, H.J., Jacob, R.A., and Ames, B.N. (1991) Ascorbic Acid Protects Against Endogenous Oxidative DNA Damage in Human Sperm, *Proc. Natl. Acad. Sci. USA 88*, 11003–11006.

49. Fraga, C.G., Motchnik, P.A., Wyrobek, A.J., Rempel, D.M., and Ames, B.N. (1996) Smoking and Low Antioxidant Levels Increase Oxidative Damage to Sperm DNA, *Mutat. Res. 351*, 199–203.

50. Aitken, R.J., Harkiss, D., and Buckingham, D. (1993) Relationship Between Iron-Catalyzed Lipid Peroxidation Potential and Human Sperm Function, *J. Reprod. Fertil. 98*, 257–265.

51. Jones, R., Mann, T., and Sherins, R. (1979) Peroxidative Breakdown of Phospholipids in Human Spermatozoa, Spermicidal Properties of Fatty Acid Peroxides, and Protective Action of Seminal Plasma, *Fertil. Steril. 31*, 531–537.

52. Alvarez, J.G., and Storey, B.T. (1989) Role of Glutathione Peroxidase in Protecting Mammalian Spermatozoa from Loss of Motility Caused by Spontaneous Lipid Peroxidation, *Gamete Res. 23*, 77–90.

53. Storey, B.T., Alvarez, J.G., and Thompson, K.A. (1998) Human Sperm Glutathione Reductase Activity *in Situ* Reveals Limitation in the Glutathione Antioxidant Defense System Due to Supply of NADPH, *Mol. Reprod. Dev. 49*, 400–407.

54. Huszar, G., and Vigue, L. (1994) Correlation Between the Rate of Lipid Peroxidation and Cellular Maturity as Measured by Creatine Kinase Activity in Human Spermatozoa, *J. Androl. 15*, 71–77.

55. Grogan, W.M., Farnham, W.F., and Szopiak, B.A. (1981) Long Chain Polyenoic Acid Levels in Viably Sorted, Highly Enriched Mouse Testis Cells, *Lipids 16*, 401–410.

56. Grogan, W.M., and Huth, E.G. (1983) Biosynthesis of Long-Chain Polyenoic Acids from Arachidonic Acid in Cultures of Enriched Spermatocytes and Spermatids from Mouse Testis, *Lipids 18*, 275–284.

57. Srivastava, A., and Olson, G.E. (1996) Studies on [^{3}H]Palmitate-Binding Proteins of Rat Spermatozoa: A Post-Translational Modification of Membrane Proteins by Fatty Acid Acylation, *J. Reprod. Fertil. 108*, 245–251.

58. Rana, A.P., Misra, S., Majumder, G.C., and Ghosh, A. (1993) Phospholipid Asymmetry of Goat Sperm Plasma Membrane during Epididymal Maturation, *Biochim. Biophys. Acta. 1210*, 1–7.

59. Aveldano, M.I. (1992) Long and Very Long Polyunsaturated Fatty Acids of Retina and Spermatozoa: The Whole Complement of Polyenoic Fatty Acid Series, *Adv. Exp. Med. Biol. 318*, 231–242.

60. Aveldano, M.I., Rotstein, N.P., and Vermouth, N.T. (1992) Lipid Remodeling during Epididymal Maturation of Rat Spermatozoa. Enrichment in Plasmenylcholines Containing Long-Chain Polyenoic Fatty Acids of the N-9 Series, *Biochem. J. 283*, 235–241.

61. Adams, C.S., and Johnson, A.D. (1977) The Lipid Content of Epididymal Spermatozoa of Rattus Norvegicus, *Comp. Biochem. Physiol. B 58*, 409–411.

62. Evans, R.W., and Setchell, B.P. (1979) Lipid Changes during Epididymal Maturation in Ram Spermatozoa Collected at Different Times of the Year, *J. Reprod. Fertil. 57*, 197–203.

63. Evans, R.W., and Setchell, B.P. (1979) Lipid Changes in Boar Spermatozoa during Epididymal Maturation with Some Observations on the Flow and Composition of Boar Rete Testis Fluid, *J. Reprod. Fertil. 57*, 189–196.

64. Parks, J.E., and Hammerstedt, R.H. (1985) Development Changes Occurring in the Lipids of Ram Epididymal Spermatozoa Plasma Membrane, *Biol. Reprod. 32*, 653–668.

65. Haidl, G., and Opper, C. (1997) Changes in Lipids and Membrane Anisotropy in Human Spermatozoa during Epididymal Maturation, *Hum. Reprod. 12*, 2720–2723.

66. Hall, J.C., Hadley, J., and Doman, T. (1991) Correlation Between Changes in Rat Sperm Membrane Lipids, Protein, and the Membrane Physical State during Epididymal Maturation, *J. Androl. 12*, 76–87.

67. Angelopoulos, T., Moshel, Y.A., Lu, L., Macanas, E., Grifo, J.A., and Krey, L.C. (1998) Simultaneous Assessment of Sperm Chromatin Condensation and Morphology before and after Separation Procedures: Effect on the Clinical Outcome after *in Vitro* Fertilization, *Fertil. Steril. 69*, 740–747.

68. Lassalle, B., Ziyyat, A., Testart, J., Finaz, C., and Lefevre, A. (1999) Flow Cytometric Method to Isolate Round Spermatids from Mouse Testis, *Hum. Reprod. 14*, 388–394.

69. Le Lannou, D., and Blanchard, Y. (1988) Nuclear Maturity and Morphology of Human Spermatozoa Selected by Percoll Density Gradient Centrifugation or Swim-Up Procedure, *J. Reprod. Fertil. 84*, 551–556.

70. Hall, J.A., Fishel, S.B., Timson, J.A., Dowell, K., and Klentzeris, L.D. (1995) Human Sperm Morphology Evaluation Pre- and Post-Percoll Gradient Centrifugation, *Hum. Reprod. 10*, 342–346.

71. Menkveld, R., Swanson, R.J., Kotze, T.J., and Kruger, T.F. (1990) Comparison of a Discontinuous Percoll Gradient Method *Versus* a Swim-Up Method: Effects on Sperm Morphology and other Semen Parameters, *Andrologia 22*, 152–158.

72. Mortimer, D., and Mortimer, S.T. (1992) Methods of Sperm Preparation for Assisted Reproduction, *Ann. Acad. Med. Singapore 21*, 517–524.

73. Pardo, M., Barri, P.N., Bancells, N., Coroleu, B., Buxaderas, C., Pomerol, J.M., Jr., and Sabater, J. (1988) Spermatozoa Selection in Discontinuous Percoll Gradients for Use in Artificial Insemination, *Fertil. Steril. 49*, 505–509.

74. Pousette, A., Akerlof, E., Rosenborg, L., and Fredricsson, B. (1986) Increase in Progressive Motility and Improved Morphology of Human Spermatozoa Following their Migration Through Percoll Gradients, *Int. J. Androl. 9*, 1–13.

75. Saad, A., and Guerin, J.F. (1992) Movement Characteristics of Human Spermatozoa Collected from Different Layers of a Discontinuous Percoll Gradient, *Andrologia 24*, 149–153.

76. Sukcharoen, N. (1995) The Effect of Discontinuous Percoll Gradient Centrifugation on Sperm Morphology and Nuclear DNA Normality, *J. Med. Assoc. Thai 78*, 22–29.

77. Van Der Zwalmen, P., Bertin-Segal, G., Geerts, L., Debauche, C., and Schoysman, R. (1991) Sperm Morphology and IVF Pregnancy Rate: Comparison Between Percoll Gradient Centrifugation and Swim-Up Procedures, *Hum. Reprod. 6*, 581–588.

78. Watkins, A.M., Chan, P.J., Patton, W.C., Jacobson, J.D., and King, A. (1996) Sperm Kinetics and Morphology before and after Fractionation on Discontinuous Percoll Gradient for Sex Preselection: Computerized Analyses, *Arch. Androl. 37*, 1–5.

79. Yao, Y.Q., Ng, V., Yeung, W.S., and Ho, P.C. (1996) Profiles of Sperm Morphology and Motility after Discontinuous Multiple-Step Percoll Density Gradient Centrifugation, *Andrologia 28*, 127–131.

80. Yue, Z., Meng, F.J., Jorgensen, N., Ziebe, S., and Nyboe Andersen, A. (1995) Sperm Morphology Using Strict Criteria after Percoll Density Separation: Influence on Cleavage and Pregnancy Rates after *in Vitro* Fertilization, *Hum. Reprod. 10*, 1781–1785.

81. Lenzi, A., Gandini, L., Maresca, V., Rago, R., Sgro, P., Dondero, F., and Picardo, M. (2000) Fatty Acid Composition of Spermatozoa and Immature Germ Cells, *Mol. Hum. Reprod. 6*, 226–231.

82. Force, A., Grizard, G., Giraud, M.N., Motta, C., Sion, B., and Boucher, D. (2001) Membrane Fluidity and Lipid Content of Human Spermatozoa Selected by Swim-Up Method, *Int. J. Androl. 24*, 327–334.

83. Awano, M., Kawaguchi, A., and Mohri, H. (1993) Lipid Composition of Hamster Epididymal Spermatozoa, *J. Reprod. Fertil. 99*, 375–383.

84. Rana, A.P., Majumder, G.C., Misra, S., and Ghosh, A. (1991) Lipid Changes of Goat Sperm Plasma Membrane during Epididymal Maturation, *Biochim. Biophys. Acta. 1061*, 185–196.

85. Huszar, G., Patrizio, P., Vigue, L., Willets, M., Wilker, C., Adhoot, D., and Johnson, L. (1998) Cytoplasmic Extrusion and the Switch from Creatine Kinase B to M Isoform Are

Completed by the Commencement of Epididymal Transport in Human and Stallion Spermatozoa, *J. Androl. 19*, 11–20.

86. Ollero, M., Gil-Guzman, E., Lopez, M.C., Sharma, R.K., Agarwal, A., Larson, K., Evenson, D., Thomas, A.J., Jr., and Alvarez, J.G. (2001) Characterization of Subsets of Human Spermatozoa at Different Stages of Maturation: Implications in the Diagnosis and Treatment of Male Infertility, *Hum. Reprod. 16*, 1912–1921.

87. Huszar, G., Sbracia, M., Vigue, L., Miller, D.J., and Shur, B.D. (1997) Sperm Plasma Membrane Remodeling during Spermiogenetic Maturation in Men: Relationship among Plasma Membrane Beta 1,4-Galactosyltransferase, Cytoplasmic Creatine Phosphokinase, and Creatine Phosphokinase Isoform Ratios, *Biol. Reprod. 56*, 1020–1024.

88. Calviello, G., Palozza, P., Piccioni, E., Maggiano, N., Frattucci, A., Franceschelli, P., and Bartoli, G.M. (1998) Dietary Supplementation with Eicosapentaenoic and Docosahexaenoic Acid Inhibits Growth of Morris Hepatocarcinoma 3924a in Rats: Effects on Proliferation and Apoptosis, *Int. J. Cancer 75*, 699–705.

89. Gustafsson, J.A., Gearing, K., Widmark, E., Tollet, P., Stromstedt, M., Berge, R.K., and Gottlicher, M. (1994) Effects of Fatty Acids on Gene Expression Mediated by a Member of the Nuclear Receptor Supergene Family, *Prog. Clin. Biol. Res. 387*, 21–28.

90. Sellmayer, A., Danesch, U., and Weber, P.C. (1996) Effects of Different Polyunsaturated Fatty Acids on Growth-Related Early Gene Expression and Cell Growth, *Lipids 31 Suppl*, S37–40.

Chapter 4

Docosahexaenoic Acid Supplementation and Male Fertility

Julie A. Conquer, Ph.D.[a] **and Francis Tekpetey, Ph.D.**[b]

[a]Human Nutraceutical Research Unit and Department of Human Biology and Nutritional Sciences, University of Guelph, Guelph, Ontario, Canada N1G 2W
[b]London Health Sciences Centre and Department of Obstetrics and Gynecology, University of Western Ontario, London, Ontario, Canada N6A 5A5

Abstract

Docosahexaenoic acid (DHA; 22:6n-3) is found in extremely high levels in human ejaculate with the majority occurring in the spermatozoa. Although serum phospholipid DHA levels are similar between fertile men and asthenozoospermic (decreased sperm motility) men, seminal plasma (3.7 vs. 3.0%) and spermatozoa (13.8 vs. 8.2%) phospholipid levels of DHA are lower in asthenozoospermic men. Total n-3 fatty acids and the ratio of n-3 to n-6 fatty acids are also lower in the asthenozoospermic men. This mini-review looks at studies investigating the levels of DHA in sperm of infertile men and the effect of oral supplementation with compounds containing DHA. Researchers agree that there are decreased levels of DHA in sperm of infertile males and that supplements containing eicosapentaenoic acid (EPA; 20:5n-3) in combination with DHA potentially increase DHA levels in human sperm. However, supplements containing DHA in the absence of EPA do not appear to be capable of increasing DHA levels in sperm of infertile men or of increasing sperm motility.

Introduction

The motility patterns of spermatozoa correlate closely with the rate of natural pregnancy (1), as well as pregnancy induced by *in vitro* fertilization (2). It is not clear which compounds in seminal plasma or spermatozoa may be involved in the regulation of sperm motility. Various compounds found naturally in the spermatozoa or seminal plasma, for example levels and/or types of antioxidant enzymes (*e.g.*, glutathione peroxidase, superoxide dismutase), oxidants (*e.g.*, nitric oxide, hydrogen peroxide, singlet oxygen), and lipids (*e.g.*, cholesterol, phospholipids, individual fatty acids), may all play a role (3–10).

Previous studies suggest that the level of docosahexaenoic acid (DHA; 22:6n-3) in human ejaculate and sperm is correlated with sperm motility (11,12). DHA levels have been shown to be lower in the total ejaculate (11,12), sperm (13,14), and seminal plasma (14) of asthenozoospermic men (men with ≤50% sperm motility) versus normozoospermic men. It is unclear how DHA may be involved in regulating sperm motility in humans.

Despite recent advances in treatment for female infertility, the ability to provide simple effective treatment for male factor infertility patients remains poor. In this mini-review, the responsiveness of seminal plasma phospholipid- and sperm phospholipid-DHA status to supplementation with dietary DHA will be discussed, as will the effect of DHA supplementation on sperm motility.

DHA in the Human Ejaculate

DHA (22:6n-3) is found in extremely high levels in human ejaculate (11,12), including the spermatozoa and the seminal plasma (14). Phospholipid from normal human spermatozoa contains approximately 14% DHA (13,14,17; see Table 4.1). This compares with much lower levels of other polyunsaturated fatty acids in sperm membrane phospholipid such as 18:2n-6 (3.2%), 20:4n-6 (2.5%), 20:5n-3 (nd), and 22:5n-3 (<1%). Although the amount of DHA in sperm may decrease during the process of sperm maturation (15), an inverse relationship can be shown between the percent of

TABLE 4.1

Fatty Acid Analysis of Sperm Phospholipid of Asthenozoospermic and Normozoospermic Men

Fatty Acids (wt% of total)	Normozoospermic	Asthenozoospermic
18:1	11.6 (0.5)	13.6 (0.4)*
18:2n-6	3.2 (0.2)	2.9 (0.1)
20:0	2.6 (0.2)	4.2 (0.2)*
20:1	0.65 (0.18)	0.85 (0.04)
20:2n-6	0.48 (0.05)	0.49 (0.03)
20:3n-6	2.5 (0.2)	2.7 (0.2)
20:4n-6	2.5 (0.2)	2.6 (0.1)
22:0	3.2 (0.2)	5.2 (0.3)*
22:1	0.39 (0.05)	0.60 (0.06)*
22:4n-6	0.38 (0.04)	0.42 (0.03)
22:5n-3	0.77 (0.05)	0.73 (0.06)
22:6n-3 (DHA)	13.8 (0.9)	8.2 (0.7)*
24:0	2.6 (0.3)	4.4 (0.2)*
24:1	2.3 (0.1)	2.5 (0.1)
Total SAT	59.5 (1.0)	61.5 (0.7)
Total MUFA	16.5 (0.5)	19.3 (0.5)*
Total PUFA	24.0 (1.2)	19.1 (1.0)*
Total n-3	14.6 (0.9)	9.3 (0.8)*
Total n-6	9.4 (0.4)	9.8 (0.4)
n-3/n-6	1.6 (0.1)	1.0 (0.1)*

Values are reported as means (SEM) for $n = 30$ (normozoospermic) and 30 (asthenozoospermic) individuals.
*Significantly different as measured by *t*-test ($P < 0.05$).
Adapted from original source: Conquer *et al.,* (1999) Fatty Acid Analysis of Blood Serum, Seminal Plasma and Spermatozoa of Normozoospermic vs. Asthenozoospermic Males, *Lipids 34,* 793–799.

atypical sperm forms in a specific layer on a Percoll gradient and the percent of DHA observed (16).

DHA is also found in seminal plasma (14; see Table 4.2) at levels that are slightly higher than shown in normal blood serum (3.7% in seminal plasma vs. 2.5% in blood serum). Other polyunsaturated fatty acids in seminal plasma include 18:2n-6 (2.5%), 20:3n-6 (2.2%), 20:4n-6 (3.3%), and very low levels of 22:4n-6 and 22:5n-3 (<1%). DHA levels can also be affected by cryopreservation (18). For example, a recent study suggested that there was a decrease in 22:6n-3 containing phosphatidylcholine in sperm that had been cryopreserved.

The role of DHA in human sperm is not clear. It is possible that DHA may contribute to the membrane fluidity necessary for the motility of sperm tails (19). Furthermore, DHA may be involved in the regulation of free fatty acid utilization by sperm (20,21) or may be converted to an active metabolite such as 19,20-dihydroxy-4,7,10,13,16-docosapentaenoic acid (22). This is an area that has been relatively unexplored.

DHA Levels and Sperm Motility

The concentration of DHA in both ejaculate and spermatozoa has been suggested to be positively associated with sperm motility in various species, including chickens (23) and humans (11–13). Furthermore, DHA levels have been shown to be lower in

TABLE 4.2

Fatty Acid Analysis of Seminal Plasma Phospholipid of Asthenozoospermic and Normozoospermic Men

Fatty Acids (wt% of total)	Normozoospermic	Asthenozoospermic
18:1	16.8 (0.4)	19.0 (0.3)*
18:2n-6	2.5 (0.3)	2.3 (0.1)
18:3n-3	0.19 (0.04)	0.19 (0.01)
20:1	1.1 (0.1)	1.1 (0.0)
20:3n-6	2.2 (0.1)	2.0 (0.1)
20:4n-6	3.3 (0.1)	3.1 (0.1)
22:1	0.33 (0.10)	0.34 (0.01)
22:4n-6	0.36 (0.02)	0.44 (0.02)
22:5n-3	0.41 (0.03)	0.44 (0.03)
22:6n-3 (DHA)	3.7 (0.3)	3.0 (0.2)*
24:1	3.1 (0.1)	3.0 (0.1)
Total MUFA	21.7 (0.3)	24.2 (0.4)*
Total PUFA	13.5 (0.7)	11.8 (0.4)*
Total n-3	4.8 (0.6)	3.6 (0.2)
Total n-6	8.7 (0.3)	8.2 (0.3)
n-3/n-6	0.54 (0.05)	0.45 (0.02)

Values are reported as means (SEM) for $n = 43$ (normozoospermic) and 30 (asthenozoospermic) individuals.
*Significantly different as measured by t-test ($P < 0.05$).
Adapted from original source: Conquer et al., (1999) Fatty Acid Analysis of Blood Serum, Seminal Plasma and Spermatozoa of Normozoospermic vs. Asthenozoospermic Males, *Lipids 34*, 793–799.

complete ejaculates (11,12), as well as certain sperm fractions from asthenozoospermic versus normozoospermic individuals (13). Furthermore, retinitis pigmentosa patients, who have decreased levels of DHA in their serum and sperm, also show decreased sperm motility (24).

Studies from our laboratory are in agreement with these studies but also suggest that DHA levels in total sperm correlate with sperm motility (14) and that DHA levels in total sperm (8.2 vs. 13.8%) and seminal plasma (3.0 vs 3.7%) are decreased in asthenozoospermic men versus normozoospermic men (Tables 4.1 and 4.2). The higher levels of monounsaturated fatty acids and lower levels of polyunsaturated fatty acids, including DHA (see Table 4.1), in the sperm of asthenozoospermic individuals versus normozoospermic individuals supports the hypothesis of an increased breakdown and/or decreased accumulation of DHA in the sperm phospholipid of asthenozoospermic males. Our results are also supported by recent results of Gulaya *et al.* (25, Chapter 5 in this book) in which they found decreased levels of DHA in sperm of infertile men with a higher number of abnormal forms of sperm.

Although levels of DHA in seminal plasma are also lower in asthenozoospermic men than in normozoospermic men (14, Table 4.2), there does not seem to be any specific correlation between seminal plasma DHA levels and sperm motility. Furthermore, it is not clear what effect, if any, an altered fatty acid composition of seminal plasma phospholipid would have on sperm motility. Decreased levels of DHA in seminal plasma of asthenozoospermic men may be indicative only of altered seminal plasma oxidant status. Although there is little data to support these findings in humans, results in bulls nearing the end of their reproductive period suggest that levels of DHA fall with age in both phosphatidylcholine and phosphatidylethanolamine fractions of both sperm and seminal plasma. A decrease in DHA in these fractions is accompanied by a marked reduction of the antioxidant enzymes glutathione peroxidase and superoxide dismutase in the seminal plasma (26).

Effect of Supplementation with n-3 Fatty Acids on Sperm Motility

There are very few studies examining the effect of n-3 fatty acid supplementation on sperm lipid levels or sperm functioning in humans or animals. In 1997, in two separate studies, male birds were supplemented with fish oil (rich in EPA and DHA; 27) or linseed oil (rich in α-linolenic acid, 18:3n-3; 28). After 30 weeks of supplementation with fish oil, sperm DHA levels increased in total phospholipid, as well as in phosphatidylcholine and phosphatidylethanolamine fractions. α-Linolenic acid supplementation resulted in a decrease in sperm 22:4n-6 and an increase in docosapentaenoic acid (22:5n-3) but had little effect on the concentration of DHA. The small increase in n-3 (as 22:5n-3) resulted in enhanced semen fertility. In a third study in broiler breeder roosters, fish oil supplementation increased DHA levels and total n-3 fatty acid levels in the sperm (29). In 1995, Paulenz *et al.* (30) reported that supplementation of fertile boars with 75 mL cod liver oil (rich in EPA + DHA) per day for 9 weeks resulted in increases in sperm phospholipid levels of DHA, whereas EPA (nondetectable) and 22:5n-3 levels did not change.

In humans, n-3 fatty acid supplementation studies are limited. In 1990, Knapp (31) fed 50 mL menhaden oil (containing DHA + EPA) per day to 10 normal male subjects for 4 weeks. There was no effect on sperm motility, but semen phospholipids were enhanced in EPA. DHA was also increased in both the phosphatidylcholine and phosphatidylethanolamine fractions.

Our laboratory has investigated the effect of supplementation of asthenozoospermic males with differing levels of DHA (400 and 800 mg/day), in the absence of EPA, on phospholipid DHA levels in sperm and on sperm motility (32). This study also examined the effect of DHA supplementation on levels of phospholipid DHA in blood serum and seminal plasma. Supplementation of asthenozoospermic men with DHA resulted in increased phospholipid DHA levels in blood serum by 71 and 131% (400 mg/day and 800 mg/day, respectively; Table 4.3). This was coupled with a rise in total n-3 fatty acids and the ratio of n-3/n-6 fatty acids. Decreases were noted in 22:4n-6 and the total levels of n-6 fatty acids. In seminal plasma phospholipid, DHA supplementation resulted in a significant decrease in 22:4n-6 (–31%) in the 800 mg/day group only and an increase in the ratio of n-3 to n-6 fatty acids (Table 4.4). A small nonsignificant increase in DHA (approximately 40%) was noted with supplementation. However, all but one subject showed some increase in DHA in seminal plasma phospholipid with supplementation. Interestingly, DHA supplementation of asthenozoospermic men had no effect on fatty acid composition of sperm phospholipid other than a slight decrease in 22:4n-6 (–37 and –31% in the 400 and 800 mg DHA per day groups, respectively; data not shown). DHA supplementation had no effect on sperm motility or concentration in the asthenozoospermic men (Table 4.5).

Conclusions

In conclusion, human sperm phospholipid is high in DHA, approximately 14% in normal men. In contrast, in asthenozoospermic men DHA levels are much lower, repre-

TABLE 4.3

Effect of DHA Supplementation On Fatty Acid Analysis of Serum Phospholipid in Asthenozoospermic Men

Fatty acids (wt%)	Placebo (n = 9)		400 mg DHA/day (n = 9)		800 mg DHA/day (n = 10)	
	Pre	Post	Pre	Post	Pre	Post
22:4n-6	0.30 (0.05)[a,b]	0.37 (0.03)[a,b]	0.39 (0.06)[a]	0.32 (0.02)[a,b]	0.40 (0.04)[a]	0.28 (0.02)[b]
22:6n-3 (DHA)	2.8 (0.4)[a]	2.6 (0.3)[a]	2.4 (0.2)[a]	4.1 (0.2)[b]	2.6 (0.2)[a]	6.0 (0.3)[c]
Total n-3	5.0 (0.4)[a]	4.8 (0.3)[a]	4.3 (0.2)[a]	6.1 (0.2)[b]	4.9 (0.3)[a]	8.2 (0.4)[c]
Total n-6	35.1 (0.5)[a,b]	34.8 (0.3)[a,b]	36.2 (0.8)[a]	34.0 (0.5)[b]	35.2 (0.7)[a,b]	31.1 (0.9)[c]
n-3/n-6	0.14 (0.01)[a]	0.14 (0.01)[a]	0.12 (0.01)[a]	0.18 (0.01)[b]	0.14 (0.01)[a]	0.27 (0.02)[c]

Values are reported as means (SEM) for a total of 28 individuals.

[a,b,c]Values not sharing a superscript within the same row are significantly different ($P < 0.05$).

Adapted from original source: Conquer *et al.*, (2000) Effect of DHA Supplementation on DHA Status and Sperm Motility in Asthenozoospermic Males, *Lipids 35*, 149–154.

TABLE 4.4

Effect of DHA Supplementation on Fatty Acid Analysis of Seminal Plasma Phospholipid of Asthenozoospermic Men

Fatty acids (wt%)	Placebo (n = 9)		400 mg DHA/day (n = 9)		800 mg DHA/day (n = 10)	
	Pre	Post	Pre	Post	Pre	Post
22:4n-6	0.42 (0.03)[a,b,c]	0.38 (0.04)[a]	0.43 (0.04)[b,c]	0.38 (0.04)[a,b,d]	0.48 (0.04)[c]	0.33 (0.02)[d]
22:6n-3 (DHA)	3.1 (0.5)	3.3 (0.5)	3.0 (0.3)	4.1 (0.7)	3.0 (0.2)	4.2 (0.3)
n-3/n-6	0.45 (0.06)[a]	0.45 (0.05)[a]	0.43 (0.04)[a]	0.58 (0.07)[b]	0.48 (0.03)[a]	0.64 (0.05)[b]

Values are reported as means (SEM) for a total of 28 individuals.

[a,b,c,d]Values not sharing a superscript within the same row are significantly different ($P < 0.05$).

Adapted from original source: Conquer *et al.*, (2000) Effect of DHA Supplementation on DHA Status and Sperm Motility in Asthenozoospermic Males, *Lipids 35*, 149–154.

TABLE 4.5

Effect of DHA Supplementation On Sperm Characterisitics in Asthenozoospermic Men

Characteristics	Placebo (n = 9)		400 mg DHA/day (n = 9)		800 mg DHA/day (n = 10)	
	Pre	Post	Pre	Post	Pre	Post
Sperm motility (% total sperm)	41.1 (3.1)	47.2 (6.2)	26.7 (4.2)	39.4 (8.1)	25.3 (4.5)	32.0 (5.1)
Sperm concentration (M/mL)	34.9 (8.5)	43.1 (13.5)	31.6 (9.8)	37.8 (12.3)	57.0 (17.6)	44.6 (13.0)

Values are reported as mean (SEM) for a total of 28 individuals. There were no significant differences as measured.

Adapted from original source: Conquer *et al.*, (2000) Effect of DHA Supplementation on DHA Status and Sperm Motility in Asthenozoospermic Males, *Lipids 35*, 149–154.

senting approximately 8% of the sperm phospholipid fraction. DHA levels are also slightly lower in seminal plasma phospholipid. Supplementation of asthenozoospermic men with DHA in the absence of EPA results in increased DHA levels in serum and possibly in seminal plasma. However, DHA supplementation in the absence of EPA has a negligible effect on DHA levels in sperm and sperm motility. In the future, research should focus on ways to increase DHA in sperm of asthenozoospermic men in order to determine whether increased DHA will play a role in sperm motility. Examples may include supplementation with α-linolenic acid, a DHA precursor, with fish oils containing DHA + EPA, and/or with certain antioxidants known to reach the seminal plasma, such as vitamin E or lycopene.

Acknowledgments

We would like to thank Martek Biosciences Corporation for funding our initial investigation.

References

1. Beauchamp, P.J., Galle, P.C., and Blasco, L. (1984) Human Sperm Velocity and Post Insemination Cervical Mucous Test in the Evaluation of Infertile Couple, *Arch. Androl. 13*, 107–112.
2. Bongso, T.A., Ng, S.C., Mok, H., Lim, M.N., Teo, H.L., Wong, P.C., and Ratnam, S.S. (1989) Effect of Sperm Motility on Human *in Vitro* Fertilization, *Arch. Androl. 22*, 185–190.
3. Nissen, H.P., and Kreysel, H.W. (1983) Superoxide Dismutase in Human Semen, *Klinische Wochenschrift 61*, 63–65.
4. Alvarez, J.G., and Storey, B.T. (1983) Role of Superoxide Dismutase in Protecting Rabbit Spermatozoa from O2 Toxicity Due to Lipid Peroxidation, *Biol. Reprod. 28*, 1129–1136.
5. Alvarez, J.G., and Storey, B.T. (1992) Evidence for Increased Lipid Peroxidative Damage and Loss of Superoxide Dismutase Activity as a Mode of Sublethal Cryo-Damage to Human Sperm During Cryopreservation, *J. Androl. 13*, 232–241.
6. Weinberg, J.B., Doty, E., Bonaventura, J., and Haney, A.F. (1995) Nitric Oxide Inhibition of Human Sperm Motility, *Fertil. Steril. 64*, 408–413.
7. Griveau, J.F., and Le Lannou, D. (1997) Reactive Oxygen Species and Human Spermatozoa: Physiology and Pathology, *Int. J. Androl. 20*, 61–69.
8. Tanphaichitr, N., Zheng, Y.S., Kates, M., Abdullah, N., and Chan, A. (1996) Cholesterol and Phospholipid Levels of Washed and Percoll Gradient Centrifuged Mouse Sperm: Presence of Lipids Possessing Inhibitory Effects on Sperm Motility, *Mol. Reprod. Devel. 43*, 187–195.
9. Hula, N.M., Tron'ko, M.D., Volkov, H.L., and Marhitych, V.M. (1993) Phospholipids of Human Seminal Plasma and Their Role in Ensuring Fertility, *Ukr. Biokhim. Zh. 65*, 75–78.
10. Hong, C.Y., Shieh, C.C., Wu, P., Huang, J.J., and Chiang, B.N. (1986) Effect of Phosphatidylcholine, Lysophosphatidylcholine, Arachidonic Acid and Docosahexaenoic Acid on the Motility of Human Sperm, *Int. J. Androl. 9*, 118–122.
11. Nissen, H.P., and Kreysel, H.W. (1983) Polyunsaturated Fatty Acids in Relation to Sperm Motility, *Andrologia 15*, 264–269.
12. Gulaya, N.M., Tronko, M.D., Volkov, G.L., and Margitich, M. (1993) Lipid Composition and Fertile Ability of Human Ejaculate, *Ukr. Biokhim. Zh. 65*, 64–70.
13. Zalata, A.A., Christophe, A.B., Depuydt, C.E., Schoonjans, F., and Comhaire, F.H. (1998) The Fatty Acid Composition of Phospholipids of Spermatozoa from Infertile Patients, *Mol. Hum. Reprod. 4*, 111–118.
14. Conquer, J., Martin, J.B., Tummon, I., Watson, L., and Tekpetey, F. (1999) Fatty Acid Analysis of Blood Serum, Seminal Plasma and Spermatozoa of Normozoospermic vs. Asthenozoospermic Males, *Lipids, 34*, 793–799.
15. Ollero, M., Powers, R.D., and Alvarez, J.G. (2000) Variation of Docosahexaenoic Acid Content in Subsets of Human Spermatozoa at Different Stages of Maturation: Implications for Sperm Lipoperoxidative Damage, *Mol. Reprod. Dev. 55*, 326–334.
16. Lenzi, A., Gandini, L., Maresca, V., Rago, R., Sgro, P., Dondero, F., and Picardo, M. (2000) Fatty Acid Composition of Spermatozoa and Immature Germ Cells, *Mol. Hum. Reprod. 6*, 226–231.
17. Zalata, A.A., Christophe, A.B., Depuydt, C.E., Schoonjans, F., and Comhaire, F.H. (1998) White Blood Cells Cause Oxidative Damage to the Fatty Acid Composition of Phospholipids of Human Spermatozoa, *Int. J. Androl. 21*, 154–162.

18. Schiller, J., Arnhold, J., Glander, H.J., and Arnold, K. (2000) Lipid Analysis of Human Spermatozoa and Seminal Plasma by MALDI-TOF Mass Spectrometry and NMR Spectroscopy—Effects of Freezing and Thawing, *Chem. Phys. Lipids 106*, 145–156.
19. Connor, W.E., Lin, D.S., Wolf, D.P., and Alexander, M. (1998) Uneven Distribution of Desmosterol and Docosahexaenoic Acid in the Heads and Tails of Monkey Sperm, *J. Lipid Res. 39*, 1404–1411.
20. Jones, R.E., and Plymate, S.R. (1993) Synthesis of Docosahexaenoyl Coenzyme A in Human Spermatozoa, *J. Androl. 14*, 428–432.
21. Jones, R.E., and Plymate, S.R. (1988) Evidence for the Regulation of Fatty Acid Utilization in Human Sperm by Docosahexaenoic Acid, *Biol. Reprod. 39*, 76–80.
22. Oliw, E.H., and Sprecher, H.W. (1991) Metabolism of Polyunsaturated (n-3) Fatty Acids by Monkey Seminal Vesicles: Isolation and Biosynthesis of Omega-3 Epoxides, *Biochim. Biophys. Acta 1086*, 287–294.
23. Cerolini, S., Kelso, K.A., Noble, R.C., Speake, B.K., Pizzi, F., and Cavalchini, L.G. (1997) Relationship Between Spermatozoan Lipid Composition and Fertility during Aging of Chickens, *Biol. Reprod. 57*, 976–980.
24. Connor, W.E., Weleber, R.G., DeFrancesco, C., Lin, D.S., and Wolf, D.P. (1997) Sperm Abnormalities in Retinitis Pigmentosa, *Invest. Opthmol. Vis. Sci. 38*, 2619–2628.
25. Gulaya, N.M., Margitich, V.M., Govseeva, N.M., Klimashevsky, V.M., Gorpynchenko, I.I., and Boyko, M.I. (2001) Phospholipid Composition of Human Sperm and Seminal Plasma in Relation to Sperm Fertility, *Arch. Androl. 46*, 169–175.
26. Kelso, K.A., Redpath, A., Noble, R.C., and Speake, B.K. (1997) Lipid and Antioxidant Changes in Spermatozoa and Seminal Plasma Throughout the Reproductive Period of Bulls, *J. Reprod. Fertil. 109*, 1–6.
27. Kelso, K.A., Cerolini, S., Noble, R.C., Sparks, N.H.C., and Speake, B.K. (1997) The Effects of Dietary Supplementation with Docosahexaenoic Acid on the Phospholipid Fatty Acid Composition of Avian Spermatozoa, *Comp. Biochem. Physiol. 118B*, 65–69.
28. Kelso, K.A., Cerolini, S., Speake, B.K., Cavalchini, L.G., and Noble, R.C. (1997) Effects of Dietary Supplementation with Alpha-Linolenic Acid on the Phospholipid Fatty Acid Composition and Quality of Spermatozoa in Cockerel from 24 to 72 Weeks of Age, *J. Reprod. Fertil. 10*, 53–59.
29. Blesbois, E., Lessire, M., Grasseau, I., Hallouis, J.M., and Hermier, G. (1997) Effect of Dietary Fat on the Fatty Acid Composition and Fertilizing Ability of Fowl Semen, *Biol. Reprod. 56*, 1216–1220.
30. Paulenz, H., Taugbol, O., Hofmo, P.O., and Saarem, K. (1995) A Preliminary Study on the Effect of Dietary Supplementation with Cod Liver Oil on the Polyunsaturated Fatty Acid Composition of Boar Semen, *Vet. Res. Commun. 19*, 273–284.
31. Knapp, H.R. (1990) Prostaglandins in Human Semen During Fish Oil Ingestion: Evidence for *in Vivo* Cyclooxygenase Inhibition and Appearance of Novel Trienoic Compounds, *Prostaglandins 39*, 407–423.
32. Conquer, J.A., Martin, J.B., Tummon, I., Watson, L., and Tekpetey, F. (2000) Effect of DHA Supplementation on DHA Status and Sperm Motility in Asthenozoospermic Males, *Lipids 35*, 149–154.

Chapter 5

Phospholipid Composition of Human Sperm and Seminal Plasma in Relation to Sperm Fertility

N.M. Gulaya

O.V. Palladine Institute of Biochemistry, National Academy of Science, Leontovich str. 9, Kiev 01030, Ukraine

Abstract

Some infertile men have idiopathic infertility with near normal spermogram and have no obvious propagations of any pathological processes. The sperm lipid composition of infertile men with normozoospermia is poorly understood. Many investigators have shown that even subnormal motile densities and morphology did not predict the infertile male. We suggested that decreased sperm fertile potential can be associated with alteration of sperm lipid composition and content. To elucidate this problem we investigated the phospholipid and fatty acid composition of human normozoospermic semen in relation to its fertility. We found an approximately threefold decrease of phosphatidylethanolamine (PE) in spermatozoa of infertile normozoospermic men. In contrast the level of phosphatidylserine (PS) and simultaneously of lysophosphatidylserine (LPS) increased nearly twofold compared to healthy subjects. As a result, the phospholipid amounts in the spermatozoa of infertile men were significantly different compared to healthy men. The level of PS in seminal plasma of infertile men was found to increase more than twofold. The phosphatidic acid was found in small amounts in seminal plasma of infertile patients only. The phospholipid percentage in the seminal plasma of infertile men was significantly different compared to healthy men. In infertile men the quantity of 18:0 decreased more than twofold. The level of docosahexaenoic acid decreased more than threefold. The value of 20:5n-3 also decreased more than twofold. The amount of 18:3n-6 doubled. The amount of 20:4n-6 showed the trend to increase. The ratio of total amount of saturated to unsaturated fatty acids was not affected. There was a significant positive correlation between 22:6n-3 content and sperm motility and a negative correlation between 18:3n-6 amount and sperm motility.

Introduction

It is known that more than 15% of reproductive age couples present with infertility (1). A number of pathological states were identified as causes of male infertility including gene mutations, aneuploidy, infectious diseases, ejaculatory duct occlusion, varicocele, radiation, chemotherapy, and erectile dysfunction (2). Nearly half of infertile men have infertility with unknown etiology identified as idiopathic. Lipids are thought to play a major role in regulating spermatozoa fertility.

Human semen is formed from the secretions of different glands, and usually two main fractions can be obtained by semen centrifugation: spermatozoa and seminal plasma. Most semen protein (about 85%) is found in soluble fraction and nearly 7% in spermatozoa. On the contrary, phospholipids are largely bound to the fraction of spermatozoa (nearly 45% of total lipid phosphorus). This fraction is poor in cholesterol and has a cholesterol-to-phospholipid molar ratio of about 0.2 (3). It was shown that cholesterol was the predominant sterol both in spermatozoa ($107 +/- 7$ nmol/10^8 spermatozoa) and in seminal plasma ($0.83 +/- 0.1$ μmol/ml) (4). As shown by many authors, all the semen fractions have specific lipid content. We studied phospholipid composition in spermatozoa of the individual semen of healthy men, which showed 32.9% phosphatidylcholine (PC), 26.6% phosphatidylethanolamine (PE), 11.7% sphingomyelin (SM), 7.3% phosphatidylserine (PS), 6.7% diphosphatidylglycerol (DPG), 3.8% phosphatidylinositol (PI), 3% lysophosphatidylcholine (lysoPC), and 2.9% lysophosphatidylethanolamine (lysoPE).

The phospholipid content of seminal plasma differed markedly from spermatozoa. It contained 32.9% SM, 19.8% PE, 11.1% PC, 8.3% PS, 5.4% lysoPE, 5.2% lysoPC, 3.6% lysophosphatidylserine (lysoPS), and 1.7% DPG (5,6).

It is well established that different lipids play a significant role in sperm functional activity. Semen analysis of mammals has shown that processing, capacitation, and acrosome reaction are associated with multiple specific modifications of phospholipid composition of spermatozoa plasma membrane (7–9).

PI is found to play a role in acrosomal reaction of human spermatozoa. After induction, PI is hydrolyzed by phospholipase C with formation of diacylglycerol and inositolphosphates (10). Progesterone is known to induce acrosomal reaction, whereas cholesterol is a major inhibitor of this reaction.

Cholesterol inhibited the progesterone-induced acrosome reaction when it was added *in vitro* to sperm during capacitation and when it was added with progesterone during the induction of acrosome reaction. Similarly acrosome reaction that was induced by db-cAMP was also inhibited by cholesterol in concentration of 0.2 μg/mL. Cholesterol's inhibition of induced acrosome reaction was independent of progesterone concentration. Cholesterol inhibited acrosome reaction in a noncompetitive manner by modifying the structure of the sperm plasma membrane, which prevented exposure of the progesterone surface receptor to progesterone binding (11).

Capacitation is also a lipid dependent process, namely, a complex series of molecular events that occurs in sperm after epididymal maturation and confers on spermatozoa the ability to fertilize an egg. Capacitation correlates with cholesterol efflux from the sperm plasma membrane, increased membrane fluidity, modulations in intracellular ion concentrations, hyperpolarization of the sperm plasma membrane, and increased protein tyrosine phosphorylation. These molecular events are required for the subsequent induction of hyperactivation and the acrosome reaction (12).

The lipid composition of the sperm membrane has a significant effect upon the functional characteristics of spermatozoa. Changes of sperm lipid composition cause alterations of sperm functional characteristics. Damage induced by reactive oxygen species generated by spermatozoa endogenously has been proposed as a major factor in male infertility (13). It is known that polyunsaturated fatty acids (PUFA) are the main substrate of lipid peroxidation. Recently, we and others have shown that docosahexaenoic acid (DHA, 22:6n-3) is a major PUFA in human spermatozoa (14,15).

The essential fatty acid DHA is a minor component of the Western diet but a major fatty acid in human testis and semen. In mature spermatozoa, the physical and fusogenic properties of the plasma membrane are probably influenced by its particular fatty acid composition. According to some authors, DHA accounts for up to 30% of fatty acids esterified in phospholipids and 73% of all PUFA (14,16). DHA is thought to play a major role in regulating membrane fluidity in spermatozoa. It serves as a main substrate of lipid peroxidation in human spermatozoa. It was shown that spermatozoa motility depends on DHA (17). We also published the results of an investigation that showed the existence of positive correlation between sperm motility and DHA amount in spermatozoa (14).

Changes in the proportions of the various lipid components in spermatozoa were investigated throughout the development and reproductive period of many male beings, including men. Sperm motility and *in vivo* fertility are known to depend on sperm lipid composition. This question was studied by many investigators and it was assumed that seminal lipid composition played a major role in providing normal realization of different processes of sperm fertile function.

It was shown that total lipid concentration was elevated in the seminal plasma of oligo- and azoospermic men. The total cholesterol content was comparatively higher in the seminal plasma of azoospermic men than in that of normo- and oligospermic men. In general, infertility was associated with increased seminal concentrations for most of the neutral lipid classes. However, total phospholipids and most of the phospholipid classes were diminished in the seminal plasma of oligo- and azoospermic men and in the spermatozoa of oligospermic men. Authors suggest that there is a positive correlation between seminal phospholipids and fertility and a negative correlation between seminal neutral lipids and fertility (18).

Unfortunately, the sperm lipid composition of infertile men with normozoospermia is poorly understood. Some authors did not find a strong correlation between abnormal sperm morphology and male infertility (19). Many investigators have shown that even subnormal motile densities and morphology did not predict the infertile male (20). It is known that some infertile men have idiopathic infertility with near normal spermogram and have no obvious propagations of any pathological processes. We suggested that decreased sperm fertile potential can be associated with alteration of sperm lipid composition and content. To elucidate this question we investigated the phospholipid and fatty acid composition of human normozoospermic semen in relation to its fertility.

Material and Methods

Semen samples were obtained by masturbation from 8 normal healthy men (22–46 years of age) who had children and 16 infertile patients (23–50 years of age) with semen characteristics similar to normal ones. However, the abnormal forms of sperm in this group was elevated.

Sperm Count and Separation

Sperm were counted immediately after liquefaction of semen according to the WHO protocol (21) with some modifications. For evaluation of the number of sperm, two counter chambers were used. Dissolved native semen was placed in one chamber. Another portion of the sperm were immobilized by treating with the solution of sulfuric acid. Quantity of immotile sperm in both chambers was compared. The difference shows the number of motile sperm. Dead sperm and abnormal cells were determined after staining by eosin and nigrosine. Sperm and seminal plasma were separated by centrifugation of the semen at 600g for 12 min at room temperature. Semen was previously diluted by 3 volumes of Krebs-Ringer phosphate buffer. The supernatant was aspirated and used for lipid extraction. Sperm pellets were washed twice by the same solution. The pellet was resuspended in 0.85% NaCl to receive the suspension, which contained 10–50 × 10^6 sperm/mL. This suspension was then homogenized and used for lipid extraction.

Lipid Analysis

Extraction of lipids was performed within 120 min after semen collection. The lipids were extracted with methanol-chloroform (2:1 vol/vol) according to Bligh and Dyer (22). The ratio of water/methanol/chloroform was close to 0.8:2:1 in the monophasic system and 0.9:1:1 in the biphasic system. The lower phase, which contained purified lipid, was aspirated. The upper phase was extracted once more in the same manner. The lower phase was combined with the first extract and dried on the rotary evaporator. For more complete extraction of anionic phospholipids, the procedure recommended by Palmer was used (23). The lipid extract was stored in a small volume of chloroform at –20°C.

Phospholipids were analyzed by two-dimensional, high-resolution, micro thin-layer chromatography on silica gel KSK-2 (Russia) by using chloroform/methanol/benzene/ammonium (28%) (65:30:10:6, by vol) and chloroform/methanol/benzene/acetone/acetic acid/water (70:30:10:5:4:1, by vol) (24) as solvent systems. For phospholipid development we used 60 × 60-mm^2 plates. To determine the quantity of the phospholipid phosphorus, the molybdate spray reagent was used (25). This method permitted us to analyze the phospholipid composition of individual samples of semen.

Individual phospholipids were revealed with molybdate (25) and malachite green reagents (26). The anthrone reagent (27) was also used to determine phospholipid, sulpholipid, and glycolipid containing spots, which were stained under special conditions in different colors. For identification of free amino groups containing phospholipids, the ninhydrin reagent was used (28). Finally, the chromatographic behavior and chemical properties of standard phospholipids were compared with those of experimental samples.

Gas–Liquid Chromatography of Fatty Acids

Fatty acid methyl esters of the total lipid extract of each semen sample obtained by the method of Bligh and Dyer (22) were prepared by reaction with 3 M HCl in methanol (29) in a boiling water bath for 1 h. Methyl esters were purified by one-dimensional, high-resolution, micro thin-layer chromatography in benzene. Methyl esters of fatty acids were quantitatively determined on a gas–liquid chromatograph (Chrom-5, Czech). The column of 2 m x 3 mm (L x i.d) containing 7.5% Silar-5CP (Serva) on Chromaton NAW-DMSC was used. For identification of fatty acids the standard fatty acid methyl esters (Sigma) were used. Temperature program was 140–250°C at the rate of 2°C/min.

Protein was measured by the method of Lowry *et al.* (30). The results were analyzed by the Student *t*-test.

Results

Two groups of men with very similar semen morphologic characteristics were investigated, healthy men ($n = 8$) and infertile men ($n = 16$). In both groups semen volume was 4.0 (SD 0.4) mL *versus* 4.2 (SD 0.4) mL; sperm count was 103 (SD 15) $\times$ 10^6/mL *versus* 103 (SD 9) $\times$ 10^6/mL; and total sperm count in whole ejaculate was 413 (SD 67) $\times$ 10^6 *versus* 415 (SD 47) $\times$ 10^6. The amount of motile sperm cells, 68 (SD 9) $\times$ 10^6 *versus* 52 (SD 7) $\times$ 10^6, and quantity of dead cells, 31 (SD 7) $\times$ 10^6 *versus* 42 (SD 6) $\times$ 10^6, were statistically the same. Only the quantity of abnormal cells was significantly higher in infertile men: 26 (SD 6) $\times$ 10^6/mL *versus* 43 (SD 5) $\times$ 10^6/mL ($P < 0.05$).

The level of total phospholipid phosphorus significantly varied in healthy and infertile men. The great deviations of these values caused the lack of the statistically significant changes of the amount of total phospholipids in infertile men (data not presented). The amounts of individual phospholipids in sperm of normal men were in the following order (Table 5.1): PC > PE > SM > PS > DPG > PI > lysoPE > lysoPC > lysoPS. We found a significant (about threefold) decrease in the PE amount in spermatozoa of infertile men. In contrast the level of PS and simultaneously of lysoPS increased nearly twofold compared to healthy subjects ($P < 0.05$). As a result the order of the phospholipid amounts in the spermatozoa of infertile men became as follows: PC > SM > PS > PE > lysoPS > DPG > lysoPC > lysoPE > PI.

We did not find changes in the level of total protein and phospholipid phosphorus and amount in seminal plasma of infertile men compared to healthy subjects (Table 5.2). However, we noted great individual deviations of these values. The main phospholipid of seminal plasma was SM. The content of individual phospholipids in seminal plasma significantly differed from that of spermatozoa and was ordered as fol-

Table 5.1

The Individual Phospholipid Content of Human Spermatozoa (μg Pi/10^9 cells, mean $\pm$ SE)

Phospholipids	Healthy men (n = 5)	Infertile men (n = 11)
Phosphatidylcholine	22.0 ± 2.2	16.1 ± 3.1
Phosphatidylethanolamine	20.0 ± 2.7	7.0 ± 1.9*
Sphingomyelin	8.5 ± 1.5	12.7 ± 2.2
Phosphatidylserine	4.4 ± 0.7	8.2 ± 1.4*
Diphosphatidylglycerol	3.0 ± 0.6	2.7 ± 0.5
Phosphadylinositol	2.2 ± 0.2	1.7 ± 0.5
Lysophosphatidylcholine	1.8 ± 0.3	2.4 ± 0.5
Lysophosphatidylethanolamine	1.9 ± 0.5	2.0 ± 0.4
Lysophosphatidylserine	1.3 (n = 1)	4.7 ± 1.2*

*$p < 0.05$, compared to healthy men.

Table 5.2

The Individual Phospholipids in Human Seminal Plasma (μg Pi/10 mL of seminal plasma, mean $\pm$ SE)

Phospholipids	Healthy men (n = 5)	Infertile men (n = 11)
Sphingomyelin	52.1 ± 11.5	57.9 ± 9.8
Phosphatidylethanolamine	35.1 ± 7.6	28.3 ± 6.0
Phosphatidylcholine	17.1 ± 4.0	28.7 ± 5.2
Phosphatidylserine	13.4 ± 1.9	29.1 ± 6.9*
Lysophosphatidylcholine	9.1 ± 1.7	12.8 ± 5.0
Lysophosphatidylethanolamine	8.8 ± 2.7	8.4 ± 1.8
Phosphadylinositol	6.6 ± 0.5	5.6 ± 0.9
Lysophosphatidylserine	5.4 ± 1.4	10.2 ± 3.8
Diphosphatidylglycerol	3.2 ± 1.3	4.9 ± 1.8
Phosphatidic acid	—	0.9 ± 0.1*

*$p < 0.05$, compared to healthy men.

lows: SM > PE > PC > PS > lysoPC > lysoPE > PI > lysoPS > DPG. The level of PS in seminal plasma of infertile men was found to increase more than twofold when compared to healthy men. It is interesting to note that phosphatidic acid was found in trace amounts in seminal plasma of infertile patients only.

The major unsaturated fatty acids in normal human semen were docosahexaenoic (22:6n-3) and oleic (18:1n-9) acids (Table 5.3). Palmitic acid (16:0) was the main saturated fatty acid; stearic acid (18:0) took second place. In infertile men the quantity of 18:0 was decreased more than twofold. The level of major n-3 PUFA of human semen, 22:6n-3, was decreased more than three times. The value of eicosapentaenoic acid (20:5n-3) also significantly decreased more than two times. At the same time the amount of γ-linolenic acid (18:3n-6) increased two times. The amount of arachidonic acid (20:4n-6) showed the trend to increase. The analysis of saturated/unsaturated

Table 5.3
Composition of the Main Fatty Acids in Ejaculate of Healthy and Infertile Men (mol% of total quantity, mean ± SE)

Fatty acid	Healthy men (n = 3)	Infertile men (n = 5)
Palmitic (c16:0)	19.0 ± 1.58	26.0 ± 2.82
Stearic (c18:0)	17.0 ± 1.39	8.0 ± 1.16*
Oleic (c18:1n-9)	16.0 ± 0.39	16.0 ± 2.57
Linoleic (c18:2n-6)	3.76 ± 0.34	4.46 ± 1.02
Linolenic (c18:3n-3)	0.4 ± 0.07	1.0 ± 0.23*
Arachidonic (c20:4n-6)	1.14 ± 0.43	3.08 ± 1.19
Eicosopentaenoic (c20:5n-3)	2.31 ± 0.37	1.04 ± 0.20*
Docosahexaenoic (c22:6n-3)	16.0 ± 3.01	5.36 ± 0.47*
Lignoceric (c24:0)	0.17 ± 0.03	0.34 ± 0.06*

*$p < 0.05$, compared to healthy men.

fatty acids ratio shows that the total amount of saturated and unsaturated fatty acids was not affected. There was a significant positive correlation between 22:6n-3 and sperm motility ($r = 0.82$, $P < 0.001$) and a negative correlation between γ-linolenic acid and sperm motility ($r = -0.58$, $P < 0.05$).

Discussion

In infertile men some common changes were found in spermatozoa and seminal plasma: an increase in the level of PS and a significant decrease of PE. PE is the main nonlamellar phospholipid, which plays an important role in membrane fusion. Hence, the changes of PE in sperm of infertile men would be expected to have a definite impact on the alteration of sperm fertilizing ability.

LysoPS is not a characteristic constituent for many mammalian cells. Bruni and other authors (31,32) found this phospholipid in noticeable amounts in some pathological cases in granulocytes, mast cells, etc., and supposed that it served as a natural autacoid that promoted intercellular communications in coordinated reactions against perturbing stimuli. The reason for lysoPS appearance in infertile sperm and the functional role of this lipid here is not clear. The significant decrease of the PE content in the sperm of infertile men could be the result of (i) the peroxidative degradation of this phospholipid and (ii) the inhibition of its synthesis from PS by decarboxylation. Reactive oxygen substances can damage the phospholipids by the free radical-induced oxidation of PUFA (33–35). Thus, the loss of PE, a highly unsaturated phospholipid, in sperm of infertile men could be due at least partly to its peroxidative decomposition. This idea is supported by the drastic fall of the major n-3 PUFA (22:6n-3 and 20:5n-3), which are important constituents of PE and other phospholipids. The last fact could be easily explained by the free radical mechanism of PUFA destruction. PS is one of the main precursors of PE (for review see (36)). Probably an inhibition of the PS-decarboxylase pathway (37) could cause the high level of PS and decreased level of PE in infertile sperm; further investigations are necessary to clarify this question. The nature of γ-linolenic acid (18:3n-6) enhancement in infertile semen is unknown. The results of these investigations show that sperm infertility is associated with the drastic loss of PE and n-3 PUFA with simultaneous enhancement of PS and some n-6 PUFA.

It is interesting to note that there were some attempts to correct male infertility by dietary 22:6n-3 (38,39, Chapter 4 in this book). The effects of supplementation with DHA on DHA levels in serum, seminal plasma, and sperm of asthenozoospermic men as well as on sperm motility were examined in a randomized, double-blind, placebo-controlled manner (38,39). Asthenozoospermic men ($n = 28$; less or $= 50\%$ motility) were supplemented with 0, 400, or 800 mg DHA per day for three months. Sperm motility and the fatty acid composition of serum, seminal plasma, and sperm phospholipid were determined before and after supplementation. There was no effect of DHA supplementation on sperm motility. The results showed that dietary supplementation resulted in increased serum and possibly seminal plasma phospholipid DHA levels without affecting the incorporation of DHA into the spermatozoa phospholipid in asthenozoospermic men. This inability of DHA to be incorporated into sperm phospholipid was most likely responsible for the observed lack of DHA supplementation effect on sperm motility.

This fact can be partly explained by the results recently published by Retterstol *et al.* (40, Chapter 2 in this book). They studied the synthesis of 22:6n-3 and 22:5n-6 in isolated human testicular cells. [1-^{14}C]20:4n-6, [1-^{14}C]20:5n-3, [1-^{14}C]22:4n-6, and [1-^{14}C]22:5n-3 were incubated in a "crude" cell suspension (consisting of a mixture of the cells in the seminiferous tubule) and in fractionated pachytene spermatocytes and round spermatids. The esterification of fatty acids in lipid and phospholipid classes and the fatty acid chain elongation and desaturation were measured. The "crude" cell suspension metabolized the fatty acids more actively than did the fractionated germ cell suspension, indicating that types of cell other than the germ cells are important for fatty acid elongation and desaturation and thus the production of [^{14}C]22:6n-3. This finding is in agreement with previous results in rats that indicated that the Sertoli cells are the most important type of cell for the metabolism of essential fatty acids in the testis. Some [1-^{14}C]20:5n-3 was elongated to [^{14}C]22:5n-3 in the fractionated germ cells, but very little was elongated further to [^{14}C]24:5n-3, possibly restricting the formation of [^{14}C]22:6n-3. In the fractionated germ cells, the fatty acid substrates were recovered primarily in the phospholipid fraction, indicating an incorporation in the membranes, whereas in the "crude" cells, more substrates were esterified in the triacylglycerol fraction. In the phospholipids, more radioactivity was recovered in PC than in PE and more radioactivity was recovered in PE than in PI or PS. These results show that many types of cells play a role in the fatty acid and phospholipid synthesis, and in many cases the deep disturbances of different lipids and particularly PUFA synthesis and metabolism cause the male infertility.

Summary

About threefold decrease of PE amount in spermatozoa of infertile normozoospermic men was found when compared to healthy men. In contrast the level of PS and simultaneously of lysoPS increased nearly twofold when compared to healthy subjects. As a result the order of the phospholipid amounts in the spermatozoa of infertile men changed significantly .

The level of PS in seminal plasma of infertile men was found to increase more than twofold. The phosphatidic acid was found in small amounts in seminal plasma of infertile patients only. The order of the phospholipid quantities in seminal plasma of infertile men significantly changed compared to healthy men.

In infertile men the quantity of 18:0 decreased more than twofold. The level of DHA decreased more than three times. The value of 20:5n-3 also significantly decreased, more than twofold. The amount of 18:3n-6 increased two times. The amount of 20:4n-6 showed the trend to increase. The ratio of total amount of saturated to unsaturated fatty acids was not affected. The significant positive correlation between 22:6n-3 content and sperm motility and negative correlation between 18:3n-6 amount and sperm motility were shown. The results of this investigation suggest that decreased sperm fertile capacity can be associated with alteration of sperm lipid composition and content.

Acknowledgments

The author is grateful to Dr. M.I. Boyko and Dr. I.I. Gorpynchenko, whose patients were investigated in this study, and to Drs. V.M. Margitich, N.M.Govseeva, and V.M. Klimashevsky for the assistance in performing the work.

References

1. Hull, M.G.R., Glazener, C.M.A., and Kelly, N.Y. *et al.* (1995) Population Study of Causes, Treatment, and Outcome of Infertility, *Br. Med. J. 291*, 1693–1697.
2. Ollero, M., Gil-Guzman, E., Lopez, M.C., Sharma, R.K., Agarwal, A., Larson, K., Evenson, D., Thomas, A.J., Alvares, Jr., and Juan, G. (2001) Characterization of Subsets of Human Spermatozoa at Different Stages of Maturation: Implications in the Diagnosis and Treatment of Male Infertility, *Human Reproduction 16(9)*, 1912–1921.
3. Arienti, G., Saccardi, C., Carlini, E., Verdacchi, R., and Palmerini, C.A. (1999) Distribution of Lipid and Protein in Human Semen Fractions, *Clin. Chim. Acta 289 (1–2)*, 111–120.
4. Sion, B., Grizard, G., and Boucher, D. (2001) Quantitative Analysis of Desmosterol, Cholesterol, and Cholesterolsulfat in Semen by High-Performance Liquid Chromatography, *J. Chromatogr. A. 935(1–2)*, 259–265.
5. Gulaya (Hula), N.M., Vaskovsky, V.E., Tronko, M.D.,Volkov, G.L., and Margitich, V.M., (1993) Phospholipids of Human Spermatozoa and Their Role in Fertile Ability, *Ukr. Biochim. Zh. 65(4)*, 70–74.
6. Gulaya (Hula), N.M., Tronko, M.D.,Volkov, G.L., and Margitich, V.M. (1993) Phospholipids of Human Seminal Plasma and Their Role in Fertile Ability, *Ukr. Biochim. Zh. 65(4)*, 75–78.

7. Breitbart, H., and Spungin, B. (1997) The Biochemistry of the Acrosome Reaction, *Mol. Hum. Reprod. 3*, 195–202.

8. Rana, A.P.S, Majumder, G.C., Misra, S., and Ghosh, A. (1991) Lipid Changes of Goal Sperm Plasma Membrane during Epididimal Maturation, *Biochim. Biophys. Acta. 1061*, 185–196.

9. Roldan, E.R.S., and Harrison, R.A.P. (1989) Phosphoinositide Breakdown and Subsequent Exocytosis in the Ca(2+)/Ionophore Induced Acrosome Reaction of Mammalian Spermatozoa, *Biochem. J. 259*, 397–406.

10. Ribbes, H., Plantavid, M., Bennet, P.J., *et al.* (1987) Phospholipase C from Human Sperm Specific for Phosphoinositides, *Biochim. Biophys. Acta. 919*, 245–54.

11. Khorasani, A.M., Cheung, A.P., and Lee, C.Y. (2000) Cholesterol Inhibitory Effects on Human Sperm-Induced Acrosome Reaction, *J. Androl. 21(4)*, 586–94.

12. Visconti, P.E., Westbrook, V.A., Chertihin, 0., Demarco, I., Sleight, S., and Diekman, A.B. (2002) Novel Signaling Pathways Involved in Sperm Acquisition of Fertilizing Capacity, *J. Reprod. Immunol. 53(1–2)*, 133–50.

13. Aitken, J., and Fisher, H. (1994) Reactive Oxygen Species Generation and Human Spermatozoa: The Balance of Benefit and Risk, *Bioessays 16 (4)*, 259–267.

14. Gulaya (Hula), N.M., Tronko, M.D., Volkov, G.L., and Margitich, V.M. (1993) Lipid Composition and Fertile Ability of Human Ejaculate, *Ukr. Biochim. Zh. 65(4)*, 64–70.

15. Poulos, A., Darin-Bennett, A., and White, I.G. (1973) The Phospholipid Bound Fatty Acids and Aldehydes of Mammalian Spermatozoa, *Comp. Biochem. Physiol. B. 46*, 541–549.

16. Alvarez, J.G., and Storey, B.T. (1995) Differential Incorporation of Fatty Acids into and Peroxidative Loss of Fatty Acids from Phospholipids of Human Spermatozoa, *Mol. Reprod. Dev. 42*, 334–346.

17. Nissen, H.P., Kreisel, H.W. (1983) Polyunsaturated Fatty Acids in Relation to Sperm Motility, *Andrologia 15*, 264–269.

18. Sebastian, S.M., Selvaraj, S., Aruldhas, M.M., and Govindarajulu, P. (1987) Pattern of Neutral and Phospholipids in the Semen of Normospermic, Oligospermic, and Azoospermic Men, *J. Reprod. Fertil. 79(2)*, 373–378.

19. Check, J.H., Bollendorf, A., Press, M., and Blue, T. (1992) Standard Sperm Morphology as a Predictor of Male Fertility Potential, *Arch. Androl. 28*, 39–41.

20. Homonnai, Z.T., Paz, G., Weiss, J.N., and David, M.P. (1980) Quality of Semen Obtained from 627 Fertile Men, *Int. J. Androl. 3 (3)*, 217–228.

21. Aitken, R.J., Comhaire, F.H., and Eliasson, R., *et al.* (1987) *WHO Laboratory Manual for the Examination of Human Semen and Semen-Mucus Interaction*, Cambridge University Press, Cambridge, UK.

22. Bligh, E.G., and Dyer, W.I. (1959) A Rapid Method of Total Lipid Extraction and Purification, *Can. J. Biochem. Physiol. 37*, 911–917.

23. Palmer, F.B.St.C. (1971) The Extraction of Acidic Phospholipids in Organic Solvent Mixtures Containing Water, *Biochim. Biophys. Acta. 231*, 134–144.

24. Vaskovsky, V.E., and Terehova, T.A. (1979) HPTLC of Phospholipid Mixtures Containing Phosphatidyl-Glycerol, *J. High. Resol. Chromatogr. & C.C. 2*, 671–672.

25. Vaskovsky, V.E., Kostetsky, E.Y., and Vasendin, I.M. (1975) A Universal Reagent for Phospholipid Analysis, *J. Chromatogr. 114*, 129–141.

26. Vaskovsky, V.E., and Latyshev, N.A. (1975) Modified Jungnickel's Reagent for Detecting Phospholipids and other Phosphorus Compounds on Thin Layer Chromatograms, *J. Chromatogr. 115*, 246–249.

27. van Gert, C.M., Rosseleur, O.J., and van Bigl, P. (1973) The Detection of Cerebrosides on Thin-Layer Chromatograms with an Antrone Spray Reagent, *J. Chromatogr. 85*, 174–176.
28. Christie, W.W. (1979) *Lipid Analysis,* Pergamon Press, Oxford, UK.
29. Carreau, I.D., and Dubaco, I.P. (1978) Adaptation of a Macro-Scale Method to the Micro-Scale for Fatty Acid Methyl Transeterification of a Biological Lipid Extraction, *J. Chromatogr. 151(3)*, 384–390.
30. Lowry, O.H., Rosebrough, N.J., Fan, A.L., and Randall, R.J. (1951) Protein Measurement with the Folin Phenol Reagent, *J. Biol. Chem. 193*, 265–275.
31. Bruni, A. (1988) Autacoids from Membrane Phospholipids, *Pharmacol. Res. Commun. 20*, 529–544.
32. Bruni, A., Monastra, G., Bellini, F., and Toffano, G. (1988) Autacoid Properties of Lysophosphatidylserine, *Prog. Clin. Biol. Res. 282*, 165–179.
33. Conte, G., Milardi, D., De Marinis, L., and Mancini, A. (1999) Reactive Oxygen Species in Male Infertility: Review of Literature and Personal Observations, *Panminerva. Med. 41(5)*, 45–53.
34. Laudat, A., Lecourbe, K., and Palluel, A.M. (1999) Lipid Peroxidation, Morphological Stress Pattern and Nuclear Maturity of Spermatozoon, *Ann. Biol. Clin. (Paris) 57 (1)*, 51–56.
35. Sebastian, S.M., Selvaraj, S., Aruldhas, M.M., Govindarajulu, P. (1987) Pattern of Neutral and Phospholipids in the Semen of Normospermic, Oligospermic, and Azoospermic Men, *J. Reprod. Fertil. 79*, 373–378.
36. Storey, B.T. (1997) Biochemistry of the Induction and Prevention of Lipoperoxidative Damage in Human Spermatozoa, *Mol. Hum. Reprod. 3*, 203–213.
37. Borkenhagen, L.F., Kennedy, E.P., and Fielding, L. (1961) Enzymatic Formation and Decarboxilation of Phosphatidylserine, *J. Biol. Chem. 236*, PC28–PC30.
38. Conquer, J.A., Martin, J.B., Tummon, I., Watson, L., and Tekpetey, F. (1999) Fatty Acid Analysis of Blood Serum, Seminal Plasma, and Spermatozoa of Normozoospermic *vs.* Asthenozoospermic Males, *Lipids 34*, 793–799.
39. Conquer, J.A., Martin, J.B., Tummon, I., Watson, L., and Tekpetey, F. (2000) Effect of DHA Supplementation on DHA Status and Sperm Motility in Asthenozoospermic Males, *Lipids 35(2)*, 149–154.
40. Retterstol, K., Haugen, T.B., and Tran, T.N., Christophersen B.O. (2001) Studies on the Metabolism of Essential Fatty Acids in Isolated Human Testicular Cells, *Reproduction 121(6)*, 881–887.

Chapter 6

Docosahexaenoic Acid-Rich Marine Oils and Improved Reproductive Efficiency in Pigs

A. Maldjian[a,b,*], P.C. Penny[a], and R.C. Noble[a]

[a]JSR Healthbred Ltd, Southburn, Driffield, Y025 9ED, UK
[b]Faculty of Veterinary Medicine, University of Milan, Milan 20133, Italy

Abstract

The lipid or fat constituents of the male gamete and associated seminal fluid are quite unique in their composition and fatty acid content. In the majority of the main tissues, long chain polyunsaturates, *i.e.*, fatty acids of 20 and 22 carbon atoms chain length containing more than two double bonds, are present to a limited extent in the lipid fractions, their levels in the lipids of the spermatozoa and seminal plasma are extremely high and show distinctive species specificity. Such lipid profiles are now increasingly suggested as playing key functions that lead to the ultimate success of the male fertilizing process. With a selection of recent investigations, a review is presented on the potential of an optimization of lipid/fatty acid parameters in the spermatozoa of the modern breeding boar with respect to a range of major determinants of semen quality and function. Significant effects across a range of gamete parameters can be observed with concomitant highly positive benefits to both male and female reproductive output and capacities. The observations are discussed in terms of major nutritional and biochemical features, comparisons with other major domesticated species, and potential economic applications to the pig-breeding sector.

Fatty Acid Composition of the Spermatozoa

The lipid composition of the spermatozoa and associated seminal fluids are very unique in their content and fatty acid constituents when compared with almost all other tissues within the animal body. Although all tissues have a requirement to maintain significant levels of essential polyunsaturated fatty acids, these are mainly present as the 18-carbon fatty acids with either two double bonds (linoleic acid, 18:2n-6) or three double bonds (α-linolenic acid, 18:3n-3), which are esterified in the phospholipids and neutral lipid fractions. Usually, very much lower concentrations of longer chain acids of higher polyunsaturation are found in these tissues. These have been obtained either directly through nutrition or indirectly through metabolism by enzymes within the tissues themselves that involve interrelated desaturation (introduction of more double bonds) and chain elongation (addition of more carbon atoms) of the precursor fatty acids, namely, linoleic and α-linolenic acids (1). This metabolism takes place principally in the liver; some evidence exists to suggest that it occurs as well in the testis of some species. As a result, 20- and 22-carbon polyunsaturated fatty acids (PUFA) are synthesized from linoleic acid as the "parent," and these are known collectively as n-6 PUFA (see Fig. 6.1). By a similar process a series of 20 and 22-carbon polyunsaturates arise from α-linolenic acid as the "parent" and are called collectively n-3 PUFA (see Fig. 6.1 for specific names, when applicable; abbreviated names; and shorthand designations of the long-chain PUFA). The major acids are arachidonic acid (AA, 20:4n-6), consisting of 20-carbon atoms with four double bonds, and docosahexaenoic acid (DHA, 22:6n-3), consisting of 22-carbon atoms with six double bonds. Contemporary interest in these long-chain PUFA is high through an increasing identification of their specific metabolic roles and associated functions in a wide range of aspects for the maintenance of human and animal health and well being (2).

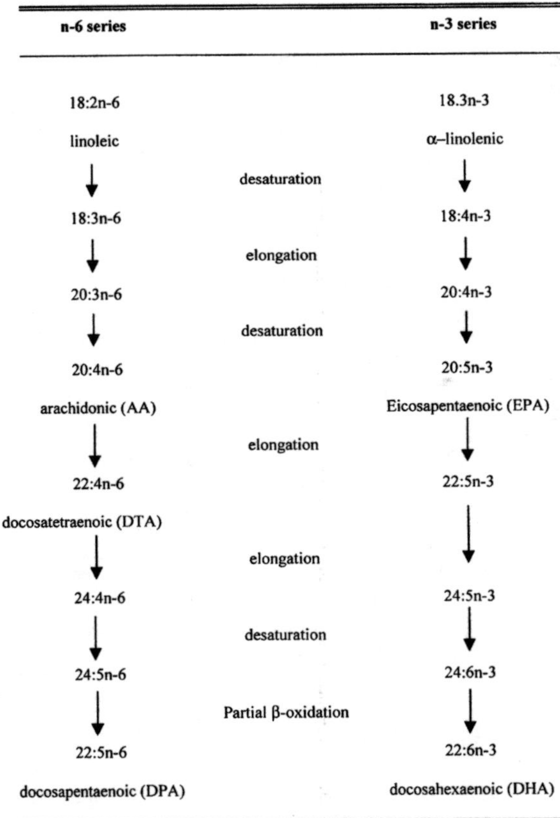

Fig. 6.1. Polyunsaturated fatty acid biosynthesis by desaturation and chain elongation in animal tissues.

Whereas in all major tissues other than the brain and retina the C20 and C22 PUFA of the n-6 and n-3 series together account for a maximum of about 6% of the total fatty acids present, in both the spermatozoa and seminal plasma their levels are strikingly elevated and in several instances account for up to 60% of the total fatty acids present (see Table 6.1). Furthermore, the lipid present in both the spermatozoa and seminal plasma consists almost wholly of phospholipids (about 70–80% of total lipids) in which polyunsaturation is directed during spermatogenesis to specific moieties and molecular configurations. All the major differentiated regions of the spermatozoan cell display their own unique lipid composition and phospholipid molecular specification involving polyunsaturation; within the regions there is also a discrete localization of the lipids in distinct domains (3,4). This specific lipid composition is regarded as being required for key functions of the spermatozoa leading to fertilization of the egg. In addition to a role in energy provision, the potential involvement of specific lipid components in wider issues of the male gamete functions, such as numbers, motility, and survivability, is increasingly being alluded to (5,6).

Even though the levels and combinations for fatty acids of both the n-6 and n-3 series within the phospholipid fractions demonstrate distinct species specificity, the total level of unsaturation of the male gamete lipid is always high (see Table 6.1). The spermatozoa of the bull and ram exhibit very high levels of DHA (major fatty acid present), which contrast most strongly with the situation of the dog and rabbit in which the levels of DHA are extremely low. The spermatozoa of the boar display an interesting fatty acid profile with similar levels of both DHA and of its n-6 counterpart docosapentaenoic acid (DPA). The question therefore arises as to the major reasons for these large variations between species. In the case of intensively farmed animal species, considerations have to be paid to the bioavailability of essential fatty acids restricted by limited dietary and environmental situations that can severely compromise "natural" tissue fatty acid supply and metabolism with the result that best fit alternatives may be an enforced situation (7).

Our observations and other reports (5) on the pig have shown that reductions in the proportions of DHA and increases in that of DPA within the spermatozoa are cor-

TABLE 6.1

Major Polyunsaturated Fatty Acids (% of total fatty acids present) of Phospholipids in the Spermatozoa of Various Animal Species (ND = not detected)

	18:2(n-6)[a]	20:4(n-6)	22:4(n-6)	22:5 (n-6)	22:6(n-3)
Boar (29)	2.1	3.2	1.6	27.9	37.7
Bull (29)	3.0	3.3	ND	6.9	55.4
Ram (29)	1.7	4.5	ND	ND	61.4
Fowl (6,30)	1.8	6.2	19.2	1.0	2.3
Man (31)	1.8	2.5	ND	ND	58.7
Dog (32)	3.2	6.6	ND	28.4	3.9
Rabbit (29)	4.8	ND	ND	39.0	ND

[a]See Fig. 6.1 for polyunsaturated fatty acid nomenclature.

related with reductions of semen quality and/or fertilizing capacity. From available evidence from the pig and other species, it would appear that whereas significant variations in the proportions of the major PUFA within the spermatozoa can be accommodated during spermatogenesis, there is a priority to sustain a required overall level of polyunsaturation.

Lipid Oxidation

The integrity of the PUFA in order to perform their specific metabolic roles requires protection from oxidation from the environment and reactive oxygen free radical attack through adequate levels of both antioxidants and specific protective enzyme systems (8,9). Under normal circumstances, a balance is maintained between the extent of free radical production and antioxidant capacity. With the loss of this balance (*e.g.,* heat stress) the accumulation of highly reactive oxygen species causes extensive fatty acid structural damage and associated interference in cellular metabolism. With high polyunsaturation and therefore an increasing double bond presence, lack of sufficient protection can result in an accumulation of lipid/fatty acid oxidation products in spermatozoa with a consequential impairment of function through a range of features arising from the loss of membrane PUFA and the concomitant accumulation of peroxides; these include decreased sperm motility and integrity and reduced capacitation (10,11). Antioxidant protection within the spermatozoa and seminal plasma is provided by a variety of molecules that embrace liposoluble components, such as vitamin E and ubiquinones; water soluble components, such as vitamin C; and major enzyme systems that include, most importantly, glutathione peroxidase, superoxide dismutase, and catalase (11).

Changes occurring to qualitative and quantitative parameters of spermatozoa quality and function in breeding males both over their productive life (12,13) and during *in vitro* storage (8) have initiated a series of investigations into the possible means to reduce such variations and thereby lead to a potential enhancement of the commercial value of the boar. Considering the importance of the C20 and C22 PUFA to a wide range of spermatozoa metabolic features, a specific interest has involved the optimization of their availability and subsequent cellular metabolism. The work has been based upon the variation of fatty acid content between mammalian farm animals, and therefore, investigations have been made to determine if this was a specie specificity or due to inadequate fatty acid content of the commercial diets. All data were obtained using modern male breeding boars (JSR Yorker-Large White) maintained under conditions appropriate to commercial artificial insemination (AI) semen production. A range of dietary supplements were examined, all designed to enhance the dietary intake of DHA, in combination with additional levels of vitamin E (alpha-tocopherol) and enzyme co-factors, for the specific purpose of increasing the spermatozoan level of DHA, at the expense of DPA, and its chemical integrity and cellular functionality. Increased levels of DHA in a breeding boar standard diet were achieved through the addition of tuna fin oil (Hi-DHA™, Clover Corporation, Australia) in which the level of DHA was about 25–27% of the total long chain fatty acids present. The boars and appropriate controls were fed the diets for 16 weeks with semen harvested according to AI commercial procedures and every 4 weeks data was recorded on a range of physiological and chemical parameters appropriate to the evaluation of the quality of the spermatozoa and their fertilizing capacities. These parameters embraced lipid composition and fatty acid analyses, tocopherol content, and a range of standard features associated with spermatozoa functions, *e.g.,* concentration, motility, and vitality.

These data were obtained by both standard and "state of the art" methodologies. Thus, following appropriate solvent extraction, lipid fraction and fatty acid analysis and quantification were performed by combinations of high-performance thin layer chromatography and capillary gas–liquid chromatography (14). Identification of fatty acids was by comparison with standard retention data and ultimately by gas–liquid chromatography, and identification of antioxidants (tocopherols) was by high-performance liquid chromatography (15). Spermatozoa viability was evaluated by the SYBR 14/propidium iodide procedure (16) and motility by a computer assisted sperm analyzer (CASA, Cell Soft™). Fertilizing capacity *in vivo* was measured by AI as for commercial practice involving 478 gilts (JSR Genepacker 90).

As has been reported in some other major animal species (6), enhancement of the diet of the boar with differing levels of n-6 and n-3 PUFA effected significant changes to the spermatozoa fatty acid composition. Thus when the diet was suitably supplemented with an appropriate DHA-rich oil, the proportion of DHA associated with the spermatozoa dramatically increased indicating effective dietary transfer. The proportion of DHA within the total fatty acid of the spermatozoa increased from 32.8 to 45.8% of total fatty acids (see Table 6.2). As can be seen, this occurred solely at the expense of a significant decrease in the proportion of DPA. The total lipid or phospholipid content and proportions within the spermatozoa were not affected; the effect was therefore confined solely to a readjustment of the two major PUFA and involved substitution of the n-6 long chain acid by its n-3 counterpart. Under these conditions and in the absence of any dramatic antioxidant supplementation above that normally associated with a standard breeder ration, positive effects were observed over 16-week trial periods on a range of parameters of spermatozoa quality that included concentration, percentage of viable spermatozoa, and overall morphology. Nevertheless, in order to observe any changes in biochemical or quality parameters of the spermatozoa, a minimum period of 6 weeks has to be considered to cover spermatogenesis and sperm maturation.

The extent of the DHA levels in the spermatozoa, and to some extent in the surrounding seminal plasma, clearly resulted in a rise in the overall level of unsaturation, which was significantly above that which is normally encountered in the boar. Under these circumstances, there existed a high risk of peroxidative stress within the cells through inadequate antioxidant protection. This could have offset any potential positive effects on spermatozoa quality parameters that the fatty acids might be effecting. Consequently, investigations were undertaken involving a dietary combination of sup-

TABLE 6.2

Fatty Acid Composition (% of total fatty acids present) of the Phospholipid Fraction of the Spermatozoa from Control ($n = 9$, standard boar diet) and Treated Boars ($n = 18$) at 16 Weeks of Supplementation (Supplemented: **1** = DHA + vitamin E supplement, **2** = DHA + vitamin E + selenium supplement)[a]

		Supplemented		
Fatty Acid:	Control	1	2	Significance
Palmitic, 16:0	14.7	16.2	14.8	NS
Palmitoleic, 16:1	<0.2	0.3	<0.2	NS
Stearic, 18:0	6.5	6.7	6.0	NS
Oleic, 18:1 (n-9)	1.8	1.4	1.6	NS
Linoleic, 18:2 (n-6)*	2.5	1.8	2.5	NS
Alpha-linolenic, 18:3 (n-3)	<0.2	<0.2	<0.2	NS
Arachidonic, 20:4 (n-6)	3.2	2.8	3.2	NS
Docosapentaenoic, 22:5 (n-6)	25.1	**11.1**	**13.8**	*
Docosahexaenoic, 22:6 (n-3)	32.8	**45.8**	**45.4**	*

aStatistical analysis, student Fisher test, *$P < 0.001$ treatment *versus* control; NS: not significant.

plemental PUFA but with enhanced vitamin E levels. Fatty acid changes within the spermatozoa and seminal plasma remained similar to those previously observed but no further promotion of indicators of fertility was observed. However, in spite of the considerable increase in the level of vitamin E supplementation, any increase in the level of vitamin E within the spermatozoa was minimal. This agreed with observations of the chicken (17), in which it was shown that, compared to body tissues, normal semen is very unresponsive to dietary increases in vitamin E supply. Also in the chicken, it was shown that there was a need for a lengthy time scale to observe even a small response. By contrast, data on the ram (18) had shown an enhancement of a range of spermatozoan characteristics, including motility and acrosomal morphology, as the result of a dietary supplementation with vitamin E.

Whereas the role of vitamin E is its chain-breaking capacity on the lipid peroxidation process, that of the cellular enzymes is their scavenging properties through the elimination of the reactive oxygen species themselves (9). Within the latter process the presence in the semen of the selenium-containing enzyme glutathione peroxidase is of major importance because of its dual role as antioxidant and an inhibitor of lipid peroxidation. With the enzyme's selenium dependency, there exists an ability to induce the enzyme's presence and therefore activity within the cell through an enhanced dietary supply of the element; potential promotion of other suggested beneficial selenoprotein cellular effects within the spermatozoa would also be accessed.

Feed manipulation of the boars with DHA-rich oil accompanied also by an increase of both vitamin E and selenium contents were therefore investigated. The qualitative effects upon spermatozoa fatty acid composition were as previously observed (see Table 6.2). However, in addition to the previous results, the effect upon a range of spermatozoa quality parameters was highly positive. Tables 6.3 and 6.4 show that the specific substitution of DHA at the expense of DPA in the presence of

TABLE 6.3

Spermatozoa Concentration and Total Sperm Numbers from Ejaculates of Control and Supplemented (fish oil + alpha tocopherol + selenium) Boars (Mean values from weeks 4–16 of feeding)

	Control	Supplemented	Significance
Sperm concentration ($\times 10^6$/ml)	502	584	$P < 0.01$
Total sperm numbers ($\times 10^9$)	74.1	83.4	$P < 0.01$

TABLE 6.4

Proportion of Live Spermatozoa (mean value of the group) in Ejaculates from Control and Supplemented (as in Table 6.3) Boars

Weeks of feeding	Control	Supplemented	Significance
0	78	75	NS
4	84	86	NS
8	73	88	$P < 0.05$
12	81	86	$P < 0.05$
16	70	89	$P < 0.01$

TABLE 6.5

Number of Artificial Inseminations per Ejaculate Collection (using a dose of 2.5×10^9 cells, volume of 75 ml)

	Control	Supplemented	Significance
AI per ejaculate collection	30	33	$P < 0.02$

proper antioxidant protection within the spermatozoa significantly promoted major features of sperm output and function. Thus it was clear that although the previous changes to the polyunsaturate composition of the spermatozoa had the potential to effect promotion of spermatozoa features, the provision of additional selenium enabled fulfillment of this potential through its cofactorial relationship to the antioxidant capacities of the cell, in particular, but possibly also through other roles in cellular metabolism and structural integrity. Table 6.5 indicates the potential economic returns arising from boars that displayed the enhancement of DHA within their spermatozoa.

Effect on Female Reproductive Output

Gilts were inseminated with semen doses from either control or supplemented boars. Results in terms of conception, born alive, and fecundity of females following artificial insemination of DHA-rich spermatozoa were highly positive (Table 6.6). These results show a clear economic benefit on the female side as well. Experiments under-

TABLE 6.6
Female Fertility Output from Gilts Serviced with Semen Doses from Control or
Supplemented (see Table 6.3) Boars (Means of fertility for semen samples collected from
week 4 to 16 of the feeding trial)

	Control	Supplemented	Significance
Conception rate (%)	83	90	$P < 0.05$
Number born alive	10.2	10.6	$P < 0.05$
Fecundity (born alive / 100 services)	846	956	$P < 0.001$

taken on the potential improvement of the fertility of the cockerel through fatty acid manipulation of the spermatozoa showed similar effects in terms of overall female reproductive output (See Chapters 7 and 8 of this book). Some evidence in the literature (19) based on a series of *in vitro* investigations has strongly suggested that the synthesis of highly unsaturated phospholipids through a supply of exogenous lipids can be achieved to some extent by boar spermatozoa.

Time to Change Dietary Lipids in Male Breeder's Feed

The boar is unique among major farm animal species in the display within its spermatozoa of a very high level of DPA. The results presented in this chapter clearly show that displacement of this acid by its n-3 counterpart DHA, in the presence of supplemental vitamin E and selenium, is of significant benefit to the overall reproductive performance of the boar under modern intensive breeding situations. Much has been said over the years about the role of the polyunsaturated essential fatty acids in farm animal nutrition, husbandry, and ultimate product quality (7,20,21). In this respect, although there has been an unqualified recognition that inadequacies exist and should be addressed, there has been an almost blanket emphasis on the C18 components but in particular linoleic acid (n-6 series) through its overwhelming presence in most of the widely available dietary oils. However, increasing recognition of the specific metabolic roles played by the longer chain C20 and C22 polyunsaturates EPA (20:5n-3) and DHA is suggesting a requirement for a far more balanced dietary strategy to be considered in the overall provision of the n-3 acids relative to those of the n-6 series.

In cells such as the spermatozoa, the need for long chain polyunsaturation appears paramount. However the composition of such PUFA will, under present modern breeding situations, be considerably influenced by the C18 precursor, which presently is very much biased toward the n-6 series (linoleic acid). As a monogastric animal, the supply of C18 PUFA has a marked effect on tissue lipid composition in the pig (22). Thus, any preferential requirement during spermatogenesis in the boar for DHA may be severely compromised by the overwhelming availability of competitive n-6 metabolites. Under these circumstances chain elongation and desaturation to achieve the required level of C22 polyunsaturation would give rise to a preponderance of the n-6 metabolite DPA with its potentially limited ability to satisfy the metabolic needs of the spermatozoa.

In the present investigations on the boar, an increase in DHA within the spermatozoa was achieved through a uniquely high DHA enriched oil (about 25–27% of total fatty acids). There is a tendency throughout farm animal experiments attempting DHA enhancement of tissues and products to involve the use of alpha-linolenic acid as the dietary fatty acid substrate and rely on the animal's inherent desaturation/chain elongation processes to provide the desired level of DHA (1). Where substantial increases in DHA are to be achieved, the efficiency of relying upon the synthetic pathway to satisfy DHA requirements has proved to be routinely inadequate with the result that there is no realistic alternative to that of supplying the DHA itself through an appropriate oil-rich source (7). Such was also the situation with respect to the present series of investigations on promoting the DHA levels in boar spermatozoa.

Spermatozoa Storage and Fatty Acid Composition

The efficiency of AI in gilts or sows depends not only on the initial fertility of the fresh ejaculate but the maintenance of this fertility during subsequent storage. The processing and storage of semen (cooled but even more so when frozen) reduces the motility and disrupts the membrane integrity of the spermatozoa (8,26) with concomitant effects upon the fertilizing capacity. In the pig, storage of semen for AI purposes presents a particular problem with loss of fertilizing capacity at ambient, sub-ambient, and freezing temperatures used in practice (23,24). Stored semen invariability has a significantly lower fertilizing capacity than fresh at equal insemination doses. Despite many suggestions to explain this, the reasons still largely remain unresolved and are probably due to many factors. However, there is recent evidence to suggest that while the majority of the spermatozoa may retain their motility during and after storage, the membranes of the motile cells undergo destabilisation to such an extent that their survival time within the female tract is reduced (24). One suggestion is that this reduced survival time post-storage is related to the composition of the plasma and organelle membranes, in particular the phospholipid composition and associated polyunsaturated components (3), and therefore to their membrane fluidity and sensibility to oxidation. Spermatozoa showing varying lipid and polyunsaturated compositions display a wide range of membrane fluidity and resistance to cold shock (25). It is a feature of cells in general that differences in the state of saturation of the membrane lipids give rise to changes in transition temperatures and resistance to membrane damage during cold exposure. The present substantial evidence for the specific role of the PUFA in unique phospholipid form for the maintenance of spermatozoa physiology and function together with their susceptibility to oxidation and therefore the need for adequate antioxidant protection, suggests that attention to a combination of these features may reduce the risk of damage to spermatozoa and their lack of survival during storage at ambient or reduced temperatures (8,26).

Fertilization processes necessitate that the spermatozoa have in place the correct membrane lipid infrastructures to maintain required membrane fluidity. Key indices for this have been identified and embrace sterol/phospholipid, phosphatidylethanolamine/-choline and unsaturated/saturated fatty acid ratios; of the phospholipid species the sn-2 ester linked DHA phospholipid species have been identified to be of particular importance (3).

In common with other species, during storage of boar semen, significant changes occur to these lipid relationships, in particular reductions in the level of polyunsaturation and associated phospholipid moieties (26). By both inference and experimental evidence such destabilizing situations can also be implicated in changes to transitional temperatures and membrane fluidity resulting in both impaired survival and spermatozoa function following storage. Because of the presence of highly unsaturated lipids, *in vitro* storage can provide a good environment for the formation of oxygen free radicals and peroxides (11,24,27).

The process of cooling, freezing, and thawing is suggested to modify and/or damage the cell membranes to such an extent that the proportion of progressively motile cells is reduced, as well as overall viability of the spermatozoa at insemination and therefore within the female tract. The promotion of antioxidant levels under situations involving semen storage has therefore been tried in a range of species (11,26,28). Of the antioxidants available for suggested protection of spermatozoa stability during storage, vitamin E has been the most studied with its twin advantages of cost and known protective abilities; its potential has been assessed following both dietary administration and addition to the fresh semen. The fat-soluble nature of vitamin E puts it at some disadvantage in terms of direct semen addition due to the requirements for a suitable carrier system to deliver to aqueous semen extender. However, where this has been achieved (26,28), appropriate benefits on spermatozoa viability and fatty acid integrity have been reported.

Considering the metabolic and physical features that the highly unsaturated phospholipids impart to spermatozoa function and survival, deliberate promotion of their presence in boar spermatozoa and protection may be beneficial when storage of semen is considered. As mentioned above, the increase by dietary means of PUFA within the spermatozoa prior to storage can be achieved in the pig providing that some appropriate safeguards are taken. Whereas storage of semen at temperatures of 18°C for 4–5 days had reduced fertility to the point of limited commercial value, semen in which the DHA levels had been deliberately increased by dietary means remained viable for periods exceeding 5 days.

Summary

Although comparative data exist from both recent and much earlier sources on the lipid composition of spermatozoa and seminal plasma from a range of animal species, particular focus on their role in aspects of spermatozoa function and survival is relatively recent. Interest in the PUFA has arisen with the recognition of the competing nature of the separate n-6 and n-3 series in a wide range of aspects of animal metabolism (e.g. immune system). Increasing number of correlations are being reported between a reduction in reproductive performance and semen lipid compositional changes. However data are limited on the consequences to semen quality of attempting to optimize the lipid content of the spermatozoa and seminal plasma. The recent awareness that under intensive production systems farm animals have suffered a distinct bias toward promoting the nutritional and metabolic importance of the n-6 relative to the n-3 PUFA necessitates an evaluation of semen lipid compositions and its polyunsaturate content.

In the pig, manipulation of the lipid composition of the spermatozoa enhanced reproductive capacity for AI purposes. The pig, by its interesting fatty acid content does present an excellent model to study the role of key long-chain PUFA on given quality parameters of the male gamete function. However, in light of potential commercial rewards and contemporary male fertility problems, the search for the optimization of the lipid content of spermatozoa in breeders from all farm animal species and of man may well be extremely rewarding.

Acknowledgment

The authors are grateful to the Department of Trade and Industry, London, for an International Secondment Award for the placement of A. Maldjian at the University of Milan, Italy. The data presented is the subject of a selection of international patents to cover future potential commercialization.

References

1. Cook, H.W. (1991) *Biochemistry of Lipids, Lipoproteins, and Membranes,* pp. 141–170, Elsevier Press, New York.
2. British Nutrition Foundation (1994) *Unsaturated Fatty Acids. Nutritional and Physiological Significance,* general reference, Chapman and Hall, London.
3. Ladha, S. (1998) Lipid Heterogeneity and Membrane Fluidity in a Highly Polarized Cell, the Mammalian Spermatozoa, *J. Memb. Biol. 165,* 1–10.
4. Wolfe, C.A., James, P.S., Mackie, A.R., Ladha, S, and Jones, R. (1998) Regionalised Lipid Diffusion in the Plasma Membrane of Mammalian Spermatozoa, *Bio. Repr. 59,* 1506–1514.
5. Rooke, J.A. Shao, C.C. and Speake, B.K (2001) Effects of Feeding Tuna Oil on the Lipid Composition of Pig Spermatozoa and in vitro Characteristics of Semen, *Repr. 121,* 315–322.
6. Kelso, K.A., Cerolini, S., Speake, B.K., Cavalchini, L.G., and Noble, R.C. (1997) Effect of Dietary Supplementation with Alpha-Linolenic Acid on the Phospholipid Fatty Acid Composition and Quality of Spermatozoa in the Cockerel from 24–27 Weeks of Age, *J. Repr. Fert. 110,* 53–59.
7. Noble, R.C. (1997) *Animal Fats–BSE and After,* pp. 43–63, P.J. Barnes and Associates, Bridgewater.
8. Cerolini, S., Maldjian, A., Gliozzi, T., Pizzi, F., Surai, P., and Noble, R.C. (1999) Relationship Between Lipid Composition and Viability of Boar Spermatozoa after Freez-

ing/Thawing, in *IV International Conference on Boar Semen Preservation*, Beltsville, Maryland.

9. Yu, B.P. (1994) Cellular Defences against Damage from Reactive Oxygen Species, *Physio. Rev. 74*, 139–162.

10. Alvarez, J.G., and Storey, B.T. (1982) Spontaneous Lipid Peroxidation in Rabbit Epididymal Spermatozoa: Its Effect on Sperm Motility, *Biol. Repr. 27*, 1102–1108.

11. Sharma, R.K., and Agarwal, A. (1996) Role of Reactive Oxygen Species in Male Infertility, *Urol. 48*, 835–850.

12. Kelso, K.A., Cerolini, S., Noble, R.C., Sparks, N.H.C., and Speake, B.K. (1996) Lipid and Antioxidant Changes in Semen of Broiler Fowl from 25 to 60 Weeks of Age, *J. Repr. Fert. 106*, 201–206.

13. Kelso, K.A., Redpath, A., Noble, R.C., and Speake, B.K. (1997) Lipid and Antioxidant Changes in Spermatozoa and Seminal Plasma Throughout the Reproductive Period of Bulls, *J. Repr. Fert. 109*, 1–6.

14. Christie, W.W. (1982) *Lipid Analysis*, general reference, Pergamon Press, Oxford.

15. McMurray, C.H., Blanchflower, W.J., and Rice, D.A. (1980) Extraction Techniques in the Determination of Tocopherol in Animal Feedstuffs, *J. Asso. Anal. Chem. 63*, 1258–1261.

16. Garner, D.L., and Johnson, L.A., (1995) Viability Assessment of Mammalian Sperm using SYBR 14 and Propidium Iodide, *Biol. Repr. 53*, 276–284.

17. Surai, P.F., Kutz, E., Wishart, G.J., Noble, R.C., and Speake, B.K. (1997) The Relationship Between the Dietary Provision of Alpha-Tocopherol and the Concentration of this Vitamin in the Semen of Chicken: Effects on Lipid Composition and Susceptibility to Peroxidation, *J. Repr. Fert. 110*, 47–51.

18. Gokcen, H., Camas, H., Erding, E., Asti, R., Cekgul, E., and Sener E., (1990) Studies on the Effects of Vitamin E and Selenium Added to the Ration on Acrosomal Morphology, Enzyme Activity, and Fertilization of Frozen Ram Sperm, *Doga-Turk-Vieterinerlik-ve Hayvancilik Dergisi 14*, 207–218.

19. Vasquez, J.M., and Roldan, E.R.S. (1997) Phospholipid Metabolism in Boar Spermatozoa and Role of Diacylglycerol Species in the *de novo* Formation of Phosphatidylcholine, *Mol. Repr. Dev. 47*, 105–112.

20. Noble, R.C. (1998) *Recent Advances in Animal Nutrition*, pp. 49–66, Nottingham University Press, Nottingham.

21. Scollan, N.D., and Wood, J.D. (2000) *Beef from Grass and Forage*, pp. 29–42, British Grassland Society (BGS), Reading.

22. Morgan, C.A., Noble, R.C., Cocchi, M., and McCartney, R. (1992) Manipulation of the Fatty Acid Composition of Pig Meat Lipids by Dietary Means, *J. Sci. Food Agri. 58*, 357–368.

23. Maxwell, W.M.C., and Salamon, S. (1993) Liquid Storage of Ram Semen: a Review, *Repr. Fert. Dev. 5*, 613–618.

24. Maxwell, W.M.C., and Watson, P.F. (1996) Recent Progress in the Preservation of Ram Semen, *Anim. Repr. Sci. 42*, 55–65.

25. Parks, J.E., and Lynch, D.V. (1992) Lipid Composition and Thermotropic Phase Behavior of Boar, Bull, Stallion and Rooster Sperm Membranes, *Cryobiol. 29*:255–266.

26. Cerolini, S., Maldjian, A., Noble, R.C., and Surai, P. (2000) Viability, Susceptibility to Peroxidation and Fatty Acid Composition of Boar Semen during Liquid Storage, *Ani. Repro. Sci. 58*, 99–111

27. Aurich, J.E., Schonherr, U., Hoppe, H., and Aurich, C. (1997) Effects of Antioxidants on Motility and Membrane Integrity of Chilled-Stored Stallion Semen, *Theriog. 48,* 185–192.
28. Maldjian, A., Cerolini, S., Surai, P., and Speake, B. (1998) The Effect of Vitamin E, Green Tea Extracts, and Catechin on the *in Vitro* Storage of Turkey Spermatozoa at Room Temperature, *Poult. Avian Biol. Rev. 9*:143–151.
29. Poulos, A., Darin-Bennett, A., and White, A.G. (1973) The Phospholipid-Bound Fatty Acids and Aldehydes of Mammalian Spermatozoa, *Comp. Bioch. Physiol. 46,* 541–549.
30. Ravie, O., and Lake, P.E (1985) The Phospholipid-Bound Fatty Acids of Fowl and Turkey Spermatozoa, *Ani. Repr. Sci. 9,* 189–192.
31. Nissen, H.P., and Kreysel, H.W. (1983) Polyunsaturated Fatty Acids in Relation to Sperm Motility, *Andro. 15,* 264–269.
32. Darin-Bennett, A., Poulos, A., and White, I.G. (1974) The Phospholipid and Phospholipid-Bound Fatty Acids and Aldehydes of Dog and Fowl Spermatozoa, *J. Repr. Fert. 41,* 471–474.

Chapter 7

Specificity of Fatty Acids in Domestic Bird Spermatozoa

E. Blesbois[a] and D. Hermier[b]

[a]SRA, INRA 37380 Nouzilly, France
[b]Laboratoire de Physiologie de la Nutrition, Centre Scientifique d'Orsay, 91405 Orsay, France

Abstract

Membrane lipids of spermatozoa contain high proportions of polyunsaturated fatty acids (PUFA) in every species studied. Bird spermatozoa contain an especially low proportion of n-3 and high proportion of n-6 PUFA (n-3/n-6 = 0.04 to 0.2). In addition, species specificity is also found. For example, n-9 PUFA are widely represented in turkey spermatozoa. The aim of the present study was to examine the specificity of PUFA of spermatozoa of domestic birds and whether the very low and high proportions of n-3 and n-6 PUFA in bird spermatozoa, sometimes associated with high proportions of n-9 PUFA, originate from deficiencies in dietary fatty acids or from reproductive specificity of avian species. Chicken and turkey adult males were fed standard diets or diets enriched in n-3 PUFA originating from fish oils. Fatty acid composition and quality parameters of fresh or stored spermatozoa were also measured. The age effect was also evaluated in turkeys. The dietary supplementation in n-3 PUFA clearly resulted in higher proportions of n-3 PUFA (22:5n-3 and 22:6n-3) in chicken and turkey spermatozoa; tissue resistance to changes was higher in chicken than in turkeys. However, percentages of n-9 PUFA (22:3n-9), 10% (SD = 3) of total fatty acids, in turkey spermatozoa were not modified by diet. Dietary supplementation in n-3 PUFA increased the n-3 PUFA of spermatozoa throughout the reproductive period in turkeys, but PUFA proportions generally decreased with male aging. Spermatozoa fatty acids were severely affected by freezing in chickens. In addition, n-3 dietary supplementation had a positive effect on fertility of fresh semen but a negative effect on frozen sperm. In conclusion, the very low proportion of n-3 PUFA in domestic bird spermatozoa partly originates from a diet effect, as dietary supplementations increased n-3 PUFA of spermatozoa and in some cases reproductive performance. However, high proportions of n-6, and n-9 PUFA for turkeys, are still clearly specific to domestic birds. The significance of such specificity is discussed with regard to nutritional needs and features of reproductive physiology in these species.

Introduction

The reproductive efficiency of the male in animal species depends on internal (genetic and physiological) and environmental factors (interactions with other animals, photoperiod, temperature, and diet). Diet is very important as most food deficiencies affect reproduction. Polyunsaturated fatty acids (PUFA) of the n-3 and n-6 series cannot be synthesized by vertebrates and must be provided by the diet in the form of either the 18-carbon plant precursor (18:3 n-3 or 18:2 n-6) or its long chain derivatives found in animal tissues (20–22 carbons, 4-double bounds) (1). These long-chain PUFA are essential components of all cell membranes and also give rise to many bioactive molecules, such as eicosanoids (2). They are especially abundant in the membrane phospholipids of spermatozoa and are believed to contribute actively to membrane fluidity, regulation of cellular movement, lipid metabolism, and fusion capacity (3). In addition, very-long-chain PUFA (24–26 carbons) have been observed in the male germ cells of mammals (4,5).

In most mammals, spermatozoa share with the brain and the retina the specificity of being very rich in n-3 LC-PUFA, especially 22:6n-3 (6–9). This is also the case for the brain and the retina in domestic birds (10,11) but not for spermatozoa, which are rich in n-6 PUFA.

C22 PUFA are the major PUFA of spermatozoa. However the nature of these PUFA depends on the species (12) and may be 22:6n-3, 22:5n-6, or 22:4n-6. The main PUFA in domestic birds is 22:4n-6 (13,14), and the proportions of respective PUFA partly depend on the diet (15,16).

These findings may have economic consequences, especially in domestic bird species in which the pressure of selection on growth has been so high during the last 30 years that the reproductive efficiency of meat type lines has decreased (17,18). The decrease in reproductive performance has a male component. In these conditions, every positive effect of environmental factors, such as diet, on semen composition and quality may be very important for the management of breeders.

The present paper examines the specific features of spermatozoa biology in domestic birds, in particular fatty acid composition. We also examine how the fatty acid composition of spermatozoa in domestic birds may be affected by diet and how these modifications may be related to physiological changes. These findings will then be related to the reproductive efficiency of breeders, to species specificity of reproductive biology, and to recommendations to the diet industry.

Specific Features of the Male Reproductive System in Domestic Birds—Specificity of Spermatozoon Fatty Acids

Reproductive Features of Domestic Birds

Like other birds, domestic birds (chickens, turkeys, guinea-fowls, Pekin and muscovy ducks, geese and quails) are oviparous species. Birds differ from numerous other oviparous species, such as fish, by internal fertilization. In addition, they are homoeothermic animals and testes are positioned inside the abdomen. The reproductive process consequently occurs at the mean body temperature, which is 41–43°C. This temperature is higher than that of most other homoeothermic species.

Spermatogenesis is a rapid process (12 days in the chicken) followed by a short period of gamete maturation in the deferent duct (1 to 3 days in the chicken) before ejaculation and natural intravaginal mating or artificial insemination.

The morphology of avian ejaculated spermatozoa (spz) is characterized by a thin cylindrical appearance with a maximum diameter of 0.5 μm at the head part and a mean length of 100 μm, including a very long flagellum (90 μm). They contain all the "classical" components of male gametes including acrosome, nucleus, and intermediate piece with 20–30 mitochondria. Ejaculates have extremely high spermatozoa concentrations (2 to 10×10^9 spz) and low volume (50 to 500 μL) leading to a mean of 2×10^9 spz per ejaculate in chickens and turkeys.

One feature of spermatozoa biology in domestic birds is their long stay (up to 3 weeks in the hen, 2 months in the turkey) in the utero-vaginal glands (UVG) of the female. Spermatozoa are released daily from these glands to reach the upper oviduct and the fertilization site. Fertilization is preceded by a classical acrosomal reaction of spermatozoa and many male gametes penetrate into the oocyte (polyspermia). However, only one of the male pronuclei fuses with the female pronucleus for embryo formation.

This reproductive system is efficient because one ejaculate usually leads to the fertilization of approximately 20 eggs in chickens.

Spermatozoon Fatty Acids in Domestic Birds

Despite the specific features of reproduction in domestic birds, the overall lipid composition of spermatozoa seems fairly classic when compared to other species (13–15,19–21). The predominance of phospholipids (70–80% of total lipids) and free cholesterol (about 20%) is indicative of the membrane origin of spermatozoon lipids in domestic birds. Most of them originate from the plasma membrane, but mitochondrial and nucleus membranes also contribute notably to spermatozoon lipids. The lack of or marginal content of triacylglycerols is in accordance with the lack of intracytoplasmic reserves of these gametes.

As in most vertebrate species, the major phospholipids of bird spermatozoa are phosphatidylcholine and phosphatidylethanolamine. Their fatty acid content (Table 7.1, 14) is highly unsaturated (65–70% of total fatty acids). This high degree of unsaturation is comparable to that found in rainbow trout and comparable to or higher than the levels found in tilapia and most mammalian species, including man (6,13,22, Table 7.2).

As in other species, most of the unsaturated fatty acids of domestic bird spermatozoa are PUFA, predominantly n-6 PUFA (22:4n-6 and 20:4n-6), and 22:4n-6 is the most abundant PUFA. This indicates a functional system of elongation/desaturation from the 18:2n-6 precursor provided by the diet. However more unsaturated PUFA such as 22:5n-6 are not detected in birds, whereas the latter PUFA is present in mammalian and fish species and is the major 22-carbon PUFA in the male germ cells of rodents (12,23). This may indicate a limitation of the elongase and desaturase activities in birds or competition with the n-3 and n-9 PUFA for these enzymes.

                                    E. Blesbois and D. Hermier

TABLE 7.1
Fatty Acid Composition of Domestic Bird Spermatozoa[a]

Fatty acids[b] (%)	Chicken	Turkey	Guinea fowl	Muscovy duck	Gander
14:0	<0.5	<0.5	0.6	1.1	0.9
14:1	<0.5	<0.5	<0.5	0.8	<0.5
16:0	9.5	12.4	15.4	21.5	17.0
17:1	<0.5	0.5	0.9	<0.5	1.1
18:0	19.1	17.7	15.8	11.5	15.4
18:1n-9	11.4	7.7	9.1	5.9	13.7
18:1n-7	2.1	2.5	2.1	2.1	2.1
18:2n-6	2.6	4.6	3.8	3.8	5.7
20:0	1.3	1.2	3.8	1.1	1.7
20:1n-9	3.6	9.2	1.2	0.7	1.1
20:2n-6	1.5	4.0	3.3	1.6	3.9
20:3n-6	1.6	0.9	<0.5	1.0	<0.5
20:3n-9	<0.5	2.7	1.0	<0.5	0.9
20:4n-6	11.7	9.4	15.8	18.9	13.3
22:1n-9	0.5	1.2	0.7	<0.5	<0.5
22:3n-9	3.8	9.2	4.3	0.6	1.4
22:4n-6	27.9	12.6	19.4	19.9	17.5
22:5n-3	<0.5	0.7	<0.5	0.6	<0.5
22:6n-3	2.1	2.7	1.7	8.0	2.8
SFA	29.9	31.3	35.6	35.2	35
Unsaturated FA	70.1	68.7	64.4	64.8	65
MUFA	17.1	20.6	14	9.5	16.9
PUFA	53.0	48.1	50.0	55.0	48.1
n-9 PUFA	3.8	10	6	1.0	2.3
n-6 PUFA	43.7	30.6	42.3	45.4	40.4
n-3 PUFA	2.6	3.4	1.7	8.6	3.2
n-3/n-6	0.05	0.1	0.04	0.2	0.09

[a]Suraï *et al.*, 1998
[b]FA, fatty acids; SFA, saturated fatty acids; MUFA, mono-unsaturated fatty acids; PUFA, polyunsaturated fatty acids.

In contrast to most mammals, with the exception of rodents, the proportion of n-3 PUFA is very low in domestic bird spermatozoa with quite wide variations depending on the species: spermatozoa of muscovy ducks have a far higher n-3/n-6 ratio (0.2) than those of chickens and guinea fowls (0.04–0.05). These differences do not originate from the n-3/n-6 ratios of the corresponding diets (n-3/n-6 ratios in the diet: 0.13 in the duck *vs.* 0.09 in the chicken, 14). They are therefore likely to be species-specific.

However, the very low n-3/n-6 ratio is a feature of the gametes of domestic birds compared to other vertebrate species. From a general point of view, fish and mammalian carnivores, and also most other mammals, have spermatozoa richer in n-3 than n-6 PUFA, (9,19,22,24–26), possibly corresponding to their general metabolic needs. On the other hand, the spermatozoon fatty acids of fish herbivore species (*e.g.*, Tilapia in fish, Table 7.2) and rodents are richer in n-6 than n-3 fatty acids. Indeed, the n-3/n-6 PUFA ratio of spermatozoa in domestic birds is even lower.

TABLE 7.2
Comparison of Fatty Acid Classes in Spermatozoa from Fish, Chicken, and Primates[a]

Fatty acids (%)	Rainbow trout	Tilapia	Chicken	Rhesus monkey	Human
SFA	30.9	52.7	29.9	38.4	59.5
Unsaturated FA	69.1	47.3	70.1	61.5	40.5
MUFA	16.3	11.2	17.1	15.5	16.5
PUFA	52.8	36.1	53.0	46.0	24.0
n-9 PUFA	nd	nd	3.8	nd	nd
n-6 PUFA	24.5	32.5	46.7	19.0	9.4
n-3 PUFA	27.6	3.6	2.4	25.1	14.6
n-3/n-6	3.6	0.36	0.05	1.3	1.5

[a]Labbé *et al.*, 1993; Bell *et al.*, 1996; Suraï *et al.*, 1998; Conquer *et al.*, 1999; Lin *et al.*, 1993

Another feature of long-chain fatty acids of domestic bird spermatozoa, especially in the turkey, is their notable n-9 long-chain fatty acids content: 20:1n-9 and 22:3n-9. These n-9 long-chain fatty acids are present in all domestic bird species with wide variations, and are generally lacking in germ cells of other species with the exception of the rat (23). From a general point of view, n-9 fatty acids are believed to be present in cases of deficiency in essential fatty acids such as n-3 PUFA. This is in accordance with findings in the spermatozoa of the muscovy duck, which contain the highest percentages of n-3 PUFA (8.6%) and the lowest percentages of n-9 long chain fatty acids (1.0%). Even when birds are compared to other species, the relationship between n-3 deficiency and increased percentages of n-9 LC-PUFA is questionable for spermatozoa: for example, a low percentage of n-3 PUFA is found in the tilapia, whereas n-9 PUFA are not detectable in the spermatozoa of this species.

Whether the specificity of PUFA in domestic bird spermatozoa (low n-3/n-6 ratio and high proportion of n-9 long chain fatty acids, and more specifically 22:3n-9 PUFA) originates from dietary deficiencies or is really species specific is therefore questionable. This will be discussed next by examining changes in dietary fatty acids in chickens and turkeys with consequences on spermatozoon composition and efficacy.

Effects of Changes in Dietary Fatty Acids on the Composition and Functions of Spermatozoa in the Chicken and Turkey

Diet Affects the Fatty Acid Composition of Chicken and Turkey Spermatozoa

Fatty acids in the diet are known to affect fatty acid composition of the tissues in all animal species. However, the effects of dietary changes are usually much more effective during cell multiplication, growth, and differentiation, which are age-dependent. For example, brain morphogenesis occurs very early, and the sensitivity of the chicken brain to diet supplementation in n-3 fatty acids is thus especially high in the newly

     E. Blesbois and D. Hermier

hatched chick (10,11). By contrast, spermatogenesis occurs in adult males, is a permanent process over the entire reproductive period, and may lead to specific dietary requirements.

The diets of adult male domestic birds are essentially based on corn, wheat, and soy. They are low lipid diets (6–7%) rich in unsaturated fatty acids (Tables 7.3 and 7.4), with a predominance of n-9 fatty acids among mono-unsaturated fatty acids, n-6 fatty acids among PUFA, and hence a very low n-3/n-6 ratio.

In the chicken (Table 7.3) and the turkey (Table 7.4), replacement of part of the corn or soy lipids by fish oil (rich in n-3 long chain PUFA) in the standard diet resulted in a significant increase in the percentage of n-3 fatty acids in spermatozoa (15, Table 7.2).

However, the efficiency of incorporation of n-3 fatty acids in spermatozoa was quite different between the two species. Indeed, resistance to n-3 incorporation was observed in chicken spermatozoa, whereas the ratio of n-3/n-6 PUFA in turkey sper-

TABLE 7.3

Effects of n-3 Supplementation in the Diet on Fatty Composition of Spermatozoa in the Adult Chicken[a]

Fatty acids[b] (%)	Diet[c] Corn oil	Diet[c] Fish oil	Spermatozoa[c] Corn oil diet		Spermatozoa[c] Fish oil diet
14:0		6.0	2.0 ± 0.2	*	3.2 ± 0.6
16:0	15. 0	19.9	17.0 ± 1.5		16.0 ± 0.9
16:1n-7			1.2 ± 0.4		1.8 ± 0.6
16:1n-9	0.2	10.0	1.4 ± 0.4		2.1 ± 0.7
18:0	1.9	2.8	20.3 ± 0.5		20.4 ± 0.9
18:1n-9	29.10	18.3	14.2 ± 0.8		15.6 ± 0.6
18:1n-7	0.95	4.3	2.7 ± 0.6		4.1 ± 0.7
18:2n-6	45.8	15.0	3.3 ± 0.3		2.1 ± 0.3
18:3n-3		1.1			
18:4n-3		3.7			
20:0		6.1			
20:1n-9		5.8	2.6 ± 0.1		2.7 ± 0.1
20:4n-6	0.2	0.4	9.0 ± 0.5	*	5.3 ± 0.6
20:5n-3		4.9			
22:1n-9		3.3			
22:3n-9		1.4	1.1 ± 0.7		1.1 ± 0.6
22:4n-6			21.0 ± 0.8	*	15.0 ± 1.2
22:5n-3		4.9	2.1 ± 1.0	*	4.10 ± 1.0
22:6n-3		4.2	2.2 ± 0.9	*	5.5 ± 1.0
SFA	23.0	28.7	39.3 ± 2.2		39.6 ± 1.6
MUFA	30.3	43.1	23.1 ± 0.80	*	27.4 ± 1.4
PUFA	51.0	33.0	36.6 ± 2.1	*	22.4 ± 2.0
n-3/n-6	0.02	0.89	0.13 ± 0.04	*	0.43 ± 0.01

[a]Blesbois et al., 1997a.
[b]SFA, saturated fatty acids; MUFA, mono-unsaturated fatty acids; PUFA, polyunsaturated fatty acids.
[c]Significant differences between the two diets ($P < 5\%$).

TABLE 7.4

Effects of n-3 Supplementation in the Diet on Fatty Composition of Spermatozoa in 34-Week-Old Adult Turkeys

Fatty acids[a] (%)	Diet[b]		Spermatozoa[b]		
	Corn oil	Fish oil	Corn oil diet		Fish oil diet
14:0					
16:0	11.2	14.0	15.90 ± 1.00		16.10 ± 0.80
16:1n-7			<0.5		<0.5
16:1n-9			<0.5		<0.5
18:0	3.4	2.8	20.00 ± 0.60		21.70 ± 0.80
18:1n-9/n-7	33.4	33.4	11.50 ± 0.70		10.80 + 0.70
18:2n-6	46.3	36.3	3.7 0 ± 0.30		3.10 ± 0.30
18:3n-3	5.4	4.4			
20:1n-9			9.90 ± 0.60		10.4 ± 0.50
20:4n-6			11.50 ± 0.60	*	8.20 ± 0.60
20:5n-3		3.5			
22:1n-9					
22:3n-9			9.10 ± 3.8		11.50 ± 2.00
22:4n-6			16.00 ± 0.8	*	9.50 ± 0.50
22:5n-3		1.0	0.65 ± 0.20	*	1.90 ± 0.30
22:6n-3		1.8	1.70 ± 0.20	*	6.50 ± 0.60
SFA	14.6	19.3	35.90 ± 1.00		37.80 ± 1.00
MUFA	33.4	33.4	21.40 ± 0.80	*	21.20 ± 0.80
PUFA	52.0	47.0	42.70 ± 2.10	*	41.00 ± 2,00
n-3/n-6	0.1	0.3	0.07 ± 0.02	*	0.40 ± 0.01

[a]SFA, saturated fatty acids; MUFA, mono-unsaturated fatty acids; PUFA, polyunsaturated fatty acids.
[b]Significant differences between the two diets ($P < 5\%$).

matozoa reflected better the ratio of these fatty acids in the diet. This could indicate that the need for n-3 supplementation is higher in the turkey than in the chicken.

The n-9 PUFA were not significantly affected by changes in n-3/n-6 PUFA in the diet in any species. This suggests that, even in turkey spermatozoa in which 22:3n-9 is a major PUFA, 22:3n-9 PUFA does not originate from the n-3 deficiency in the diet. It is more probable that a high percentage of n-9 PUFA in spermatozoa could be specific to birds.

However, in view of the changes in spermatozoon fatty acids with the increased dietary content of n-3 fatty acids, the existence of n-3 deficiency in the standard diet of domestic bird species must be examined independently of n-9 PUFA. This will be discussed later.

Is Spermatozoon Composition Still Sensitive to Dietary Fatty Acids in Animals at the End of the Reproductive Period?

Domestic birds are seasonal species. In standard breeding conditions, the reproductive efficiency of chicken and turkey males is optimal between 30 and 40 weeks of age and then decreases to cease transitorily around 50–65 weeks of age (27). Antioxidant defenses become less efficient during the decreasing phase of the reproductive period and lipid peroxidation increases (20,28). The percentage of n-6 PUFA decreases in aging chickens (29), and these changes seem not to be related only to lipid peroxidation but suggest a decrease in the ability of domestic bird germ cells to synthesize or incorporate PUFA in their cell membranes. It is also debatable whether dietary PUFA supplementation is effective to change the fatty acid composition of spermatozoa in "old" animals.

The results obtained in the chicken (30) indicated that 60-week-old males fed either n-3 (tuna orbita oil) or n-6 PUFA-enriched diets (arasco oil) increased the level of spermatozoon PUFA, especially when the diet was also massively supplemented with vitamin E.

The results obtained in turkeys (Table 7.5) were based on a comparison between the standard soy-corn diet and a fish oil diet (n-3 supplemented diet, Table 7.4) with the usual content of the antioxidant vitamin E in the diet (30 mg/kg). Supplementation started at 27 weeks of age. This supplementation was clearly effective during the optimal part of the reproductive period (34 weeks of age) and also in its decreasing part (50 weeks of age), and the n-3/n-6 ratio of spermatozoon fatty acids was as changed by the diet supplementation at 50 as at 34 weeks of age.

This indicates that in both turkeys and chickens the metabolic function of transfer of n-3 fatty acids into reproductive tissues is effective, even when the reproductive function is affected by aging.

However, according to earlier results published by our laboratory (28), the percentage of n-9 PUFA is affected by aging irrespective of the diet. Whether this decrease with aging has a biological significance has not yet been established.

TABLE 7.5

Effects of n-3 Dietary Supplementation on Polyunsaturated Fatty Acid Composition of Turkey Spermatozoa Throughout the Reproductive Period

Sperm fatty acids[a] (%)	27 weeks[a]		34 weeks[b]			50 weeks[b]		
	Corn diet	Fish diet	Corn diet		Fish diet	Corn diet		Fish diet
SFA	36.9	36.2	35.9		37.8	37.4		35.7
MUFA	22.0	19.7	21.4		21.2	21.4		22.5
18:2n-6	4.5	4.0	3.7		3.1	4.1		4.0
20:4n-6	11.4	11.4	11.50	*	8.2	12.50	*	8.7
22:4n-6	10.4	12.9	16.0	*	9.5	13.0	*	10.1
22:3n-9	12.4[a]	12.6[a]	9.1[b]		11.5[ab]	9.7[b]		10.8[b]
22:5n-3	0.6	0.7[b]	0.6	*	1.9[a]	0.7	*	2.8[a]
22:6n-3	1.3	1.5[c]	1.7	*	6.5[a]	0.5[d]	*	4.6[b]
PUFA	41.1	44.1	42.7		41.0	41.2		41.8
n-3/n-6	0.07[b]	0.07[b]	0.07[b]	*	0.40[a]	0.04[b]	*	0.32[a]

[a]SFA, saturated fatty acids; MUFA, mono-unsaturated fatty acids; PUFA, polyunsaturated fatty acids.
[b]Significant differences between the two diets ($P < 5\%$, t test). Roman superscript a, b, c, d represent significant differences on the same line (for one fatty acid or on fatty acids class) with age.

In conclusion, the PUFA composition of chicken and turkey spermatozoa reflects the dietary components when the animals are in the first half of their reproductive period and also at the end of this period when the efficacy of reproduction starts to decrease. However, turkey spermatozoa seem more susceptible to these changes than chicken spermatozoa. Whether these changes have significant effects on reproductive efficiency will be examined next.

Effects of Dietary PUFA on the Biological Function of Domestic Bird Spermatozoa

Spermatozoon fatty acids are major components of the membrane phospholipids and have long been believed to have major functions in gamete biology (31). With their high PUFA content, they are thought to be involved in the regulation of membrane fluidity; high membrane fluidity is generally necessary to ensure the movement of motile cells. Spermatozoa are flagellar cells, and motility is necessary for them to reach the fertilization site. Membrane fluidity may also have an active function in the membrane destabilization that precedes the fusion at the time of fertilization. By their capacity to modulate the liquid crystal state of lipids and the temperatures of phase transition, fatty acids and especially PUFA of the membrane phospholipids may also have a considerable impact on resistance to osmotic and cold shock during *in vitro* semen storage, including cryopreservation. The composition of spermatozoon fatty acid and its modifications by the diet may therefore have a real effect on semen biology.

Despite these important activities, dietary manipulation of fatty acids, and especially n-3 supplementation, have often failed to have a major impact on the functions of fresh sperm in species where spermatozoon fatty acids have naturally high n-3/n-6 ratios. For example, variations in n-3/n-6 ratio in the diet modified n-3/n-6 ratio in the spermatozoa of the rainbow trout but did not affect spermatozoon membrane fluidity or the fertility rates obtained with fresh semen (24,32). An increase in the n-3/n-6 ratio in the diet combined with vitamin E and selenium supplementation had a positive effect on semen quality in the boar (22). However, the effect of antioxidant supplementation could not be separated from the possible effect of n-3 supplementation.

In domestic birds in which n-3/n-6 ratios are very low, the situation seems quite different: supplementation of the adult chicken diet with n-3 PUFA increases the fertility rates obtained with fresh semen (Table 7.6) in 35–47-week-old adults (15,16).

The situation may be complicated in chickens at the end of their reproductive period by a greater need for antioxidant supplementation (20). This is also currently under investigation in turkeys in our laboratory. However, the initial results confirm the findings in chickens with enhancement of reproductive performance when the diet of aging males is supplemented with n-3 PUFA.

Taken together, these results indicate that standard diets of adult male chickens and turkeys may need enhancement with n-3 PUFA for the reproductive functions when semen is used "fresh."

TABLE 7.6

Effects of n-3 Supplementation in the Diet of Adult Male Chicken 42–47 Weeks of Age on the Fertility Rates[a]

Fertility rates: % n fertile/incubated eggs	Corn oil diet	Salmon oil diet
Fresh semen	91.6 %[b]	96.0 %[a]
(n incubated eggs)	(955)	(980)
Frozen-thawed semen	35.0 %[c]	9.6 %[d]
(n incubated eggs)	(931)	(845)

[a]Blesbois *et al.*, 1997b.

[b]Roman superscript a, b, c, d represent significant differences at the rate 0.05

The reproductive efficiency and requirements are very different when semen is used frozen: spermatozoa are damaged by freezing in all species studied. The changes observed include membrane modifications with increasing membrane permeability, deformations, and ruptures (33). Freezing-thawing is accompanied by a severe decrease in fluidity in mammals (34) and by a considerable reduction in the proportions of PUFA in the spermatozoon fatty acids in chickens (35).

Under these conditions, modification of spermatozoon PUFA by the diet, including n-3 supplementation, may alter membrane rigidification of gametes during freezing with consequences on semen quality after thawing. In addition an increase in the number of double bonds in the fatty acids may also increase the number of rupture points of molecules.

Thus, in the chicken, and contrary to results obtained with fresh semen, n-3 supplementation of the diet decreases the fertility rates obtained with frozen semen (Table 7.6). These results are consistent with those obtained on species where n-3 PUFA are usually major PUFA, such as the rainbow trout: in this species, n-3 rich diets enhanced the freezing damage of spermatozoa (32).

However the effects of composition of spermatozoon fatty acids on semen cryopreservation may not be limited to the equilibrium of n-3/n-6 PUFA. Rates of unsaturation of fatty acids, spermatozoon regionalization of the phospholipids components, and equilibrium between membrane cholesterol, phospholipids, and proteins are also very important and must be further investigated in domestic birds.

Conclusion

As in other vertebrate species, in domestic birds the proportions of spermatozoon PUFA may be affected by diet. These changes may affect fertility: n-3 supplementation in the diet increases the fertility obtained with fresh semen in birds but decreases the fertility obtained with frozen-thawed semen. This means that the diet of male breeders must be adapted to the use of their semen.

However, we have also reported that spermatozoa of male birds, especially chickens, have a certain resistance to changes in their fatty acids by diet. This could indicate specificity of the fatty acid composition of these gametes. For example, n-6 PUFA are still predominant even after n-3 supplementation, and chicken spermatozoa seem more resistant to n-3 changes than turkey spermatozoa.

The predominance of n-6 PUFA involves principally 22:4n-6 PUFA. This PUFA is still the main PUFA in domestic birds. By contrast, it is very minor in the spermatozoa of most nonbird species. In addition, n-9 PUFA 22:3n-9 is also present in all domestic bird species but is not present in most mammalian and fish species. 22:3n-9 is the second most abundant PUFA in turkeys.

The origin and function of the predominance of n-6 PUFA and high representation of n-9 PUFA in domestic birds have not yet been elucidated.

One hypothesis includes specific regulation of the enzymes necessary for PUFA production: elongase and delta 5 and delta 6 desaturase. Their roles in the domestic bird reproductive tract, with possible preferences of these enzymes for n-6 and n-9 fatty acids, have to be explored.

Another hypothesis could take into account the reproductive temperature specificity of birds, which are homoeothermic animals. The mean *in vivo* temperature of reproduction in birds is 41–43°C. This is higher than in other species. For example, in most mammals the mean body temperature is close to 37°C, and spermatogenesis needs a lower temperature than the body temperature to be active. In fish, which are not homoeothermic species, the body temperature and hence the temperature of the internal reproductive tract depends on the water temperature, which is generally lower or far lower than 37°C, even in the tropical rivers from which Tilapia originate.

It can be speculated that, with their "high" reproductive temperature, the cell membranes of bird spermatozoa have naturally higher membrane fluidity than mammal and fish spermatozoa. In these conditions of high natural fluidity, the need for high specificity in the degree of fatty acid unsaturation and n-3 fatty acid levels could be less important than in species where acquisition of fertilizing power of spermatozoa needs lower temperatures. Under these conditions, bird spermatozoa might prefer less peroxidative PUFA, such as n-6 and n-9 PUFA. However even if the need for n-3 PUFA is lower in birds than in other species, a small but significant quantity of these fatty acids appears necessary to ensure an optimal reproductive rate. This must be taken into account in the formulation of diets for adult male birds.

References

1. Cook, H.W. (1996) Fatty Acid Desaturation and Chain Elongation in Eucaryotes, in *Biochemistry of Lipids, Lipoproteins and Biomembranes,* Vance, D.E. and Vance, J., Elsevier, Amsterdam, pp. 129–152.
2. Sardesai, V.M. (1992) Biochemical and Nutritional Aspects of Eicosanoids, *J. Nutr. Biochem. 3,* 562–579.
3. Stubbs, C.D., and Smith, A.D. (1984) The Modification of Mammalian Polyunsaturated Fatty Acid Composition in Relation to Membrane Fluidity and Function, *Biochim. Biophys. Acta. 779,* 89–137.

4. Grogan, W.M., and Huth, E.G. (1983) Biosynthesis of Long-Chain Polyenoïc Acids from Arachidonic Acid in Culture of Enriched Spermatocytes and Spermatids from Mouse Testis, *Lipids, 18,* 275–284.

5. Grogan, W.M., and Lam, J.W. (1982) Fatty Acids Synthesis in Isolated Spermatocytes and Spermatids of Mouse Testis, *Lipids 17,* 604–611.

6. Poulos, A., Darin Benett, A., White, I.G., and Hoskin, D.O. (1973) The Phospholipid Bound Fatty Acids and Aldehydes of Mammalian Spermatozoa, *Comp. Biochem. Physiol. 46,* 541–549.

7. Neuringer, M., Connor, W., Lin, S., Barstad, L., and Luck, S.J. (1986) Biochemical and Functional Effects of Prenatal and Postnatal Omega-3 Fatty Acids Deficiency on Retina and Brain in Rhesus Monkey, *Proc. Nat. Acad. Sci. 83,* 4021–4025.

8. Yamamoto, N.M., Saitoh, A., Moriuchi, A., Nomura, M., and Okuyama, H. (1987) Effect of Dietary Alpha Linolenate/Linoleate Balance on Brain Lipid Composition and Learning Ability of Rats, *J. Lipid Res. 28,* 144–151.

9. Lin, D.S., Connor, W.E., Wolf, D.P., Neuringer, M., and Hachey, D.L. (1993) Unique Lipids of Primate Spermatozoa: Desmosterol and Docosahexaenoïc Acid, *J. Lipid Res. 34,* 491–499.

10. Anderson, G.J., Connor, W.E., Corliss, J.D., and Lin, D.S. (1989) Rapid Modulation of the n-3 Docosahexaenoic Acid Levels in the Brain and Retina of the Newly Hatched Chick, *J. Lipid Res, 30,* 433–441.

11. Anderson, G.J. (1994) Developmental Sensitivity of the Brain to Dietary n-3 PUFA, *J. Lipid Res. 35,* 105–111.

12. Rettersol, K., Haugen, E.B., and Christopherson, B.O. (2000) The Pathway from Arachidonic to Docosapentaenoic Acid (20:4n-6 to 22:5n-6) and from Eicosapentaenoic to Docosahexaenoic and from Eicosapentaenoïc to Docosahexaenoïc Acid (20:5n-3 to 22:6n-3) Studied Intesticular Cells from Immature Rats, *Bioch. Biophys. Acta 1483,* 119–131.

13. Darin-Benett, A., Poulos, A., and White, I.G. (1974) The Phospholipids and Phospholipid-Bound Fatty Acids and Aldehydes of Dog and Fowl Spermatozoa, *J. Reprod. Fert. 47,* 471–474.

14. Suraï, P.F., Blesbois, E., Garsseau, I., Chalah, T., Brillard, J.P., Wishart, G.J., Cerolini, S., and Sparks N.H.C. (1998) Fatty Acid Composition, Glutathione Peroxidase, Superoxide Dismutase, and Total Antioxidant Activity of Avian Semen, *Comp. Biochem. Physiol. 120,* 527–533.

15. Blesbois, E., Lessire, M., Grasseau, I., Hallouis, J.M., and Hermier, D. (1997a) Effect of Dietary Fat on the Fatty Acids Composition and Fertilizing Ability of Fowl Semen, *Biol. Reprod. 56,* 1216–1220.

16. Kelso, K.A., Cerolini, S., Noble, R.C., Speake, B.K. Cavalchini, L.G., and Noble, R.C.(1997) Effects of Dietary Supplementation with Alpha-Linolenic Acid on the Phospholipid Fatty Acids Composition and Quality of Spermatozoa in Cockerels from 24 to 72 Weeks of Age, *J. Reprod. Fert. 110,* 53–59 1997.

17. Reddy, R.P.K., and Sajadi, I. (1990) Selection for Growth and Semen Traits in the Poultry Industry: What Can We Expect in the Future?, in *Control of Fertility in Domestic Birds,* Ed INRA, Paris, pp. 47–59.

18. Barbato, G.F. (1999) Genetic Relationships Between Selection for Growth and Reproductive Effectiveness, *Poult. Sci. 78,* 444–450.

19. Parks, J.E., and Lynch, D.V. (1992) Lipid Composition and Thermotropic Phase Behavior of Boar, Bull, Stallion and Roosters Sperm Membranes, *Cryobiol. 29,* 255–266.

20. Kelso, K.A., Cerolini, S., Noble, R.C., Sparks, N.H.C., and Speake, B.K. (1996) Lipid and Antioxidant Changes in Semen of Broiler Fowl from 25 to 60 Weeks Old, *J. Reprod. Fert. 106*, 201–206.

21. Douard, V., Hermier, D., Blesbois, E. (2000) Changes in Turkey Semen Lipids During Liquid *in Vitro* Storage, *Biol. Reprod. 63*, 1450–1456.

22. Penny, P.C., Noble, R.C., Maldjian, A., and Cerolini, S. (2000) Potential Role of Lipids for the Enhancement of Boar Fertility, *Pigs News Inf. 21*, 119–126.

23. Rettersol, K., Haugen, T.B., Woldseth, B., and Christopherson, B.J. (1998) A Comparative Study of the Metabolism of n-9, n-6, and n-3 Fatty Acids in Testicular Cells from Immature Rats, *Biochem. Biophys. Acta 1392*, 59–72

24. Labbé, C., Loir, M., Kaushick, S., and Loir, M. (1995) Thermal Acclimation and Dietary Lipids Alters the Composition but not the Fluidity of Trout Sperm Plasma Membranes, *Lipids 30*, 23–33.

25. Bell, M.V., Dick, J.R., Thrush, M., and Navarro, J.C. (1996) Decreased 20:4n-6/20:5n-3 Ratio in Sperm from Cultured Sea Bass, *Dicentrarchus labrax*, Broodstock Compared with Wild Fish, *Aquaculture 144*, 189–199.

26. Conquer, J.A., Martin, J.B, Tummon, I., Watson, L., and Tekpetey, F. (1999) Fatty Acids Analysis of Blood Serum, Seminal Plasma and Spermatozoa of Normospermic *Versus* Asthenozoospermic Males, *Lipids 34*, 793–799.

27. Noiraud, J., and Brillard, J.P. (1999) Effects of Frequency of Semen Collection on Quantitative and Qualitative Characteristics of Semen in Turkey Breeder Males, *Poult. Sci. 78*, 1034–1039.

28. Douard, V., Hermier, D., Magistrini, M., and Blesbois, E. (2002) Reproductive Period Affects Lipid Composition and Quality of Fresh and Stored Spermatozoa in Turkey, *Theriogenol. 8677*, 1–12

29. Cerolini, S., Kelso, K.A., Noble, R.C., Speake, B.K., Pizzi, F., and Cavalchini, L.G. (1997) Relationship between Spermatozoan Lipid Composition and Fertility during Aging in Chicken, *Biol. Reprod. 57*, 976–980.

30. Suraï, P.F., Noble, R.C., Spark, N.H.C., and Speake, B.K. (2000) Effect of Long Term Supplementation with Arachidonic or Docosahexaenoic Acids on Sperm Production in the Broiler Chicken, *J. Reprod. Fert. 120*, 257–264.

31. Mann, T., and Lutwak-Mann, C. (1981) *Male Reproductive Function and Semen*, Springer-Verlag, Berlin, Heidelberg, New-York.

32. Pustowska, C., McNiven, M.A., Richardson, G.P., and Lall, S. (2000) Source of Dietary Lipid Affects Sperm Plasma Membrane Integrity and Fertility in Rainbow Trout *Oncorhynchus mykiss* (Waldbaum) after Cryopreservation, *Aquaculture 31*, 297–305.

33. Watson, P.F. (1995) Recent Developments and Concepts in the Crypreservation of Spermatozoa in the Assessment of their Post-Thawing Function, *Reprod. Fert. Develop. 7*, 871–891.

34. Giraud, M.N., Motta, C., Boucher, D., and Grizard, G. (2000) Membrane Fluidity Predicts the Outcome of Cryopreservation of Human Spermatozoa, *Human Reprod. 15*, 2160–2164.

35. Blesbois, E., Lessire, M., and Hermier, D. (1997b) Effects of Cryopreservation and Diets on Lipids of Fowl Sperm and Fertility, *Poultry and Avian Biology Review 8*, 149–154.

Chapter 8

Lipid Composition of Chicken Semen and Fertility

Silvia Cerolini

Dipartimento di Scienze e Tecnologie Veterinarie per la Sicurezza Alimentare, Facoltà di Medicina Veterinaria, University of Milan, via Trentacoste 2, 20134 Milan, Italy

Abstract

Lipids are a basic component of semen; they contribute to the structure of spermatozoan membrane and are involved in sperm metabolism and functions. Lipid components are present in both spermatozoa and seminal plasma, probably playing different specific roles. The total amount of lipid in chicken semen ranges from 0.43 to 0.90 mg/109 spermatozoa and from 0.14 to 1.49 mg/mL seminal plasma. Phospholipid is by far the most important lipid class; it accounts for 60 to 70% of total lipids in chicken and turkey spermatozoa and for 34% in chicken seminal plasma. In chicken spermatozoa, phosphatidylcholine and phosphatidylethanolamine are generally the most important phospholipid classes and a range of minor classes have also been identified (*i.e.*, phosphatidylserine, sphingomyelin). Avian spermatozoa are characterized by high levels of long-chain n-6 polyunsaturated fatty acids, mainly arachidonic and docosatetraenoic acid. Changes in fatty acid composition of sperm total phospholipid are observed according to the avian species and the strains within species. In the chicken, sperm phospholipids and polyunsaturates are related to gamete functions and fertility. The total amount of total phospholipid is positively correlated with fertility values recorded for 14 days after artificial insemination. Also, the proportion of a few phospholipid classes is correlated with fertility. Docosatetraenoic acid might be considered the most important functional fatty acid of sperm phospholipid because it is positively correlated with the proportion of motile spermatozoa, the linearity of sperm movement, and fertility. Also the proportion of arachidonic acid is positively correlated with fertility. According to their relevance to sperm fertility, dramatic changes in the lipid composition of spermatozoa are described during aging.

Introduction

Lipids are a basic component of semen. In particular, they contribute to the structure of spermatozoan membrane and are involved in vital aspects of sperm metabolism and function. Lipid components are present in both the spermatozoa and seminal plasma, probably playing different specific roles. Originally, the interest in sperm lipid began because lipids were supposed to be an energy substrate for spermatozoan metabolism. At the present time, it is clear that lipids are involved not only in sperm energy metabolism (1–4) but also in all the main functions and events that lead to fertilization.

In mammalian spermatozoa that have been widely studied, the biochemical and functional role of lipids in fertilization has been proved. Lipid components are involved in the capacitation event (5,6) and the acrosome reaction (7); lipid domains characterize the fusigenic part of the sperm plasma membrane (8,9); and the major polyunsaturate of sperm phospholipid, 22:6n-3, has been directly associated with sperm motility in the man (10,11) and with sperm concentration and motility in the boar (12). In general, sperm polyunsaturated fatty acids are suggested as markers of fertility disorders in men (13).

In birds, the lipid and fatty acid compositions of male gametes have been reported for different species and strains. The relationship between lipids and fertility has been shown in chicken spermatozoa, and a specific effect of polyunsaturated fatty acids on sperm activities has been also found.

Lipid Composition in Chicken Spermatozoa

The total amount of lipid in chicken semen has been reported to range from 0.43 to 0.90 mg/10^9 spermatozoa (14–16) and from 0.14 to 1.49 mg/mL of seminal plasma (14,15).

In spermatozoa, phospholipid is by far the most important lipid class and accounts for 60 to 70% of total lipids in the chicken and the turkey (15,17). Free cholesterol is usually the second major lipid class in spermatozoa of broiler and turkey breeders and accounts for 20–22% of total lipids. In contrast, free fatty acids represent a higher proportion (14% of total lipid) compared to free cholesterol, reduced to 10%, in spermatozoa of egg-type chicken breeders. Other minor lipid classes (free fatty acids, triacylglycerols, and cholesteryl ester) have been also identified in all fowl strains (15).

Phosphatidylcholine (PC) and phosphatidylethanolamine (PE) are generally the most important phospholipid classes in chicken spermatozoa and account for more than 60% of total phospholipid. They are routinely accompanied by a wide range of minor moieties, *e.g.,* phosphatidylserine (PS) and sphingomyelin (15,17,18), which nevertheless may also play a significant role in aspects of spermatozoa metabolism and function. The proportion of PS is particularly high and represents the second major phospholipid class after PC in spermatozoa of ROSS broiler breeders compared to other avian strains (15).

Avian spermatozoa are characterized by a predominant presence of the long chain n-6 polyunsaturated fatty acids, mainly arachidonic acid (20:4n-6, AA) and docosatetraenoic acid (22:4n-6, DTA) (18). The ratio of polyunsaturated to saturated fatty acids in chicken and turkey spermatozoa is 0.9 and 1.1, respectively (19). The proportions of long-chain polyunsaturated fatty acids (LCPUFA) show some variations according to the avian species and the strains within species (Table 8.1). Spermatozoa from egg-type chicken breeders display the highest level of 22:4n-6

TABLE 8.1

Fatty acid composition (%) of total phospholipids in spermatozoa at different avian species and strains.

Fatty acid (% of total)	Egg-type chicken breeder[a]		Broiler breeder[a]		Turkey[a,b]	Guinea fowl[b]	Duck[b]	Goose[b]
	ISA	RIR	COBB	ROSS	NICHOLAS[a,b]			
saturates								
16:0	8.3	16.9	13.2	12.8	11.2–12.4	15.4	21.5	17
18:0	20.6	17.4	21.5	21.6	21–17.7	15.8	<0.5	15.4
20:0	3.9	nd	nd	<1	1.0–1.2	3.8	1.1	1.7
monounsaturates								
18:1n-9	13.7	15.6	13.0	12.6	4.9–7.7	9.1	5.9	13.7
18:1n-7	nd	2.2	1.70	1.4	2.3–2.5	2.1	2.1	2.1
20:1n-9	<1	3.6	3.37	3.7	10.6–9.2	1.2	<0.5	1.1
22:1n-9	<1	nd	<1	<1	1.5–1.2	0.7	<0.5	<0.5
n-6 polyunsaturates								
18:2	2.7	2.1	3.55	2.6	1.4–4.6	3.8	3.8	5.7
20:2	<1	<1	1.11	<1	2.1–4.0	3.3	1.6	3.9
20:3	1.5	1.31	2.0	1.8	<1–<1	<0.5	1	0.5
20:4	12.5	10.7	12.6	12.3	12.6–9.4	15.8	18.9	13.3
22:4	30.5	16.6	22.3	22.1	15.1–12.6	19.4	19.9	17.5
n-9 polyunsaturates								
22:3	<1	nd	<1	nd	7.1–9.2	4.3	0.6	1.4
n-3 polyunsaturates								
22:5	<1	<1	<1	<1	1.1–<1	<0.5	0.6	<0.5
22:6	1.3	2.5	2.8	4.6	3.0–2.7	1.7	8	2.8

[a]From reference 15.
[b]From reference 20; nd = not detected.

(31%) and turkey spermatozoa the lowest (13%), whereas guinea fowl, duck, and goose sperm display intermediate levels, from 18 to 20%. The proportion of 20:4n-6 also varies according to the species, *e.g.*, 10 and 19%, respectively, in the turkey and duck (15,20) (Table 8.1). In comparison, mammalian spermatozoa contain much higher levels of n-3 LCPUFA, in particular docosahexaenoic acid (22:6n-3, DHA), and therefore in general terms are far more unsaturated compared to avian species (21,22).

Ninety percent (by weight) of the lipids extracted from the whole sperm are obtained from cell membranes including plasma, acrosomal, nuclear, and mitochondrial membrane; differences may occur between the four membrane types (23). The plasma membrane contains less than 35% of the total cellular lipid (24), therefore its lipid composition may greatly differ from that of the whole spermatozoon. Plasma membrane of chicken spermatozoa display a higher free cholesterol/phospholipid ratio (0.47 *vs.* 0.34) compared to the whole spermatozoon. The fatty acid composition of chicken plasma membrane phospholipid is also more saturated compared to the composition of spermatozoan phospholipid. The proportion of total polyunsaturates is reduced from 44 to 33% of total fatty acids, and in particular both 22:4n-6 and 20:4n-6 are significantly reduced (25). In mammals, different results have been found according to the species; the free cholesterol/phospholipid ratio in spermatozoan plasma membrane compared to the whole cell is increased in the ram (26) and reduced in the rabbit (27) and the boar (28), and discordant results have been reported in the bull (27,29). Differences in fatty acid composition between plasma membrane and cellular total phospholipid have been shown in boar spermatozoa (28).

In chicken spermatozoa, the proportions of LCPUFA bound to phospholipid classes have been reported for PE and PC (14,30,31) and variations have been found again among chicken strains (15). PE is the most unsaturated phospholipid moiety and shows the largest differences between strains. For example, whereas 20:4n-6 and 22:4n-6 account for some 55% of PE-bound fatty acids in spermatozoa from highly selected egg-type strains, such as ISA and ROSS, the level of the same fatty acids is only 30% in spermatozoa from less selected strains such as RIR. The difference in polyunsaturated fatty acid content is compensated by differing levels of the monounsaturated fatty acid, oleic (18:1n-9) (15). The major proportions of total fatty acids in chicken sperm PC are represented by the saturated fatty acids 16:0 and 18:0, and the monounsaturate 18:1n-9 (14,15,30).

In chicken seminal plasma, phospholipid is still the major class (46–47%) of total lipid, even if its level is much lower than that found in spermatozoa. The proportion of the other lipid classes changes according to the strain considered, and free cholesterol (32%) or free fatty acids (34%) account for the second major class in broiler and egg-type chicken breeders, respectively (15).

Stearic acid, 18:0, is the major fatty acid (23–36% of total fatty acids) in total phospholipid of chicken seminal plasma; however, relatively high proportions of n-6 LCPUFA, 20:4, and 22:4 (8–15% and 11–14% of total fatty acids respectively) are also present (15).

Lipid Composition, Semen Characteristics, and Fertility in the Chicken

Deep investigations have been able to demonstrate a clear relationship between the level of phospholipid and polyunsaturated fatty acids in chicken spermatozoa and their functions and fertility.

The development of spermatogenesis is undoubtedly accompanied by an increase of 22:4n-6 within the testis, which reaches a maximum at 15 weeks of age (32).

Fertility rate is negatively affected after an induced alteration of the phospholipid moieties present in spermatozoan plasma membrane (33).

The characteristic LCPUFA of chicken spermatozoa, 22:4n-6, has been suggested being both quantitatively and functionally the most important of the fatty acids. Its proportion is positively directly associated to the proportion of motile spermatozoa (Fig. 8.1) and to the linear progressive movement (Fig. 8.2) of the male gamete (12). The result might suggest a specific function of DTA on fluidity of sperm membrane in the chicken.

The fatty acid composition of PE in spermatozoa of broiler breeder males displays distinctive differences according to the reproductive performance of the males. The proportion of PE-bound 20:4n-6 and 22:4n-6 increases in spermatozoa of high-fertility males from 24 to 54 weeks of age, and as a consequence the polyunsaturate/saturate ratio also increases (3.98 *vs.* 2.49). By contrast, the opposite trend is found in spermatozoa from low-fertility males and the same ratio greatly decreases (0.69 *vs.* 2.89) (34).

Semen characteristics greatly change in chicken breeders from 25 to 60 weeks of age. Traditional semen parameters, such as concentration and viability, are significantly reduced; furthermore, metabolic and enzymatic antioxidant activities, and the content of other important players in anti-oxidant protection, *e.g.,* vitamin E and A and selenium, display a large decrease (14,35). Such changes are associated with dra-

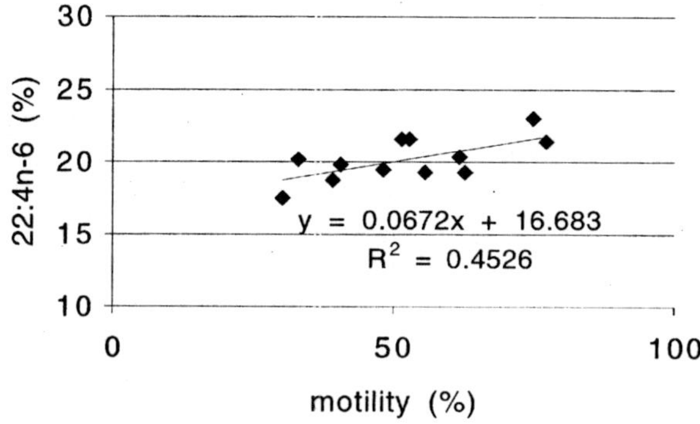

Fig. 8.1. Linear regression between sperm motility (%) and 22:4n-6 proportion of sperm phospholipid in the chicken (from reference 12).

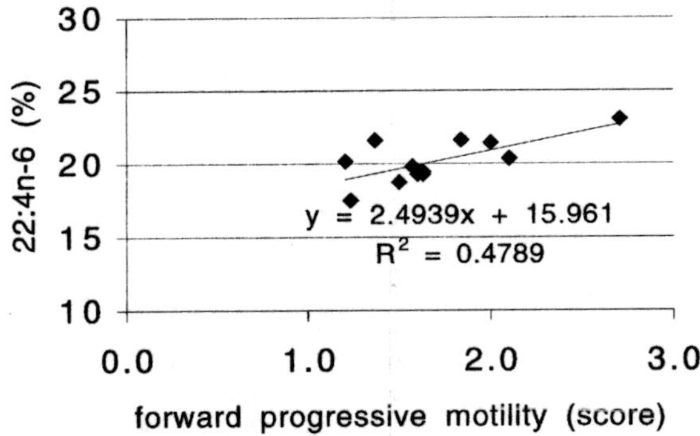

Fig. 8.2. Linear regression between forward progressive motility (score) and 22:4n-6 proportion of sperm phospholipid in the chicken (from reference 12).

matic and extensive changes in the lipid components of semen. Thus the total lipid content of both spermatozoa and seminal plasma is more than doubled in old breeders, whereas the proportions of PE and PS are reduced and the greatest changes occur in spermatozoa (PE from 30 to 17%, PS from 24 to 6%) compared to seminal plasma. Great changes occur also in the polyunsaturated fatty acid composition of the sperm PE fraction, 20:4n-6 and 22:4n-6 proportions are decreased by 52 and 30%, respectively (14).

During the whole reproductive period of broiler breeders from 24 to 72 weeks of age, fertility follows a characteristic trend and a clear aging effect occurs. The best fertility value is recorded on 39 weeks of age and then it progressively decreases. The aging effect is more evident on the fertility values recorded the second week compared to the first week after artificial insemination (AI). Some lipid components of spermatozoa display the same pattern of fertility during aging and significant positive correlations have been shown (Table 8.2) (36). The amount of total phospholipid is positively correlated to the proportion of motile sperm and to the fertility values recorded the second week after AI. The proportions of PC and PS are correlated to fertility values recorded on both weeks after AI with the opposite trend, the correlation is negative for PC and positive for PS. Phospholipid-bound 20:4n-6 and 22:4n-6 are positively correlated to the fertility values recorded the second week after AI.

Phospholipid-bound 22:4n-6 and 22:6n-3 are also positively correlated with the proportion of motile spermatozoa (Table 8.2) (36). DHA is present at a very low level in chicken spermatozoa (Table 8.1); however, such a low content is already able to play a positive effect on sperm motility, as clearly shown in the mammalian species (10,11,12).

Conclusion

The lipid, phospholipid, and fatty acid compositions of chicken semen have been studied in different strains. The specie-specific characteristic of chicken spermatozoa is

TABLE 8.2

Correlation Coefficients Between Age, Sperm Motility, Fertility, Lipid and Phospholipid Classes, and Polyunsaturated Fatty Acids in Spermatozoa of Chicken Broiler Breeders[a]

Lipids	Age	Sperm motility	Fertility week 1 after AI	Fertility week 2 after AI
Total lipids	0.563***	0.118	−0.102	−0.254
Lipid classes				
phospholipid	−0.639***	0.39***	0.139	0.409***
free cholesterol	0.175	−0.279*	0.034	−0.064
free fatty acids	0.616***	−0.237	−0.078	−0.187
triacylglycerols	0.017	−0.149	−0.161	−0.163
cholesteryl ester	0.433***	−0.126	−0.082	−0.330**
Phospholipid classes				
phosphatidylcholine	0.478***	−0.174	−0.351**	−0.287*
phosphatidylethanolamine	−0.284*	−0.077	0.167	0.036
phosphatidylserine	−0.428***	0.189	0.316*	0.399***
sphingomyelin	0.135	0.206	−0.056	−0.012
cardiolipin	0.085	−0.215	−0.040	−0.318***
Polyunsaturates in phospholipid				
20:4n-6	−0.386*	0.243	−0.058	0.254*
22:4n-6	−0.552***	0.333*	0.089	0.303*
22:6n-3	−0.599***	0.276*	0.006	0.239

[a]AI, artificial insemination; *, $P < 0.05$; **, $P < 0.01$; ***, $P < 0.001$. (Modified from reference 36.)

the unique high content of n-6 long-chain polyunsaturated fatty acids in the phospholipid moieties. The different chicken strains are characterized by different lipid and fatty acid compositions of semen. Considering that chicken commercial diets supply standard lipid components, such differences should be considered to be associated with biochemical features linked to physiological characteristics unique to the strains. According to the standards of performance for commercial breeder birds, egg-type strains are considered superior to broiler breeder strains. The classification of the strains according to their DTA content in sperm phospholipid, and in the PE fraction in particular, reflects the established standard breeding performance of the strains. Therefore, sperm DTA might be suggested as a marker of the reproductive efficiency of the male birds.

Lipid components have been clearly associated with sperm metabolic and functional activities and finally to fertility. Such associations occur in breeders of the same age but with different reproductive performance and during aging of the birds when the reproductive performance undergoes a physiological reduction.

Phospholipid, and in particular PS, and C20-22 carbon n-6 polyunsaturates in spermatozoa are the most important lipid components in relation to sperm functions and fertility. As already shown in mammalian spermatozoa, they might play functional and biochemical roles related to the biophysical properties of the sperm membrane, such as fluidity and permeability (37,38), or even related to more specific reactions involved in the fertilization process (8,39). PS in brain and retina is highly enriched in

C20-22 polyunsaturates (40,41) and it has been suggested to play a major role in regulating membrane fluidity, ionic interactions, and membrane excitation (39). Furthermore, it has been proposed that the interaction of Ca^{2+} with PS in membranes can trigger phase transitions that begin membrane fusion events similar to that of acrosome reactions (42).

The reduction of phospholipid moieties and their content in C20-22 carbon polyunsaturates associated with low fertility performance might be related to the reduction in the capacity of testicular enzymes to synthesize C20-22 polyunsaturates from their C18 precursor or to a failure to incorporate the polyunsaturates into the phospholipid fraction during spermatogenesis.

It is of interest that total phospholipid and the relative AA and DTA content are correlated with fertility levels on the second, not the first, week after AI. The result might suggest that phospholipid and its peculiar LCPUFA may affect the storability of spermatozoa after mating within the female during the fertile period. They might play a role in maintaining the positive environment or contribute to the required cell metabolism for the long survival of spermatozoa within the sperm storage tubules in the utero-vaginal junction of the female reproductive tract prior to proceeding up the oviduct and reaching the infundibulum, where fertilization takes place.

Further investigations are required to improve the knowledge on the roles played by lipids in the physiology of avian spermatozoa in order to be able to study new strategies to improve the reproductive performance of domestic birds and prevent the negative effect of aging.

Acknowledgments

The author wishes to thank Prof. Ray C. Noble for his important scientific assistance and supervision.

References

1. Scott, T.W. (1973) Lipid Metabolism of Spermatozoa, *J. Reprod. Fert. suppl. 18*, 65–76.
2. Scott, T.W., and Dawson, R.M.C. (1968) Metabolism of Phospholipids by Spermatozoa and Seminal Plasma, *J. Biochem. 108*, 457–463.
3. Howarth, B. (1980) The Role of Lipids in Avian Sperm Survival, *Proc. 9th Int. Cong. An. Reprod.*, Madrid, Spain, vol. 2, 505–509.
4. Resseguie, W.D., and Hughes, B.L. (1984) Phospholipid and Cholesterol Profiles from Chicken Seminal Components during *in Vivo* Storage at 5C, *Poul. Sci. 63*, 1438–1443.
5. Davis, B.K. (1981) Timing of Fertilization in Mammals: Sperm Cholesterol/Phospholipid Ratio as a Determinant of the Capacitation Interval, *Proc. Nat. Acad. Sci., 75(12)*, 7560–7564.
6. Tesarik, J., and Flechon, J.E. (1986) Distribution of Sterols and Anionic Lipids in Human Sperm Plasma Membrane: Effects of *in Vitro* Capacitation, *J. Ultrast. Mol. Struc. Res. 97*: 227–237.
7. Roldan, E.R.S., and Murase, T. (1994) Polyphosphoinositide-Derived Diacylglycerol Stimulates the Hydrolysis of Phosphatidylcholine by Phospholipase C during Exocytosis of the Ram Sperm Acrosome, *J. Biol. Chem. 269(38)*, 23583–23589.

8. Bearer, E.L., and Friend, D.S. (1982) Modifications of Anionic-Lipid Domains Preceding Membrane Fusion in Guinea Pig Sperm, *J. Cell Biol. 92*, 604–615.

9. Ladha, S. (1998) Lipid Heterogeneity and Membrane Fluidity in a Highly Polarized Cell, the Mammalian Spermatozoon, *J. Memb. Biol. 165*, 1–10.

10. Nissen, H.P., Kreysel, H.W., and Schirren, C. (1981) The Significance of Fatty Acids in Human Sperm and Impared Fertility, *Andrologia 13*, 444–451.

11. Nissen, H.P., Kreysel, H.W., and Schirren, C. (1983) PUFA's in Relation to Sperm Motility, *Andrologia 15*, 264–269.

12. Cerolini, S., Gliozzi, T.M., Pizzi, F., Parodi, L., Maldjian, A., and Noble, R. (2002) Relationship Between Lipid Components and Cell Functions in Spermatozoa of Domestic Animals, *Prog. Nutr. 4(2)*, 1–4.

13. Lenzi, A., Picardo, M., Gandini, L., and Dondero, F. (1996) Lipids of the Sperm Plasma Membrane: From Polyunsaturated Fatty Acids Considered as Markers of Sperm Function to Possibile Scavenger Therapy, *Hum. Reprod. Up. 2(3)*, 246–256.

14. Kelso, K.A., Cerolini, S., Noble, R.C., Sparks, N.H.C., and Speake, B.K. (1996) Lipid and Antioxidant Changes in Semen of Broiler Fowl from 25 to 60 Weeks of Age, *J. Reprod. Fert. 106*, 201–206.

15. Cerolini, S., Surai, P., Maldjian, A., Gliozzi, T., and Noble, R. (1997) Lipid Composition of Semen in Different Fowl Breeders, *Poul. Av. Biol. Rev. 8(3/4)*, 141–148.

16. Howarth, B. (1981) The Phospholipid Profile of Cock Spermatozoa before and after *in Vitro* Incubation for 24 Hours at 41C, *Poul. Sci. 60*, 1516–1519.

17. Howarth, B., Torregrossa, D., and Britton, W.M. (1977) The Phospholipid Content of Ejaculated Fowl and Turkey Spermatozoa, *Poul. Sci. 56*, 1265–1268.

18. Darin-Bennet, A., Poulos, A., and White, I.G. (1974) The Phospholipids and Phospholipid-Bound Fatty Acids and Aldehydes of Dog and Fowl Spermatozoa, *J. Reprod. Fert. 41*, 471–474.

19. Ravie, O., and Lake, P.E. (1985) The Phospholipid-Bound Fatty Acids of Fowl and Turkey Spermatozoa, *An. Reprod. Sci. 9*, 189–192.

20. Surai, P.F., Blesbois, E., Grasseau, I., Chalah, T., Brillare, J.P., Wishart, G.J., Cerolini, S., and Sparks, N.H.C. (1998) Fatty Acid Composition, Glutathione Peroxidase and Superoxide Dismutase Activity and Total Antioxidant Activity of Avian Semen, *Comp. Biochem. Physiol. 120B*, 527–533.

21. Poulos, A., Darin-Bennet, A., and White, I.G. (1973) The Phospholipid-Bound Fatty Acids and Aldehydes of Mammalian Spermatozoa, *Comp. Biochem. Physiol. 46B*, 541–549.

22. Neill, A.R., and Masters, C.J. (1972) Metabolism of Fatty Acids by Bovine Spermatozoa, *Biochem. J. 127*, 375–385.

23. Clegg, E.D. (1983) Mechanisms of Mammalian Sperm Capacitation, in *Mechanism and Control of Animal Fertilization*, Hartman, J.F., Academic Press, New York, pp. 184–212.

24. Lunstra, D.D., Clegg, E.D., and Moore, D.J. (1974) Isolation of Plasma Membrane from Porcine Spermatozoa, *Prep. Biochem. 4*, 341–352.

25. Cerolini, S., Surai, P., Gliozzi, T., and Noble, R. (1998) Fatty Acid Composition of the Sperm Plasma Membrane in Broiler Breeders Fed a n-3 Polyunsaturated Fatty Acid Supplemented Diet, *Proc. Serono Symp. Gametes: Development and Function*, Milano, Italy, pp. 518.

26. Holt, W.V., and North, R.D. (1985) Determination of Lipid Composition and Thermal Phase Transition Temperature in an Enriched Plasma Membrane Fraction from Ram Spermatozoa, *J. Reprod. Fert. 73*, 285–294.

27. Hinkovska-Galcheva, V., and Srivastava, P.N. (1993) Phospholipid of Rabbit and Bull Sperm Membranes: Structural Order Parameters and Steady-State Fluorescence Anisotropy of Membranes and Membranes Leafleats, *Molec. Reprod. Develop. 35*, 209–217.

28. Nikolopoulou, M.N., Soucek, D.A., and Vary, J.C. (1985) Changes in the Lipid Content of Bosr Sperm Plasma Membranes during Epididymal Maturation, *Bioch. Bioph. Acta 815*, 486–498.

29. Parks, J.E., Arion, J.W., and Foote, R.H. (1987) Lipids of Plasma Membrane and Outer Acrosomal Membrane from Bovine Spermatozoa, *Biol. Reprod. 37*, 1249–1258.

30. Kelso, K.A., Cerolini, S., Noble, R.C., Sparks, N.H.C., and Speake, B.K. (1997) The Effect of Dietary Supplementation with Docosahexaenoic Acid on the Phospholipid Fatty Acid Composition of Avian Spermatozoa, *Comp. Biochem. Physiol. 118B*, 65–69.

31. Cerolini, S., Kelso, A.K., Noble, R.C., Sparks, N.H.C., and Speake, B.K. (1997) Phospholipid Fatty Acid Composition of Semen in Broiler Breeders Fed a Fish Oil Supplemented Diet, *Brit. Poul. Sci. 38 suppl.*, S48–S49.

32. Nugara, D., and Edwards, H.M. Jr. (1970) Changes in Fatty Acid Composition of Cockerel Testes Due to Age and Fat Deficiency, *J. Nutr. 100*, 156–160.

33. Froman, D.P., and Thurston, R.J. (1984) Decreased Fertility Resulting from Treatment of Fowl Spermatozoa with Neuraminidase or Phospholipase C, *Poul. Sci. 63*, 2479–2482.

34. Cerolini, S., Kelso, K., Pizzi, F., Noble, R., Speake, B., Cavalchino, L.G., and Sparks, N.H. (1996) Fatty Acid Composition of Sperm Phospholipids in High and Low-Fertility Broiler Breeder Males, *Proc. 13th Int. Cong. An. Reprod.* Vol. 2, pp. 12–14.

35. Speake, B.K., Kelso, K., Cerolini, S., Noble, R.C., and Sparks, N.H.C. (1995) Changes in the Polyunsaturated Fatty Acid Composition and Antioxidant Capacity of Spermatozoa During Ageing in the Avian: A Relationship with Reduced Fertility, *Proc. 2nd Int. Cong. ISSFAL*, Maryland, USA, abstract n. 64.

36. Cerolini, S., Kelso, K.A., Noble, R.C., Speake, B.K., Pizzi, F., and Cavalchini, L.G. (1997) Relationship Between Spermatozoan Lipid Composition and Fertility During Aging of Chickens, *Biol. Reprod. 57*, 976–980.

37. Hammerstedt, R.H., (1993) Maintenance of Bioenergetic Balance in Sperm and Prevention of Lipid Peroxidation: A Review of the Effect on Design of Storage Preservation Systems, *Reprod. Fert. Develop. 5*, 675–690.

38. Stubbs, C.D., and Smith, A.D. (1984) The Modification of Mammalian Membrane Polyunsaturated Fatty Acid Composition in Relation to Membrane Fluidity and Function, *Bioch. Bioph. Acta 779*, 89–137.

39. Roldan, E.R.S., and Harrison, R.A.P. (1993) Diacylglycerol in the Exocytosis of the Mammalian Sperm Acrosome, *Biochem. Soc. Trans. 21*, 284–289.

40. Salem, N., Kim, H.Y., and Yergey, J.A. (1986) Docosahexaenoic Acid: Membrane Function and Metabolism, in *Health Effect of Polyunsaturated Fatty Acids in Seafoods*, Simopoulos, A.P., Kifer, R.R., and Martin, R.E., Academic Press, New York, pp. 263–317.

41. Maldjian, A., Cristofori, C., Noble, R.C., and Speake, B.K. (1996) The Fatty Acid Composition of Brain Phospholipids from Chicken and Duck Embryos, *Comp. Biochem. Physiol. 115B*, 153–158.

42. Cullis, P.R., and Hope, M.J. (1991) Physical Properties and Functional Roles of Lipids in Membranes, in *Biochemistry of Lipids, Lipoproteins, and Membranes*, Vance, D.E., and Vance, J., Elsevier, Amsterdam, pp. 1–41.

Chapter 9

Regulation of Avian and Mammalian Sperm Production by Dietary Fatty Acids

Brian K. Speake[a], Peter F. Surai[a], and John A. Rooke[b]

[a]Avian Science Research Centre, Scottish Agricultural College, Auchincruive, Ayr KA6 5HW, United Kingdom
[b]Applied Physiology Department, Scottish Agricultural College, Craibstone Estate, Aberdeen, AB21 9YA, United Kingdom

Abstract

Lipids of spermatozoa from many mammalian species are very enriched with docosahexaenoic acid (DHA), the most highly unsaturated fatty acid found in animal cells. Current evidence suggests that this n-3 polyunsaturate may endow the plasma membrane of the sperm tail with a high degree of flexibility and compressibility, enabling the lipid bilayer to withstand the stresses of flagellar movement. Avian sperm, by contrast, generally contain much lower levels of DHA and are instead enriched with the n-6 docosatetraenoic acid (DTA). Age-related changes in spermatogenesis and sperm quality in mammals and birds are associated with changes in the fatty acid composition of sperm phospholipid. Aging in the bull is accompanied by decreasing levels of DHA in the phospholipids of sperm, and aging in the boar is accompanied by increases in the 22:5n-6/DHA ratio. Inclusion of fish oil in the diet of boars increased the proportion of DHA in sperm at the expense of 22:5n-6, abolished the relationship between the 22:5n-6/DHA ratio and boar age, stimulated spermatogenesis, and improved sperm quality. In the chicken, the later stages of the reproductive cycle are characterized by reductions in testis weight, spermatogenesis, and the level of DTA in sperm phospholipid. All these reductions were effectively counteracted by dietary supplementation of the birds with arachidonic acid, the biosynthetic precursor of DTA. Surprisingly, dietary fish oil, rich in DHA, also prevented the fall in testis weight and spermatogenesis in these birds, even though this supplementation caused a reduction in sperm DTA content. The mechanisms of these beneficial effects of dietary polyunsaturates are not known but could include effects on sperm assembly, anti-apoptosis, eicosanoid synthesis, and hormone secretion.

Introduction

Importance of Lipids for the Structure and Function of Spermatozoa

The stimulus for the research described in this chapter, and indeed the premise for much of this book, originates from the discovery that sperm lipids contain extremely high proportions of long-chain polyunsaturated fatty acids (1–4), thus establishing a link between lipid biochemistry and male fertility. Moreover, the fact that polyunsaturated fatty acids must, in some form, be supplied in the diet suggests a relationship between fertility and nutrition and raises the possibility of improving male fertility by dietary means. In this chapter, we discuss possible reasons why sperm lipids are so unsaturated, describe how dietary supplementation with appropriate polyunsaturated fatty acids can improve the output and quality of sperm, and suggest potential mechanisms for these effects.

The unique structure of spermatozoa reveals why lipids are quantitatively such important structural components. The relatively large surface area resulting from the elongated shape, the presence of the acrosome, the abundance of mitochondria, and the minimal amount of cytoplasm all contribute to the predominance of membranous structures in these cells. Thus, phospholipid is the major lipid class, forming approximately 70% (w/w) of the total lipids of spermatozoa of the chicken (5), bull (6), and boar (7); the other main membrane lipid, free cholesterol, forms most of the remainder. The nonpolar lipids, triacylglycerol and cholesteryl ester, are relatively minor constituents of spermatozoa.

Mature spermatozoa are highly specialized cells consisting of three distinct regions, the head, midpiece, and tail, each performing defined roles during the events leading to fertilization. Accordingly, the functions of membrane lipids in sperm differ between these regions. For instance, the lipids of the sperm head are intimately involved in the mechanism by which the outer membrane of the sperm fuses with the plasma membrane of the egg. To achieve fertilization, the membranes of the sperm head must first enact a series of dramatic modifications. These occur during the successive stages of capacitation, the acrosome reaction, and membrane fusion, all of which are characterized by profound rearrangements of the sperm head lipids (8,9). Moreover, capacitation and acrosomal exocytosis are triggered by complex signal transduction cascades mediated by lipid-derived messengers such as inositol trisphosphate, diacylglycerol, lysophospholipids, and free fatty acids. Generation of these molecular signals within the cell is achieved by the action of phospholipases C and A_2 on membrane lipids of the head region and follows the stimulation of the spermatozoon by zona pellucida proteins and other agents present in the female tract (8,9).

In contrast to the dynamic behavior of the lipids of the head region, those of the midpiece and tail may appear at first sight to have a more passive, structural role. However, it should be noted that the structural properties of the lipids in these regions are likely to be extremely important for sperm function, especially in the tail, where the plasma membrane has to adapt to the physical stresses of the rapid whiplash movements. In fact, it seems that the lipids of the tail are highly specialized for this purpose.

Docosahexaenoic Acid and Mammalian Sperm Function

For many mammalian species, the most striking feature of the fatty acid composition of sperm phospholipid is the very high proportion of docosahexaenoic acid (DHA;

22:6n-3). For example, DHA forms approximately 61, 61, 38, 24, and 35% (w/w) of the phospholipid fatty acids of the spermatozoa of the bull, ram, boar, rhesus monkey, and human, respectively (10,11). In some species, other long-chain polyunsaturates, such as 22:5n-6, are also present in large amounts (7,10). The exceedingly high proportions of DHA that are achieved in the sperm of the bull and ram are particularly impressive since this fatty acid is usually absent from the diets of these species. Moreover, much of the dietary α-linolenic acid (18:3n-3), which could serve as a precursor for the biosynthesis of DHA, is destroyed in the rumen of these animals by biohydrogenation. The testes of the bull and ram must, therefore, be highly efficient in using the limited amount of 18:3n-3 for DHA formation during spermatogenesis.

Why do sperm phospholipids display such high levels of DHA? Of the 300 or so cell types in the body, the phospholipids of only 3 are notable for being so enriched with DHA: the neurons of the brain, the rod outer segments of the retina, and sperm (10,12). Apart from this extraordinary distribution, DHA is also unique in being the most highly unsaturated fatty acid to be found in cellular lipids, a feature that presumably has great functional significance. Since the synthesis and maintenance of a long-chain fatty acid with six double bonds represents a substantial investment of biological energy and also demands a high degree of antioxidant protection, cells must have a good reason for incorporating DHA into their phospholipid (10).

A major advance in understanding the role of polyunsaturates in sperm has been provided by the discovery that almost all of the DHA in monkey sperm is located in the tail, whereas the head region is almost devoid of this fatty acid (13). In that study, DHA accounted for 19.6% (w/w) of fatty acids of the tail phospholipids but only 1.1% of those of the head, and it was estimated that the tail contained 99% of the total DHA of the cell (13). Since the tail and head have distinctive functions, this highly polarized distribution strongly implies that DHA is not involved in the membrane fusion and signal transduction events associated with fertilization. Rather, it seems likely that the presence of this polyunsaturate in sperm phospholipids somehow relates to the ability of the tail to provide motility by flagellar action (13).

Important insights into the role of DHA-rich lipids in cell membranes have been provided by the application of a range of advanced biophysical techniques. These have shown that the DHA acyl-chain in phospholipid bilayers is highly flexible and can rapidly convert between an extended and a looped conformation. This confers a springy quality to the membrane, allowing it to accommodate and recover from compressive forces in the lateral plane of the bilayer. Membranes with a high content of DHA in their phospholipids are, therefore, distinguished by high levels of flexibility, compressibility, deformability, and elasticity (14–17).

A series of elegant studies involving the reconstitution of elements of the photoreceptor signal transduction system within phospholipid bilayers differing in acyl-chain composition are beginning to provide a conceptual framework for the role of DHA in vision and possibly in brain function (16–18). The first step in the detection of light by the retina is the photoactivation of the visual pigment protein, rhodopsin, located in the disk membranes of the rod outer segments. The conformational change performed by rhodopsin on conversion from the M I form to the photoactivated M II form involves an expansion of the volume of the protein molecule, thus increasing the lateral pressure on the lipids of the bilayer. In reconstituted bilayers, the M I to M II transition was greatly facilitated by the degree of unsaturation of the acyl-chains, with phospholipids containing DHA being the most effective. It appears that the exceptional compressibility exhibited by phospholipids that contain DHA enables the lipid matrix to accommodate major structural transitions of membrane-embedded proteins. This unique attribute derives from the ability of DHA to contract and expand the area it occupies in the membrane (via transitions between the extended and looped forms), thereby compensating for the fluctuations in lateral pressure caused by conversions between M I and M II.

The subsequent stages of the visual transduction system within the disk membrane, involving the interaction of M II with a G-protein, which in turn activates a cGMP-phosphodiesterase, have also been studied in reconstituted systems (17). Both the association of M II with G-protein and the resultant activation of phosphodiesterase were greatly enhanced in reconstituted bilayers consisting of DHA-rich phospholipids (17). Thus, the exceptionally high concentrations of DHA in the disk phospholipids of the rod outer segment facilitate protein-protein interactions as well as protein conformational changes in the membrane as part of the chain of events that generate the response of the retina to light. These insights into the function of DHA in membranes can be extended to the brain, since neurotransmission requires many proteins of the synaptic membranes to perform conformational transitions and protein-protein interactions (17).

Biophysical properties such as compressibility, flexibility, and deformability, imparted to membranes by DHA, immediately seem to provide an explanation for the abundance of this polyunsaturate in the phospholipid of sperm tails. It should, however, be noted that these attributes, as inferred from biophysical measurements and theoretical considerations and applied in the context of photoreception in disk membranes, refer to molecular events *within* membranes at the Ångstrom scale. In the case of sperm, by contrast, these terms take on their more familiar meaning, relating to actual movements of the membrane as a whole, performed over the μm range. Nevertheless, it is possible that these two situations derive from the same underlying molecular properties of DHA, although expressed at different scales. It may, therefore, be suggested that the role of DHA in sperm phospholipid is to endow the membrane of the tail with physical properties compatible with the rapid flexing and bending movements required for motility (13).

Provision of Docosahexaenoic Acid for Spermatogenesis

The differentiation of immature germ cells into mature spermatozoa during human spermatogenesis is accompanied by a progressive increase in the proportion of DHA in the cellular lipid (19). In the rat, where 22:5n-6 is the main polyunsaturate of sperm, the proportion of this fatty acid increased from 10 to 20% during the differentiation of spermatocytes into spermatids (20). When rats were raised on a diet deficient in essential fatty acids, their seminiferous tubules contained spermatogonia but few spermato-cytes and no spermatids or spermatozoa, dramatically illustrating that spermatogenesis is dependent on the appropriate provision of fatty acids (26).

Consideration of the origin of the long-chain polyunsaturates required for sper-matogenesis raises a series of questions. For instance, does this process depend on the provision of the "preformed" C22-polyunsaturate from the circulation, or is spermato-genesis normally supported by the uptake of precursors, such as 18:3n-3 or 20:5n-3, into the testis followed by their conversion to DHA? This point may be relevant to the design of dietary fatty acid supplements intended to improve male fertility. Secondly, does the testis obtain its polyunsaturates from the nonesterified fatty acid fraction of the plasma, as is the case for the brain (21), or are plasma lipoproteins involved in their provision? The extracellular matrix layers that separate the seminiferous tubules from the blood capillaries appear to exclude any access of very low density lipopro-teins and low density lipoproteins to the germ cells, although some high density lipoprotein particles can permeate this barrier and deliver cholesterol to Sertoli cells (22). Thirdly, do the non-germ cells of the testis play any role in the synthesis and delivery of polyunsaturates to the differentiating sperm?

With regard to this last question, a salient feature common to the three cell types that display high DHA contents is their association with other cells that specifically perform a supporting role. Since neurons, photoreceptor cells, and spermatozoa are all highly differentiated cells performing extremely specialized functions, certain tasks related to nutrient provision, removal of waste products, and metabolite interconver-sions are delegated to such helper cells. Thus, astrocytes, retinal pigment epithelial cells, and Sertoli cells, respectively, provide sustenance for neurons, photoreceptor cells, and developing sperm cells, mediating the supply of nutrients from the blood-stream. Most notably, astrocytes are able to convert 18:3n-3 to DHA and transfer the latter fatty acid to the neurons, which are unable to perform this conversion them-selves (23). Also, the retinal pigment epithelium performs an important role in the turnover and recycling of DHA in the rod photoreceptor outer segment (24,25). By analogy, it may therefore be expected that the Sertoli cells will be involved in the pro-vision of DHA to the developing sperm.

Throughout their differentiation, from spermatogonia via the spermatocyte and spermatid stages to the maturing spermatozoa, the male germ cells remain in intimate contact with the Sertoli cells. During this process, the germ cells migrate from the basal to the inner face of the Sertoli cell, where the mature spermatozoa are then released into the lumen of the seminiferous tubule (26). With the exception of sper-matogonia, the maturing germ cells are tightly sandwiched between adjacent pairs of Sertoli cells or embedded in crypts at the luminal surface. Thus, once a germ cell has become committed to spermatogenesis, all the nutrients required by these differentiat-ing cells must first transit part of the Sertoli cell.

There is considerable evidence that the Sertoli cell plays an important role in delivering the requisite polyunsaturates to the developing sperm (27). For example, whereas spermatocytes and spermatids isolated from rat testes were almost incapable of converting radioactive C20-polyunsaturates to their C22-derivatives, isolated Sertoli cells were very effective in synthesizing DHA from radioactive 20:5n-3 (28). Also, a rat testicular cell preparation enriched in Sertoli cells actively synthesized both DHA and 22:5n-6 from their respective C18-precursors (29). These results imply that Sertoli cells take up 18:3n-3 from the circulation and convert it to DHA for transfer to the developing sperm. Thus, it appears that the role of the Sertoli cell in relation to the sperm cell is, to some extent, analogous to the role of the astrocyte in relation to the neuron. Even when "preformed" DHA is provided in the diet and/or abundant in the circulation, obviating the need for its synthesis from 18:3n-3, the long chain polyunsaturate will still have to pass through part of the Sertoli cell to gain access to the sperm.

The Distinctive Fatty Acid Composition of Avian Sperm

Whereas DHA is usually the predominant polyunsaturate in the sperm of mammals, avian spermatozoa are instead characterized by very high proportions of the n-6 polyunsaturate, docosatetraenoic acid (DTA; 22:4n-6), with substantial levels of arachidonic acid (AA; 20:4n-6) also present (3,5,30). DTA was the major polyunsaturate in the sperm lipid of five species of domestic birds, AA was the next most common polyunsaturated fatty acid, but only low levels of DHA were present (31). As yet, there is no information on the fatty acid compositions of spermatozoa from birds in the wild. It would be interesting to see if the predominance of n-6 polyunsaturates is conserved in the spermatozoa of birds, such as the king penguin, that consume large amounts of DHA in their fish-based diet (32).

Since, in the lipids of the brain, the accumulation of long-chain n-6 fatty acids is usually regarded as a sign of n-3 deficiency (10,12), it could be argued that the preponderance of these polyunsaturates in the spermatozoa of domestic birds might simply be due to the very high n-6/n-3 ratio of their manufactured feeds. If this were the case, the disparity between the fatty acid profiles of avian and mammalian spermatozoa would be an artefact, resulting from the current feeding regimes for domestic birds rather than a true phylogenetic difference between these two classes of vertebrate. However, the proportions of DTA and AA in sperm phospholipid were not reduced by supplementing the diet of male chickens with an oil rich in 18:3n-3 (33). Furthermore, dietary supplementation of male chickens with fish oil, while causing a substantial increase in the proportion of DHA in sperm phospholipid, did not dislodge DTA from its preeminence as the major polyunsaturate of these cells (34). The use of n-6, rather than n-3, fatty acids for the formation of avian sperm lipids therefore represents a true distinction between birds and mammals and cannot be explained merely as an artefact of the diets given to domestic animals.

Although the reason for this clear difference between avian and mammalian sperm is not known, it is possible that the distinct fatty acid profiles could represent an adaptation to body temperature (34). The higher body temperature of birds compared to mammals (43°C *vs.* 37°C), coupled with the fact that the testes of many mammals are 4–7°C cooler than the body core due to their scrotal location, indicates that avian spermatozoa develop in an environment that may be at least 10°C warmer than that of their mammalian counterparts. Since the lipid dynamics and physical properties of membranes are highly sensitive to temperature, the difference in the degree of unsaturation between DTA and DHA could represent a means of maintaining the appropriate biophysical features of the spermatozoan membranes despite this temperature divergence. Thus, the fact that DTA has the same chain length but two fewer double bonds than DHA may offset the membrane effects of the higher temperature experienced by avian sperm. This scenario is, to some extent, analogous to the compensatory decrease in the unsaturation of membrane lipids displayed by some ectothermic animals on acclimation to higher environmental temperatures, thereby preventing major changes in membrane fluidity (35). A comparative approach could provide a test for this theory since several mammals (*e.g.,* elephants, marine mammals) have undescended testes, providing a warmer environment for sperm development, whereas the body temperature of some birds (*e.g.,* penguins) is much lower than the typical avian values (26). Such comparisons could, however, be confounded by dietary effects, particularly since marine mammals and penguins have a high intake of DHA.

Results

This section describes a series of studies on the consequences of aging on spermatogenesis, sperm quality, and sperm fatty acids and on the effects of dietary polyunsaturates on these parameters. Details of materials, methods, and statistics can be found in the indicated references.

Age-Related Changes in Spermatogenesis, Sperm Quality, and Fatty Acid Composition

The importance of DHA in mammalian spermatozoa is underlined by observations that several types of human subfertility, variously characterized by impaired sperm number, motility, and fertilizing ability, are associated with marked reductions in the level of this fatty acid in the sperm phospholipid (36–38). Aging is another situation that may affect the production of viable sperm. Although the males of many species remain fertile into old age, there is often a gradual decline in spermatogenesis, possibly related to a decrease in the concentration of free testosterone in the plasma (26). Several studies have shown that such age-related reductions in the number and quality of the spermatozoa are accompanied by decreased levels of DHA (or DTA in the case of birds) in the sperm phospholipid. For instance, spermatozoa from old bulls displayed reduced motility and contained significantly less DHA in their phosphatidylcholine and phosphatidylethanolamine fractions compared with spermatozoa from younger animals (Table 9.1) (6).

The phospholipid of boar sperm is characterized by high proportions of both DHA and 22:5n-6 (7,39). A comparison of semen from boars of different ages (age range: 395–761 days) demonstrated a significant positive correlation between the 22:5n-6/DHA ratio in sperm phospholipid and the age of the boar ($y = 0.03 + 0.0014x$,

TABLE 9.1

Semen Characteristics and Spermatozoan Fatty Acids[a] from Bulls of Different Ages[e]

	Age of bulls (years)	
	2–3	>9
Sperm concentration[b]	1.4 ± 0.1	0.9 ± 0.1[d]
Motility[c]	5.0	2.0
Phosphatidylcholine		
16:0	5.5 ± 0.4	4.8 ± 0.4
18:0	1.8 ± 0.7	3.4 ± 1.4
18:1n-9	1.0 ± 0.1	1.3 ± 0.2
22:5n-3	1.2 ± 0.1	1.3 ± 0.1
22:6n-3	91.1 ± 1.2	76.0 ± 3.8[d]
Phosphatidylethanolamine		
16:0	8.6 ± 1.2	13.8 ± 0.5[d]
18:0	14.8 ± 1.5	12.9 ± 0.9
18:1n-9	4.3 ± 0.1	10.9 ± 1.5[d]
18:1n-7	3.4 ± 1.2	3.7 ± 0.3
20:4n-6	15.0 ± 0.4	9.9 ± 1.0[d]
22:6n-3	47.3 ± 4.6	30.9 ± 1.7[d]

[a]Wt% of FA in the lipid class; values are mean ± SE, $n = 4$.
[b]10^9 cells/mL.
[c]Scale of 0–5.
[d]$P < 0.05$; comparison with young bulls.
[e]Data from (6).

where y = ratio 22:5n-6/DHA and x = days of age; $r = 0.781$; $P = 0.008$; $n = 10$) (Fig. 9.1). This replacement of DHA by 22:5n-6 with advancing age is accompanied by a fall in sperm quality, as the percent of spermatozoa with a normal acrosome was negatively correlated with the 22:5n-6/DHA ratio ($y = 62.5 - 23.1x$, where y = % with normal acrosome and x = ratio 22:5n-6/DHA; $r = -0.636$; $P = 0.048$; $n = 10$).

These same boars were then allocated into two groups matched for age, one maintained on a control diet and the other supplemented with fish oil (7). After six weeks on these treatments, the control group continued to show a strong positive correlation between the 22:5n-6/DHA ratio in sperm phospholipid and the age of the boar ($y = 0.0016x - 0.09$, where y = the ratio and x = days of age; $r = 0.923$; $P = 0.025$; $n = 5$). However, this correlation disappeared for the boars supplemented with fish oil ($r = -0.28$; $P > 0.1$, $n = 5$) as this diet tended to reduce the ratio to a fairly constant value that was not dependent on age (Fig. 9.2).

Spermatogenesis in the male chicken was far lower at 72 weeks than at 39 weeks of age (Table 9.2), and this fall in sperm output was accompanied by a significant decrease in the level of DTA in the total phospholipid of the spermatozoa (33). A comparison between four ages (24, 39, 54, and 72 weeks) revealed that the proportion of DTA in spermatozoan phospholipid was negatively correlated with age and positively correlated with the motility and fertilizing ability of the sperm (40). Another

                                    B.K. Speake et al.

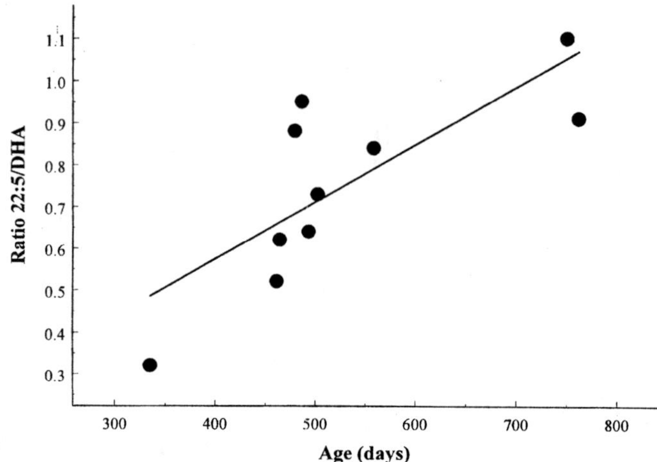

Fig. 9.1. Relationship between boar age and the 22:5n-6/DHA ratio of sperm phospholipid prior to dietary supplementation.

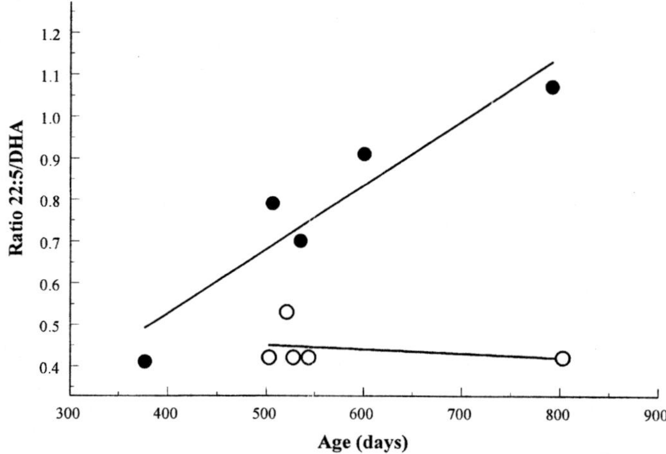

Fig. 9.2. Relationship between boar age and the 22:5n-6/DHA ratio of sperm phospholipid after 6 weeks on a fish oil-supplemented (○) or control (●) diet.

study, comparing cockerels at 25 and 60 weeks of age, indicated that the decline in sperm DTA with age occurred mainly in the phosphatidylethanolamine fraction, where the level of this fatty acid decreased from 33.5 to 23.1% (w/w) (5). By contrast, the proportion of this polyunsaturate in the phosphatidylcholine fraction remained relatively constant with age, at around 12–15% (w/w) (5).

TABLE 9.2
Semen Characteristics and Spermatozoan[a] Fatty Acids from Chickens of Different Ages[d]

	Age of chickens (weeks)	
	39	72
Sperm concentration[b]	7.7 ± 0.4	1.9 ± 0.7[c]
Fatty acids		
16:0	14.0 ± 1.0	15.1 ± 1.0
18:0	19.5 ± 1.1	20.4 ± 1.1
18:1n-9	12.2 ± 0.6	16.2 ± 0.6[c]
18:2n-6	3.4 ± 0.5	6.0 ± 0.8[c]
20:1n-9	3.1 ± 0.1	3.0 ± 0.1
20:4n-6	11.8 ± 0.8	11.0 ± 0.8
22:4n-6	22.9 ± 1.2	17.8 ± 1.2[c]
22:6n-3	2.5 ± 0.2	1.7 ± 0.1[c]

[a]Wt% of FA in total sperm phospholipid; values are means ± SE, $n = 5$.
[b]10^9 cells/mL.
[c]$P < 0.05$: comparison with 39 weeks.
[d]Data from (33).

These studies suggest that a decrease in the level of DHA (or DTA in birds) in spermatozoan phospholipid may be a characteristic of advancing age and is associated with reductions in sperm number and quality. Other age-related changes in sperm lipids appear to be common to birds and mammals. For instance, aging in the bull was accompanied by an increased proportion of phosphatidylcholine at the expense of phosphatidylethanolamine in the total phospholipid of the spermatozoa (6). Similarly, an increased level of phosphatidylcholine, together with decreased contributions from phosphatidylethanolamine and phosphatidylserine, were reported in the spermatozoa of older chickens (5,33,40).

In these examples, the composition of the diets was constant throughout the duration of the investigations. The reduced levels of DHA or DTA in spermatozoa from the older animals are not, therefore, due to any dietary effects. Possibly, such changes arise from a reduced ability of the Sertoli cells to synthesize C22 polyunsaturates from their C18 precursors. The age-related decline in δ6-desaturase activity in rat testes is consistent with this view (41). Alternatively, the loss of highly polyunsaturated fatty acids could be a consequence of inadequate protection by antioxidants at the later ages. In particular, the activity of glutathione peroxidase in semen decreased dramatically with age in the bull (6) and the chicken (5). Moreover, the levels of DTA and AA in sperm phospholipid of the cockerel were shown to be proportional to the concentration of vitamin E in the semen (42).

It should be noted that the changes described here for the chicken, in contrast to the situation for the bull and boar, are not strictly consequences of old age but rather represent the effects of different stages of the reproductive cycle. Birds are seasonal breeders, and in the wild their reproductive cycle is initiated by photostimulation due to increasing day-length. This environmental cue instigates a chain of physiological events that result in rapid testis growth and intense spermatogenesis. The reproductive cycle is terminated by the onset of photorefractoriness, when the bird becomes insensitive to the stimulatory effects of the long days, resulting in the cessation of spermatogenesis and regression of the testes. Usually, a period of short day-length is required to regain photosensitivity in preparation for the next breeding season the following spring (43). Although the reproductive cycle of the domestic chicken is extended by use of appropriate lighting regimes, the birds eventually become refractory and require a period of recovery on short day-lengths before starting a new cycle (44). Since many species of birds are very long-lived (45), with the potential to complete a large number of breeding seasons, the age-difference between the peak and the end of their first reproductive cycle is trivial in comparison with the prospective longevity. Nevertheless, the decline in spermatogenesis and the reduction in the level of DTA in sperm phospholipid observed in the cockerel at 72 weeks of age (*i.e.,* at the end of the first reproductive cycle) (33) may represent an accelerated and exaggerated version of the changes that occur during the true aging of nonseasonal animals.

Effect of Dietary DHA on Sperm Number and Quality in the Boar

The effectiveness of dietary fish oil in reducing the 22:5n-6/DHA ratio of boar sperm and in rescinding the age-dependence of this ratio has already been described (Fig. 9.2). In this study (7), boars were maintained for six weeks on either a control diet or a diet supplemented with Tuna Orbital Oil. The control diet contained no DHA; the main polyunsaturates were 18:2n-6 and 18:3n-3 forming 36 and 8% (w/w), respectively, of the total fatty acids. By contrast, DHA formed 8.5% (w/w) of fatty acids in the supplemented diet. The main effect of supplementation with fish oil on the fatty acid profile of the boars' spermatozoa was to increase the proportion of DHA in phospholipid from 33 to 41% while simultaneously reducing the level of 22:5n-6 from 25 to 16% (Fig. 9.3). This reciprocal change was not apparent by three weeks of supplementation but was clearly evident after five weeks, consistent with spermatogenesis in the boar requiring 34 days (46). The number of spermatozoa per ejaculate after six weeks of supplementation was almost double the value observed in the controls (Table 9.3).

Dietary supplementation with fish oil also improved the quality of the boar spermatozoa (Table 9.3). The percentage of viable spermatozoa, the proportion of those displaying forward motility, and the percent with a normal acrosome were significantly increased by the DHA diet. Conversely, the percent of spermatozoa with abnormal morphological characteristics was significantly reduced by the dietary supplementation.

There is considerable variation among previous studies in the proportions of 22:5n-6 and DHA reported in boar sperm phospholipid (1,39,47,48). The current findings suggest that these discrepancies probably arise from differences in the age and/or the diet of the boars under study. It is also clear from our work that the levels of these two polyunsaturates in boar sperm are reciprocally related: an increase in one is accompanied by a commensurate decrease in the other. Although this was particularly

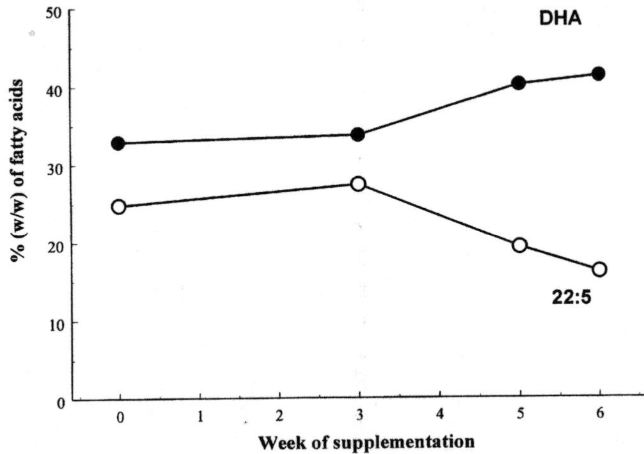

Fig. 9.3. Changes in the proportions of DHA (●) and 22:5n-6 (○) (% w/w of phospholipid fatty acids) of boar sperm during dietary supplementation with fish oil. Values are means from $n = 5$ boars.

TABLE 9.3

Effect of Dietary DHA[a] on the Quality of Boar Spermatozoa[d]

	Diet	
	Control	Fish oil
Sperm number ($\times 10^{10}$)	6.8	12.1[c]
Viable sperm (%)	71.3	80.4[c]
Progressive motility (%)	72.0	76.6[c]
Normal acrosome (%)	44.6	53.7[c]
Abnormal morphology (%)[b]	7.7	3.3[c]

[a]Results after 6 weeks of supplementation; $n = 5$ boars on each diet.
[b]Includes detached, abaxial or malformed head, bent or coiled tail, presence of cytoplasmic droplets.
[c]$P < 0.05$; comparison with control.
[d]Data from (7).

illustrated by the effects of DHA supplementation (Fig. 9.3), there was also a highly significant inverse relationship between the proportions of these two fatty acids ($r = -0.98$; $P < 0.001$; $n = 12$) in sperm obtained from the boars before the start of the experiment (7). It is noteworthy that these two polyunsaturates together form a very high proportion (57–67%) of the total fatty acids of boar sperm phospholipid.

The diets offered to domestic pigs typically have a very high n-6/n-3 ratio and do not contain DHA. Possibly this results in an unnaturally high 22:5n-6/DHA ratio in spermatozoa and prevents the achievement of optimal fertility. The present results clearly demonstrate the potential for improving the fertility of the domestic boar by including a source of DHA in the diet.

Effect of Dietary Polyunsaturated Fatty Acids on Sperm Number and Quality in the Chicken

Since the decline in spermatogenesis toward the end of the chicken's reproductive cycle is accompanied by a decreased level of DTA in sperm lipid (Table 9.2), we tested the possibility that dietary supplementation with appropriate fatty acids could offset this loss of DTA and thereby forestall the reduction in sperm output (50). Because oils enriched in DTA are currently unavailable, the diets of male chickens were supplemented with Arasco Oil, a rich source of ARA, the direct biosynthetic precursor of DTA. It was anticipated that the conversion of AA to DTA in the Sertoli cells of the testis might provide sufficient amounts of the latter polyunsaturate to sustain spermatogenesis beyond its usual duration.

In the same experiment, another group of male chickens was supplemented with Tuna Orbital Oil as a source of DHA. The purpose of this was twofold. Firstly, the incorporation of DHA into chicken sperm lipids causes a commensurate reduction in the level of DTA in the sperm (34), thus providing a contrast to the effects of Arasco Oil. Secondly, it has previously been shown that dietary n-3 fatty acids can improve the fertilizing ability of avian semen. For example, supplementation of the diet of male chickens with 18:3n-3, while having no effect on the proportion of DHA in sperm phospholipid at 39 weeks of age, caused a modest increase in the level of 22:5n-3 and significantly improved the fertilizing ability of the semen (33). Similarly, the fertilizing ability of the semen of chickens at the peak of the reproductive cycle was enhanced by dietary fish oil (49).

The effects of the fish oil diet (DHA forms 19% of fatty acids) and Arasco Oil Diet (AA forms 28% of fatty acids) were compared with a control diet supplemented with an equivalent amount of maize oil (18:2n-6 forms 53% of fatty acids). The birds were maintained on these diets from 26 to 60 weeks of age. The effects of the different dietary oils on the fatty acid composition of spermatozoan phospholipid at 60 weeks of age are shown in Table 9.4. The proportion of DTA in the sperm lipid was significantly increased (27% w/w of fatty acids compared with 22% in the control) as a result of the Arasco Oil supplementation, although the level of AA in the phospholipid was not altered. This suggests that the AA from the diet is converted to DTA in the Sertoli cells prior to incorporation of the latter fatty acid into the developing spermatozoa. Thus, the level of the characteristic polyunsaturate of avian sperm can indeed be enhanced by dietary means. The control diet was highly enriched in 18:2n-6, which is also a precursor of DTA. However, the conversion of 18:2n-6 to DTA requires 4 enzymatic steps, the first of which, catalyzed by δ-6 desaturase, is regarded as rate-limiting. AA is, therefore, likely to be more effective than 18:2n-6 as a precursor for the synthesis of DTA since only one enzymatic step is needed for the conversion and the rate-limiting stage is bypassed. As expected, consumption of the fish oil diet increased the proportion of DHA in the sperm lipid and concomitantly reduced the level of DTA and ARA.

The number of spermatozoa per ejaculate declined by 50% between 26 and 60 weeks of age for the birds on the control diet (Fig. 9.4). Most remarkably, this age-

TABLE 9.4
Fatty Acid Compositions[a] of Spermatozoan Phospholipid From Chickens at 60 Weeks of Age Supplemented With Different Dietary Oils[b]

	Dietary oil[c]		
	Maize oil	Arasco oil	Tuna oil
16:0	12.8 ± 0.5[a]	12.7 ± 0.3[a]	13.9 ± 0.6[a]
18:0	21.6 ± 0.7[a]	21.4 ± 0.5[a]	20.2 ± 0.6[a]
18:1n-9	12.6 ± 0.3[a]	11.7 ± 0.4[a]	16.7 ± 0.5[b]
18:2n-6	2.6 ± 0.3[a]	1.0 ± 0.1[b]	1.1 ± 0.2[b]
20:1n-9	3.7 ± 0.3[a]	3.8 ± 0.2[a]	4.5 ± 0.5[a]
20:4n-6	12.3 ± 0.3[a]	13.4 ± 0.6[a]	8.3 ± 0.3[b]
22:4n-6	22.1 ± 0.3[a]	27.0 ± 0.4[b]	15.5 ± 0.3[c]
22:6n-3	4.6 ± 0.3[a]	3.7 ± 0.4[a]	13.1 ± 0.4[b]

[a]Wt% of FA; values are means ± SE, $n = 5$.
[b]Data from (50).
[c]Values within a row that do not share a common superscript are significantly different; $P < 0.05$.

related reduction in spermatogenesis was completely averted by dietary supplementation with either Arasco Oil or Tuna Orbital Oil. Another dramatic finding was that the testis mass at 60 weeks was twice as high for the birds supplemented with AA or fish oil than for those on the control diet (Fig. 9.5), even though the total body weights did not differ between the dietary groups (50). In a separate study, dietary supplementation with evening primrose oil also resulted in a testis mass at 60 weeks that was double that in birds on a control (maize oil) diet, although no difference in the fatty acid composition of testis phospholipid was observed (51). It is notable that dietary DHA and AA achieve similar enhancements of spermatogenesis and testis mass despite having opposite effects on the level of DTA in sperm lipid.

The Importance of Antioxidants When Supplementing Diets With Polyunsaturated Fatty Acids

Because of their highly unsaturated lipids, spermatozoa are very susceptible to peroxidative damage resulting from the action of free radicals and reactive oxygen species. This heightened vulnerability is regarded as a major cause of male infertility (52) and it is, therefore, of great importance that the semen contains sufficient antioxidants to protect the spermatozoa from such harmful effects (53). Dietary supplementation with antioxidants such as vitamin E and selenium has been shown to improve the quality, motility, and fertilizing ability of spermatozoa in a number of species (53).

Although, as described above, certain dietary oils can improve the polyunsaturate status of spermatozoa, these beneficial effects could potentially be offset by the increased peroxidative susceptibility of these cells. It is, therefore, suggested that any elevation of dietary polyunsaturates should be accompanied by supplementary vitamin E (and possibly selenium) in the feed. These concerns are illustrated by the effects of dietary Arasco Oil and Tuna Orbital Oil on lipid peroxidation in chicken

                      B.K. Speake et al.

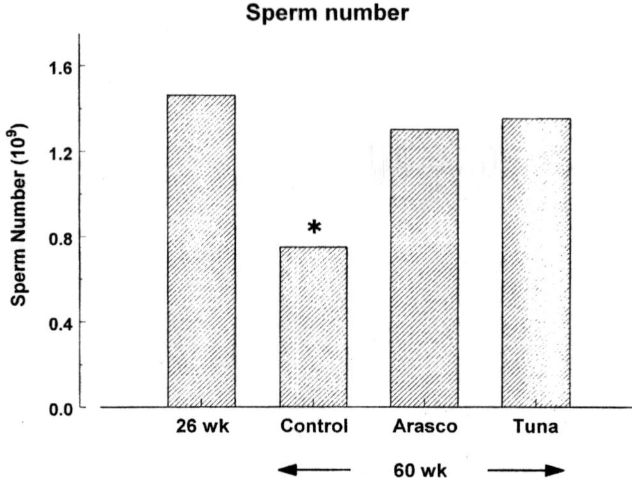

Fig. 9.4. Effect of dietary supplementation with Tuna Orbital Oil or Arasco Oil on sperm number per ejaculate (_109) from chickens at 60 weeks of age. Values are means from *n* = 10 birds in each group. *Comparison with 26 weeks: *P* < 0.05.

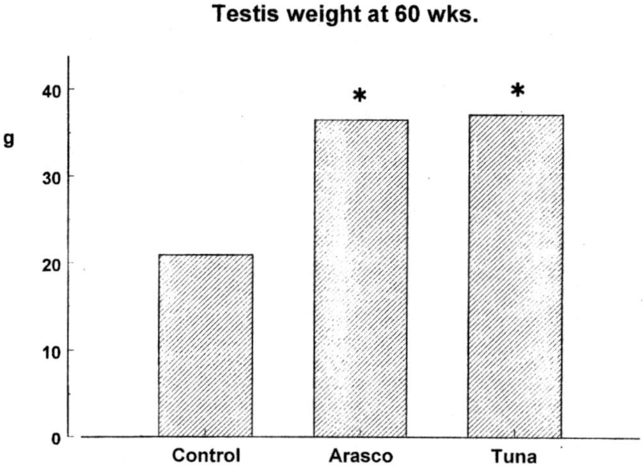

Fig. 9.5. Effect of dietary supplementation with Tuna Orbital Oil or Arasco Oil on testis wt (g) in chickens at 60 weeks of age. Values are means from *n* = 10 birds in each group. *Comparison with control: *P* < 0.05.

semen (50). The *in vitro* rate of peroxidation was significantly higher in semen from birds supplemented with either of these two oils compared with those on the maize oil diet. However, this effect was completely reversed by the inclusion of a higher level (200 *vs.* 40 mg/kg feed) of vitamin E in the diets. Moreover, the long-term (34 weeks) consumption of Tuna Orbital Oil was found to drastically deplete the tissues (heart, kidney, lung, liver, testis) of vitamin E unless the higher level of this vitamin was present in the diet.

Discussion

The studies described previously demonstrated that dietary supplementation with appropriate polyunsaturated fatty acids can produce major increases in spermatogenesis and improvements in sperm quality, at least in the pig and the chicken. In this section, we discuss possible mechanisms for these beneficial effects. The enhancement of sperm quality in boars fed fish oil is probably due to the increased level of DHA and the optimization of the 22:5n-6/DHA ratio in sperm phospholipid. These changes may be expected to promote successful spermatozoan development and to facilitate the flagellar movements of the tail. The explanation for the improved fertilizing ability of chicken semen following supplementation with oils rich in 18:3n-3 (33) or DHA (49) is less obvious given that the n-6 fatty acids, DTA and AA, are the characteristic spermatozoan polyunsaturates in this species. Conceivably, a mixture of phospholipid molecular species, with both n-6 and n-3 fatty acids represented, may be compatible with optimal flexibility of the avian sperm tail membrane. It is possible that the free-living ancestor of the domestic chicken would have experienced a more equitable intake of n-3 and n-6 fatty acids than is provided by today's commercial feeds. The "natural" n-6/n-3 ratio for spermatozoa of this species may, therefore, be slightly lower (and possibly more attuned to optimum fertility) than the values obtained under domestication.

Four mechanisms for the effect of dietary polyunsaturates on spermatogenesis can be suggested. The first mechanism assumes that DHA and DTA are obligatory structural components for the formation of mammalian and avian sperm, respectively. Inadequate provision of the relevant fatty acid could, therefore, result in impaired differentiation or, in severe cases, in the physical inability to construct a spermatozoon. This view is consistent with the effects of fish oil on boar spermatogenesis and with those of Arasco Oil on sperm production in the chicken. It does not, however, readily explain the stimulation of avian spermatogenesis by fish oil.

Secondly, polyunsaturated fatty acids could promote net spermatogenesis by inhibiting apoptosis during germ cell maturation. DHA has been shown to be highly effective in preventing apoptosis of cultured neurons (54) and retinal photoreceptors (55). Although extensive degeneration of germ cells can occur at several stages during spermatogenesis (26), the effectiveness of DHA in rescuing the maturing sperm from this fate has not been tested.

A third suggestion is that spermatogenesis may be stimulated by eicosanoids derived from the dietary polyunsaturated fatty acids. Arasco Oil provides large amounts of AA for potential conversion to type 2 prostaglandins and type 4 leukotrienes, whereas Tuna Orbital Oil provides substrate for the synthesis of type 3 prostaglandins and type 5 leukotrienes after the retroconversion of DHA to 20:5n-3 (56). Since both oils were effective in increasing sperm production in the chicken, this explanation requires the derived eicosanoids from n-3 as well as n-6 fatty acids to be equally stimulatory in this regard. Although prostaglandins in seminal plasma regulate various aspects of sperm function (57), their relevance to the present findings is unclear, particularly since a range of prostaglandins has been shown to inhibit spermatogenesis in rodents (58).

A fourth consideration is the potential interaction of polyunsaturated fatty acids, or their derived eicosanoids, with the hypothalamo-pituitary-gonadal axis and the hormonal control of spermatogenesis. Since testis growth and the maintenance of spermatogenesis are controlled by a cascade of hormonal events involving GnRH, FSH, LH, and testosterone (59,60), the effects of dietary polyunsaturates on the secretion and action of these hormones may be worthy of investigation. As dietary DHA is known to affect many aspects of brain function (12,17,61), it is reasonable to suggest that this fatty acid might play a regulatory role in the neural events that lead to the release of GnRH from the hypothalamus. The timing of puberty and seasonal breeding in mammals is coupled to photoregulatory environmental cues by the action of the pineal gland (62). Melatonin, released from the pineal gland in relation to the light-dark cycle, generally has an inhibitory effect on GnRH secretion from the hypothalamus and consequently on the plasma levels of FSH, LH and testosterone (62). It is, therefore, of considerable interest that DHA deficiency was found to produce a substantial increase in the daytime melatonin level in the pineal gland of the rat (63). If, on this basis, dietary supplementation with DHA could be shown to inhibit pineal melatonin synthesis, the consequent elevation of plasma FSH, LH, and testosterone would explain the stimulatory effects of this fatty acid on spermatogenesis.

The astounding (up to 500-fold) changes in testis weight of free-living birds at both the onset and the termination of each breeding season are accompanied by major alterations of plasma FSH, LH, and testosterone and are entrained by the increasing day-length (43,64,65). The mechanism of the avian photoperiodic response is, however, different from that of mammals since birds use nonretinal photoreceptors for this purpose (66). These are located in the hypothalamus and respond to photons that pass through the skull (67). Evidence for the presence of rhodopsinlike proteins in these encephalic photoreceptors (67) may be suggestive of a need for high local concentrations of DHA, possibly providing a link to the interactions between dietary fatty acids and avian spermatogenesis.

The increasingly speculative nature of this discussion illustrates the potential for further investigations into the mechanisms by which polyunsaturated fatty acids affect fertility. The effects of dietary fatty acids on spermatogenesis in the chicken are particularly of interest since they seem to represent an adjustment to the timing of the reproductive cycle. The maximum period that the cycle can be extended by such means is a topic for future study.

Summary

The spermatozoon is one of a select group of cell types (the others being the neuron and the retinal photoreceptor) whose phospholipids contain exceptionally high proportions of C20-22-polyunsaturated fatty acids. It is suggested that the high representation of DHA in the membrane lipids of the mammalian sperm tail enhances the flexibility and compressibility of the bilayer, thereby facilitating the flagellar movements. The presence of DTA instead of DHA in avian spermatozoa may be an adaptation to the higher body temperature of birds. The gradual decline in spermatogenesis during aging of some nonseasonal mammals (bull, boar) is accompanied by reduced levels of DHA in the sperm lipid. Similarly, the more rapid loss of spermatogenic capacity at the end of the avian reproductive cycle is characterized by a fall in the DTA content of the sperm.

Inclusion of a source of DHA into the diet of boars produced major improvements in the production and quality of spermatozoa. Supplementation of the diet of the male chicken with either DHA or with AA, a precursor of DTA, prevented the fall in testis weight and spermatogenesis that normally occurs at the end of the reproductive cycle. The mechanism of these effects is not known, but various roles for polyunsaturated fatty acids in spermatozoon assembly, anti-apoptosis, eicosanoid formation, and hormone action can be suggested. It may seem surprising that such major improvements in fertility can be achieved by simple changes to the diet. The application of these findings to livestock production, captive breeding, wildlife conservation, and human fertility is anticipated.

Acknowledgments

We thank Karen Kelso, Silvia Cerolini, Ray Noble, and C-C. Shao for their major contributions to the work described here from our laboratory. We are also grateful to the Scottish Executive Environment and Rural Affairs Department for financial support and to Scotia Pharmaceuticals (Carlisle, UK) for their gifts of Tuna Orbital Oil and Arasco Oil.

References

1. Ahluwalia, B., and Holman, R.T. (1969) Fatty Acid Composition of Lipids of Bull, Boar, Rabbit, and Human Semen, *J. Reprod. Fert. 18*, 431–437.
2. Poulos, A., Darin-Bennett, A., and White, I.G. (1973) The Phospholipid-Bound Fatty Acids and Aldehydes of Mammalian Spermatozoa, *Comp. Biochem. Physiol. 46B*, 541–549.
3. Darin-Bennett, A., Poulos, A., and White, I.G. (1974) The Phospholipids and Phospholipid-Bound Fatty Acids of Dog and Fowl Spermatozoa, *J. Reprod. Fert. 41*, 471–474.
4. Jain, Y.C., and Anand, S.R. (1976) Fatty Acids and Fatty Aldehydes of Buffalo Seminal Plasma and Sperm Lipid, *J. Reprod. Fert. 47*, 261–267.
5. Kelso, K.A., Cerolini, S., Noble, R.C., Sparks, N.H.C., and Speake, B.K. (1996) Lipid and Antioxidant Changes in Semen of Broiler Fowl From 25 to 60 Weeks of Age, *J. Reprod. Fert. 106*, 201–206.
6. Kelso, K.A., Redpath, A., Noble, R.C., and Speake, B.K. (1997) Lipid and Antioxidant Changes in Spermatozoa and Seminal Plasma Throughout the Reproductive Period of Bulls, *J. Reprod. Fert. 109*, 1–6.
7. Rooke, J.A., Shao, C-C., and Speake, B.K. (2000) Effects of Feeding Tuna Oil on the Lipid Composition of Pig Spermatozoa and *in vitro* Characteristics of Semen, *Reproduction 121*, 315–322.

8. Flesch, F.M., and Gadella, B.M. (2000) Dynamics of the Mammalian Sperm Plasma Membrane in the Process of Fertilization, *Biochim. Biophys. Acta 1469*, 197–235.

9. Roldan, E.R.S. (1998) Role of Phospholipases During Sperm Acrosomal Exocytosis, *Front. Biosci. 3*, D1109–D1119.

10. Salem, N. Jr., Kim, H-Y., and Yergey. J.A. (1986) Docosahexaenoic Acid: Membrane Function and Metabolism, in *Health Effects of Polyunsaturated Fatty Acids in Seafoods*, Simopoulos, A.P., Kifer, R.R., and Martin, R.E., Academic Press, New York, pp. 263–321.

11. Lin, D.S., Connor, W.E., Wolf, D.P., Neuringer, M., and Hachey, D.L. (1993) Unique Lipids of Primate Spermatozoa: Desmosterol and Docosahexaenoic Acid, *J. Lipid Res. 34*, 491–499.

12. Neuringer, M., Anderson, G.J., and Connor, W.E. (1988) The Essentiality of n-3 Fatty Acids for the Development and Function of the Retina and Brain, *Annu. Rev. Nutr. 8*, 517–541.

13. Connor, W.E., Lin, D.S., Wolf, D.P., and Alexander, M. (1998) Uneven Distribution of Desmosterol and Docosahexaenoic Acid in the Heads and Tails of Monkey Sperm, *J. Lipid Res. 39*, 1404–1411.

14. Holte, L.L., Separovic, F., and Gawrisch, K. (1996) Nuclear Magnetic Resonance Investigation of Hydrocarbon Chain Packing in Bilayers of Polyunsaturated Phospholipids, *Lipids 31*, S199–S203.

15. Salem N. Jr., and Niebylinski, C.D. (1995) The Nervous System has an Absolute Molecular Species Requirement for Proper Function, *Mol. Membr. Biol. 12*, 131–134.

16. Mitchell, D.C., Gawrisch, K., Litman, B.J., and Salem, N. Jr. (1998) Why is Docosahexaenoic Acid Essential for Nervous System Function?, *Biochem. Soc. Trans. 26*, 365–370.

17. Salem, N. Jr., Litman, B., Kim, H.-Y., and Gawrisch, K. (2001) Mechanisms of Action of Docosahexaenoic Acid in the Nervous System, *Lipids 36*, 945–949.

18. Litman, B.J., and Mitchell, D.C. (1996) A Role for Phospholipid Polyunsaturation in Modulating Membrane Protein Function, *Lipids 31*, S193–S197.

19. Lenzi, A., Gandini, L., Maresca, V., Rago, R., Sgro, P., Dondero, F., and Picardo, M. (2000) Fatty Acid Composition of Spermatozoa and Immature Germ Cells, *Mol. Hum. Reprod 6*, 226–231.

20. Beckman, J.K., Gray, M.E., and Coniglio, J.G. (1978) The Lipid Composition of Isolated Rat Spermatids and Spermatocytes, *Biochim. Biophys. Acta 530*, 367–374.

21. Rapoport, S.I., Chang, M.C., and Spector, A.A. (2001) Delivery and Turnover of Plasma-Derived Essential PUFA in Mammalian Brain, *J. Lipid Res. 42*, 678–685.

22. Maboundou, J-C., Fofana, M., Fresnel, J., Boquet, J., and Le Goff, D. (1995) Effect of Lipoproteins on Cholesterol Synthesis in Rat Sertoli Cells, *Biochem. Cell Biol. 73*, 67–72.

23. Moore, S.A., Yoder, E., Murphy, S., Dutton, G.R., and Spector, A.A. (1991) Astrocytes, Not Neurones, Produce Docosahexaenoic Acid (22:6n-3) and Arachidonic Acid (20:4n-6), *J. Neurochem. 56*, 518–524.

24. Chen, H., and Anderson, R.E. (1993) Differential Incorporation of Docosahexaenoic and Arachidonic Acids in Frog Retinal Pigment Epithelium, *J. Lipid Res. 34*, 1943–1955.

25. Jeffrey, B.G., Weisinger, H.S., Neuringer, M., and Mitchell, D.C. (2001) The Role of Docosahexaenoic Acid in Retinal Function, *Lipids 36*, 859–871.

26. Setchell, B.P. (1982) in *Reproduction in Mammals 1: Germ Cells and Fertilization*, Austin, C.R., and Short, R.V., Cambridge University Press, Cambridge, pp. 63–101.

27. Coniglio, J.G. (1994) Testicular Lipids, *Prog. Lipid Res. 33*, 387–401.

28. Retterstøl, K., Tran, T.N., Haugen, T.B., and Christopherson, B.O. (2001) Metabolism of Very Long Chain Polyunsaturated Fatty Acids in Isolated Rat Germ Cells, *Lipids 36*, 601–606.

29. Retterstøl, K., Haugen, T.B., Woldseth, B., and Christopherson, B.O. (1998) A Comparative Study of the Metabolism of *n*-9, *n*-6 and *n*-3 fatty acids in testicular cells from immature rat, *Biochim. Biophys. Acta 1392*, 59–72.

30. Ravie, O., and Lake, P.E. (1985) The Phospholipid-Bound Fatty Acids of Fowl and Turkey Spermatozoa, *Anim. Reprod. Sci. 9*, 189–192.

31. Surai, P.F., Blesbois, E., Grasseau, I., Chalah, T., Brillard, J-P., Wishart, G.J., Cerolini, S., and Sparks, N.H.C. (1998) Fatty Acid Composition, Glutathione Peroxidase and Superoxide Dismutase Activity and Total Antioxidant Activity of Avian Semen, *Comp. Biochem. Physiol. Part B 120*, 527–533.

32. Decrock, F., Groscolas, R., McCartney, R.J., and Speake, B.K. (2001) Transfer of n-3 and n-6 Polyunsaturated Fatty Acids From Yolk to Embryo During Development of the King Penguin, *Am. J. Physiol. Regul. Integr. Comp. Physiol. 280*, R843–R853.

33. Kelso, K.A., Cerolini, S., Speake, B.K., Cavalchini, L.G., and Noble, R.C. (1997) Effects of Dietary Supplementation with α-Linolenic Acid on the Phospholipid Fatty Acid Composition and Quality of Spermatozoa in Cockerel from 24 To 72 Weeks of Age, *J. Reprod. Fert. 110*, 53–59.

34. Kelso, K.A., Cerolini, S., Noble, R.C., Sparks, N.H.C., and Speake, B.K. (1997) The Effects of Dietary Supplementation with Docosahexaenoic Acid on the Phospholipid Fatty Acid Composition of Avian Spermatozoa, *Comp. Biochem. Physiol. 115B*, 65–69.

35. Thompson, G.A. Jr. (1992) *The Regulation of Membrane Lipid Metabolism*, 2nd edn., pp. 201–220, CRC Press, Boca Raton.

36. Nissen, H.P., and Kreysel, H.W. (1983) Polyunsaturated Fatty Acids in Relation to Sperm Motility, *Andrologia 15*, 264–269.

37. Zalata, A.A., Christophe, A.B., Depuydt, C.E., Schoonhans, F., and Comhaire, F.H. (1998) The Fatty Acid Composition of Phospholipids of Spermatozoa from Infertile Patients, *Mol. Hum. Reprod. 4*, 111–118.

38. Conquer, J.A., Martin, J.B., Tummon, I., Watson, L., and Tekpety, F. (1999) Fatty Acid Analysis of Blood Serum, Seminal Plasma, and Spermatozoa of Normozoospermic *Versus* Asthenozoospermic Males, *Lipids 34*, 793–799.

39. Paulenz, H., Taugbøl, O., Hofmo, P.O., and Saarem, K. (1995) A Preliminary Study on the Effect of Dietary Supplementation with Cod Liver Oil on the Polyunsaturated Fatty Acid Composition of Boar Semen, *Vet. Res. Commun. 19*, 273–284.

40. Cerolini, S., Kelso, K.A., Noble, R.C., Speake, B.K., Pizzi, F., and Cavalchini, L.G. (1997) Relationship Between Spermatozoan Lipid Composition and Fertility During Aging of Chickens, *Biol. Reprod. 57*, 976–980.

41. Brenner, R.R. (1989) in *The Role of Fats in Human Nutrition*, Vergroesen, A.J., and Crawford, M.A., Academic Press, London, 2nd edn., pp. 46–79.

42. Surai, P.F., Kutz, E., Wishart, G.J., Noble, R.C., and Speake, B.K. (1997) The Relationship Between the Dietary Provision of α-Tocopherol and the Concentration of this Vitamin in the Semen of Chicken: Effects on Lipid Composition and Susceptibility to Peroxidation, *J. Reprod. Fert. 110*, 47–51.

43. Nicholls, T.J., Goldsmith, A.R., and Dawson, A. (1988) Photorefractoriness in Birds and Comparison with Mammals, *Physiol. Rev. 68*, 133–176.

44. Sharp, P.J. (1993) Photoperiodic Control of Reproduction in the Domestic Hen, *Poult. Sci.* 72, 897–905.

45. Holmes, D.J., and Austad, S.N. (1995) The Evolution of Avian Senescence Patterns: Implications for Understanding Primary Aging Processes, *Amer. Zool. 35*, 307–317.

46. Swierstra, E.E. (1968) Cytology and Duration Cycle of the Seminiferous Epithelium of the Boar: Duration and Spermatozoan Transit Through the Epididymis, *Anat. Rec. 161*, 171–186.

47. Johnson, L.A., Pursel, V.G., and Gerrits, R.J. (1972) Total Phospholipid and Phospholipid Fatty Acids of Ejaculated and Epididymal Semen and Seminal Vesicle Fluids of Boars, *J. Anim. Sci. 35*, 398–403.

48. Evans, R.W., and Setchell, B.P. (1979) Lipid Changes in Boar Spermatozoa During Epididymal Maturation with Some Observations on the Flow and Composition of Boar Rete Testis Fluid, *J. Reprod. Fert. 57*, 189–196.

49. Blesbois, E., Lessire, M., Grasseau, I., Hallouis, J.M., and Hermier, D. (1997) Effect of Dietary Fat on the Fatty Acid Composition and Fertilizing Ability of Fowl Semen, *Biol. Reprod. 56*, 1216–1220.

50. Surai, P.F., Noble, R.C., Sparks, N.H.C., and Speake, B.K. (2000) Effect of Long-Term Supplementation with Arachidonic or Docosahexaenoic Acids on Sperm Production in the Broiler Chicken, *J. Reprod. Fert. 120*, 257–264.

51. Surai, P.F., Cerolini, S., and Speake, B.K. (2000) Effect of Supplementing the Diet of Male Chickens with Oils Rich in n-6 Polyunsaturated Fatty Acids on the Fatty Acid Profiles of the Testis and Liver, *Asian-Aus. J. Anim. Sci. 13*, 1518–1522.

52. Aitken, R.J. (1994) A Free Radical Theory of Male Infertility, *Reprod. Fert. Dev. 6*, 19–24.

53. Surai, P.F., Fujihara, N., Speake, B.K., Brillard, J-P., Wishart, G.J., and Sparks, N.H.C. (2001) Polyunsaturated Fatty Acids, Lipid Peroxidation and Antioxidant Protection in Avian Semen, *Asian-Aust. J. Anim. Sci. 14*, 1024–1050.

54. Kim, H.Y., Akbar, M., Lau, A., and Edsall, L. (2000) Inhibition of Neuronal Apoptosis by Docosahexaenoic Acid (DHA): Role of Phosphatidylserine in Antiapoptotic Effect, *J. Biol. Chem. 275*, 35215–35233.

55. Rotstein, N.P., Aveldaño, M.I., Barrantes, F.J., Roccamo, A.M., and Politi, L.E. (1997) Apoptosis of Retinal Photoreceptors During Development *in Vitro*: Protective Effect of Docosahexaenoic Acid, *J. Neurochem. 69*, 504–513.

56. Sardesai, V.M. (1992) Biochemical and Nutritional Aspects of Eicosanoids, *J. Nutr. Biochem. 3*, 562–579.

57. Gottlieb, C., and Bygdeman, M. (1988) Prostaglandins in Sperm Function, *Prostagland. Leukot. Essent. Fatty Acids 34*, 205–214.

58. Abbatiello, E.R., Kaminsky, M., and Weisbroth, S. (1976) The Effect of Prostaglandins $F_{1\alpha}$ and $F_{2\alpha}$ on Spermatogenesis, *Int. J. Fert. 21*, 82–88.

59. De Kretser, D.M. (1984) in *Reproduction in Mammals 3: Hormonal Control of Reproduction*, Austin, C.R., and Short, R.V., Cambridge University Press, Cambridge, pp. 76–90.

60. Etches, R.J. (1996) *Reproduction in Poultry*, 1st edn., CAB International, Wallingford, pp. 209–233.

61. Chalon, S., Vancassel, S., Zimmer, L., Guillotaue, D., and Durand, G. (2001) Polyunsaturated Fatty Acids and Cerebral Function: Focus on Monoaminergic Neurotransmission, *Lipids 36*, 937–944.

62. Lincoln, G.A. (1984) in *Reproduction in Mammals 3: Hormonal Control of Reproduction*, Austin, C.R., and Short, R.V., Cambridge University Press, Cambridge, pp. 52–75.

63. Zhang, H., Hamilton, J.H., Salem, N. Jr., and Kim, H-Y. (1998) N-3 Fatty Acid Deficiency in the Rat Pineal Gland: Effects on Phospholipid Molecular Species Composition and Endogenous Levels of Melatonin and Lipoxygenase Products, *J. Lipid Res. 39*, 1397–1403.

64. Romanoff, A.L. (1960) *The Avian Embryo*, 1st edn., Macmillan, New York, pp. 5–72.

65. Follett, B.K. (1984) in *Marshall's Physiology of Reproduction*, Lamming, G.E., Churchill Livingstone Press, Edinburgh, pp. 283–350.

66. Follett, B.K. (1982) in *Biological Timekeeping*, Brady, J., Cambridge University Press, Cambridge, pp. 83–100.

67. Silver, R. (1990) in *Endocrinology of Birds: Molecular to Behavioral*, Wada, M., Ishii, S., and Scanes, C.G., Japan Scientific Societies Press, Tokyo, pp. 261–272.

Chapter 10

Neutral Sterols in the Epididymis: High Concentrations of Dehydrocholesterols

G. Haidl[a], B. Lindenthal[b], and K. von Bergmann[c]

[a]University of Bonn, Department of Dermatology/Andrology Unit, Sigmund-Freud-Str. 25. 53105 Bonn, Germany
[b]Schering AG, Female Health Care, Muellerstr. 170–178, 13342 Berlin, Germany
[c]University of Bonn, Department of Clinical Pharmacology, Sigmund-Freud-Str. 25, 53105 Bonn, Germany

Abstract

Changes in the membrane lipids and membrane fluidity of spermatozoa during epididymal maturation have been described in several species, including humans. These studies focused on the role of phospholipids, cholesterol, and fatty acids in different sperm functions. Much less is known about the significance of cholesterol precursors. High amounts of 7- and 8-dehydrocholesterol and desmosterol have been found in the caput epididymidis of rats, and desmosterol has been found in the cauda as well. Moreover, these sterols were detected in spermatozoa from the caput epididymidis, whereas high amounts of desmosterol were present only in spermatozoa from the cauda epididymidis. With regard to desmosterol, similar distribution patterns in different species have been reported. In contrast, high amounts of 7- and 8-dehydrocholesterol have not been described in other species. The role of these cholesterol precursors in sperm or receptor functions is still unknown.

Lipids and Epididymal Maturation—General Remarks

The role of the epididymis in sperm maturation has been demonstrated by numerous fundamental research studies. It comprises various functions, for example, the development of progressive motility, capability of capacitiation with subsequent undergoing of the acrosome reaction and binding to the zona pellucida, as well as fusion with the oolemma (1). Maturation of spermatozoa in the epididymis involves remodeling of many protein and lipid components of the plasma membrane. Changes in the membrane lipids of spermatozoa during epididymal transit have been reported on several animal species as well as in the human (2,3). Membrane fluidity depends on the amounts of phospholipids, the fatty acid composition of the phospholipids, and the amount of cholesterol in the membrane, among other things. A high fluidity is achieved by a low cholesterol/phospholipid ratio as well as a high percentage of unsaturated fatty acids. It has been shown that membrane fluidity of the sperm membrane increases during the passage from caput to cauda epididymidis, which is accompanied by a decrease of the cholesterol/phospholipid ratio and a change in the pattern of the fatty acids (4). These modifications go in parallel with the development of progressive motility of spermatozoa but are obviously important for further sperm functions as well. The environment of the female tract provides conditions that promote efflux of cholesterol from the sperm plasma membrane as well as the loss of membrane asymmetry. The loss of cholesterol has been demonstrated to be a prerequisite for the capacitation of spermatozoa with subsequent sperm-egg interaction (5,6). In addition it has been shown that bovine seminal vesicles secrete a family of proteins called bovine seminal plasma proteins that stimulate cholesterol and phospholipid efflux from the sperm membrane during capacitation (7,8).

The Role of Neutral Sterols in Epididymal Function

Whereas the major interest in the role of lipids for sperm maturation in the epididymis and sperm functions is concentrated on phospholipids and cholesterol (demonstrating the function of cholesterol as membrane stabilizer and enzyme inhibitor to provide protection against the premature release of proteolytic enzymes, such as acrosin), little attention has been drawn to the occurrence and potential functions of precursors of cholesterol. Cholesterol synthesis comprises at least 19 steps from the first sterol, lanosterol, to cholesterol with desmosterol and 7-dehydrocholesterol as ultimate cholesterol precursors (Fig. 10.1) (9). Although the importance of cholesterol for membrane functions (as a precursor for bile salts and steroid hormones as well as a membrane stabilizer) has been studied extensively, considerably less is known about the sterol precursors of cholesterol in biological systems. For a long time they were regarded as intermediates, appearing only in very low amounts compared with cholesterol and without association to major biological functions. However, recent findings give rise to a more distinct view of this class of sterols.

Cholesterol precursors have been investigated in different animal species. The lipid composition of hamster epididymal spermatozoa showed little difference in the amount of total sterol between caput and cauda sperm. However, sterol composition changed markedly during epididymal transit: the amount of cholesterol decreased, while there was an increase in the amount of desmosterol and cholesta-7,24-dien-3-β-ol (10). This 3-β-hydroxysterol is also found in hamster epididymal tissue (11). The sterol composition of hamster cauda epididymal spermatozoa was demonstrated to be remarkably different from that of several other mammalian spermatozoa. Cholesterol and desmosterol represent the major components of mouse cauda epididymal spermatozoa and rabbit, boar, and bull ejaculated spermatozoa as well, whereas cholesta-7,24-dien-3-β-ol was not detected in these species. Higher concentrations of desmosterol were also detected in whole tissues of cauda epididymidis of humans compared to caput (12). In contrast, desmosterol is present in ram spermatozoa entering the epididymis but negligible in sperm after epididymal transit (cauda sperm) (13). Moreover, it has been shown that desmosterol is nearly exclusively confined to the flagella of monkey spermatozoa, thus proposing a role for this sterol in motility of spermatozoa (14,15). Most recently, the normal appearance of high concentrations of

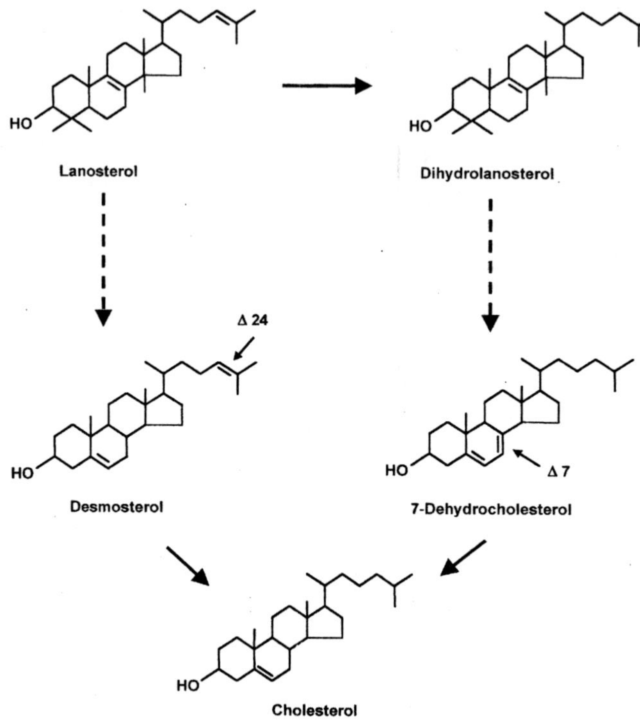

Fig. 10.1. The late steps of cholesterol synthesis

the cholesterol precursors 7- and 8-dehydrocholesterol in caput epididymidis of rats was reported (16). The caput epididymidis of Sprague-Dawley rats contained three noncholesterol sterols in considerable concentrations. These were identified as desmosterol and 7- and 8-dehdyrocholesterol. Interestingly, the appearance of 7- and 8-dehydrocholesterol was strictly confined to the caput epididymidis, whereas desmosterol was also present in cauda epididymidis (Fig. 10.2).

The same pattern was observed in Wistar rats, the dehydrocholesterols comprise up to 30% of total sterols. In prepubertal rats 7-dehydrocholesterol was also present in caput epididymidis but not in the cauda. Desmosterol was measured in caput as well as in cauda epididymidis and was again lower in caput epididymidis, as was the case in adult rats. To further localize the appearance of dehydrocholesterols, neutral sterols were investigated in spermatozoa obtained from testis, caput and cauda epididymidis, and in the remaining tissue after sperm preparation. High concentrations of dehydrocholesterols were found in both spermatozoa and the remaining tissue of caput epididymidis. However, the ratio of these sterols to cholesterol is higher in the spermatozoa compared to the remaining tissue. It is unlikely that the marked change of the sterol composition of spermatozoa during epididymal maturation is accomplished by changes of cholesterol synthesis in the spermatozoa alone. Therefore, it might be

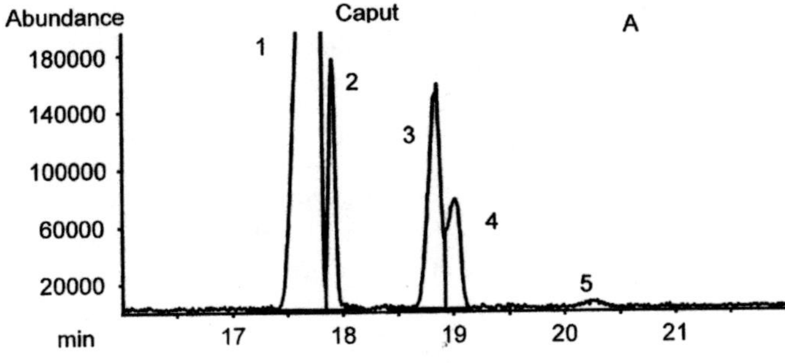

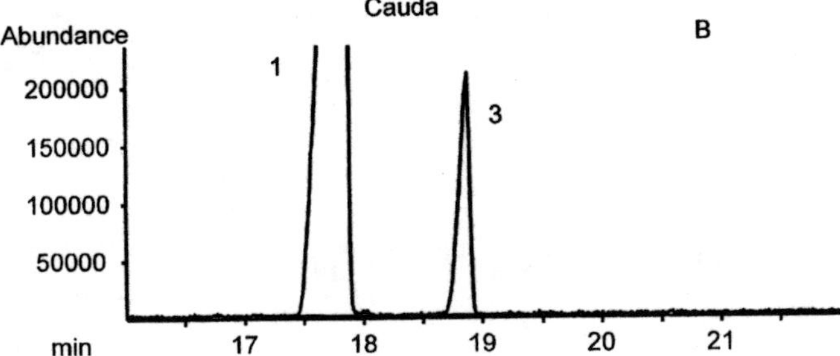

Fig. 10.2. Neutral sterols of caput (A) and cauda (B) epididymidis of an adult Sprague-Dawley rat. Full scan chromatogram of a GC–MS analysis; peak identification: 1) cholesterol; 2) 8-dehydrocholesterol; 3) desmosterol; 4) 7-dehydrocholesterol, and 5) triunsaturated sterol.

assumed that other cells of the caput epididymidis have a markedly altered biosynthesis providing dehydrocholesterols and desmosterol for spermatozoa. Moreover, cauda epididymidis cells must also possess marked changes in cholesterol biosynthesis compared to other tissues in order to provide high amounts of desmosterol.

Changes of Cholesterol Precursors in Cells and Tissues Might be the Result of Various Processes

Inhibitors may affect distinct enzymes of cholesterol synthesis. The possibility has to be considered that an inhibitor might affect more than one enzyme, since cholesterol precursors are closely related, and enzymes metabolizing this class of sterols might also have related substrate binding sites. Therefore, the same compound might affect multiple enzymes in this pathway at different concentrations as described for triparanol (17).

If one enzyme in cholesterol biosynthesis is inhibited, another enzymatic step in this pathway might become the bottleneck for further synthesis, and cholesterol precursors upstream of this particular step might accumulate. Products such as 8-dehydrocholesterol might also appear from the activity of a Δ7-Δ8 isomerase, which uses 7-dehydrocholesterol as a substrate. This might lead to the wrong impression that this step is directly affected.

Sterols are transported forth and back from the endoplasmic reticulum (ER), where synthesis takes place, and the cell membrane, where most of the cholesterol resides. It has been shown that disturbances of these transport systems also lead to an accumulation of cholesterol precursors. Interestingly, it has been shown that the cholesterol precursor zymosterol is transported faster from the ER to the cell membrane than cholesterol (18).

In contrast, in spermatozoa from testis, cauda epididymidis and the remaining tissues, dehydrocholesterols, were virtually absent. Interestingly, the cholesterol content of testicular spermatozoa was markedly increased compared with spermatozoa obtained from caput and cauda, whereas in the remaining tissue, cholesterol was only slightly higher in the testis compared with caput and cauda epididymidis. The concentration of desmosterol increased not only in the epididymal tissue from caput to cauda but also in spermatozoa during epididymal transit. As already pointed out desmosterol and 7-dehydrocholesterol are the ultimate precursors of cholesterol in the process of cholesterol synthesis. They cannot be converted into each other in the cholesterol biosynthetic pathway, and they originate from two different routes of cholesterol synthesis (Fig. 10.1). High levels of 7- and 8-dehydrocholesterol normally do not occur in mammalian tissues except in pathophysiological conditions, drug interventions, or in human skin serving as a precursor for vitamin D formation. Desmosterol is also a known constituent of spermatozoa of human, rhesus monkey, hamster, boar, rabbit, goat, and mouse. Its amount increases from caput to cauda epididymidis in some but not all species investigated. Desmosterol and docosahexaenoic acid are nearly exclusively confined to the flagella in monkey sperm, and a role for desmosterol in sperm motility has been postulated (15). The appearance of desmosterol together with cholesta-7,24-dien-3-β-ol, which can be converted to desmosterol, has been described. It might, therefore, be regarded as a desmosterol precursor. Desmosteryl-sulfate has been shown to increase markedly from hamster caput to cauda epididymidis spermatozoa, with a proposed role in membrane stabilization and the capacitation process (19). Therefore, cholesterol precursors, such as desmosterol, seem to play an important role in sperm maturation and function. However, because 7- and 8-dehydrocholesterol were virtually absent in cauda epididymidis, any potential function of these two sterols in sperm maturation seems to be different from the putative functions of desmosterol. Because 7-and 8-dehydrocholesterol cannot be converted to desmosterol, they cannot serve as a precursor pool for desmosterol synthesis. The simultaneous appearance of desmosterol together with 7- and 8-dehydrocholesterol in the caput of rat epididymis is a unique precursor pattern not reported previously; 7- and 8-dehydrocholesterol were not detected in the epididymis of other mammalian species investigated so far. The function of this unique pattern of high concentrations of dehydrocholesterols has still to be elucidated. As active metabolites of vitamin D and vitamin D receptors have been described in rat epididymis as well, which is suggestive of a regulatory role for vitamin D in Ca^{2+}

and phosphate transport, one could speculate that the dehydrocholesterols may act as precursors for vitamin D synthesis similar to the situation in human skin (20–22).

Another possibility is that marked changes of cholesterol precursors in cell membranes influence the properties of lipid rafts. Lipid rafts contain high amounts of cholesterol and may serve as areas of receptor and enzyme assemblies. Pioneering work in studying the effects of different sterols in cell membranes on receptor properties has been performed on the oxytocin receptor (23). Besides different effects on lipid raft associated receptors, cholesterol precursors might be different from cholesterol in regard to desorption from the plasma membrane (*e.g.,* desmosterol) (24) or in the velocity of intracellular transport (*e.g.,* zymosterol) (18). At high concentrations cholesterol precursors might even effect cell morphology (25).

Conclusion

Taken together, the high amounts of desmosterol, dehydrocholesterol, and cholesta-7,24-dien-3-β-ol in mammalian epididymis and spermatozoa and the recent discovery of meiosis-activating sterols, which also belong to the class of cholesterol precursors (26), show that in the reproductive system late cholesterol synthesis is markedly changed and deserves the attention of devoted scientists. Possible effects might exist on such heterogeneous processes as sperm motility, sperm maturation, receptor functions within lipid rafts, or effects on meiosis and still wait to be elucidated.

References

1. Bedford, J.M., Calvin, H.I., and Cooper, G.W. (1973) The Maturation of Spermatozoa in the Human Epidydimis, *J. Reprod. Fertil. 18 (Suppl.)*, 199–213.
2. Nikolopoulou, M., Soucek, D.A., and Vary, J.C. (1985) Changes in the Lipid Content of Boar Sperm Plasma Membranes During Epididymal Maturation, *Biochim. Biophys. Acta 815*, 486–498.
3. Haidl, G., Badura, B., Hinsch, K.D., Ghyczy, M., Gareiss, J., and Schill, W.B. (1993) Disturbances of Sperm Flagella Due to Failure of Epididymal Maturation and Their Possible Relationship to Phospholipids, *Hum. Reprod. 8*, 1070–1073.
4. Haidl, G., and Opper, C. (1997) Changes in Lipids and Membrane Anisotropy in Human Spermatozoa During Epididymal Maturation, *Hum. Reprod. 12*, 2720–2723.
5. Nikolopoulou, M., Soucek, D.A., and Vary, J.C. (1986) Lipid Composition of the Membrane Released After an *in Vitro* Acrosome Reaction of Epididymal Boar Sperm, *Lipids 21*, 566–570.
6. Nolan, J.P., and Hammerstedt, R.H. (1997) Regulation of Membrane Stability and the Acrosome Reaction in Mammalian Sperm, *FASEB J. 11*, 670–682.
7. Therien, I., Moreau, R., and Manjunath, P. (1998) Major Proteins of Bovine Seminal Plasma and High Density Lipoprotein Induce Cholesterol Efflux from Epididymal Sperm, *Biol. Reprod. 59*, 768–776.
8. Manjunath, P., and Therien,I. (2002) Role of Seminal Plasma Phospholipid-Binding Proteins in Sperm Membrane Lipid Modification that Occurs During Capacitation, *J. Reprod. Immunol. 53*, 109–119.
9. Schroepfer, G.J., Jr.(1982) Sterol Biosynthesis, *Ann. Rev. Biochem. 51*, 555–585.

10. Awano, M., Kawaguchi, A., and Mohri, H. (1993) Lipid Composition of Hamster Epididymal Spermatozoa, *J. Reprod. Fertil. 99*, 375–383.

11. Legault, Y., van den Heuvel, W.J., Arison, B.H., Bleau, G., Chapdelaine, A., and Roberts, K.D. (1978) 5alpha-Cholesta-7,24-dien-3betaol as a Major Sterol of the Male Hamster Reproductive Tract, *Steroids 32*, 649–658.

12. Lindenthal, B., Aldaghlas, T.A., Haidl, G., Tolba, R., von Bergmann, K., and Kelleher, J.K. (2000) Cholesterol and Cholesterol Precursors in the Caput and Cauda Epididymidis of Humans and Rats, *Andrologia 32*, 370.

13. Parks, J.E., and Hammerstedt, R.H. (1985) Development Changes Occurring in the Lipids of Ram Epididymal Spermatozoa Plasma Membrane, *Biol. Reprod. 32*, 653–668.

14. Lin, D.S., Connor, W.E., Wolf, D.P., Neuringer, M., and Hachey, D.L. (1993) Unique Lipids of Primate Spermatozoa: Desmosterol and Docosahexaenoic Acid, *J. Lipid Res. 34*, 491–499.

15. Connor, W.E., Lin, D.S., Wolf, P., and Alexander, M. (1998) Uneven Distribution of Desmosterol and Docosahexaenoic Acid in the Heads and Tails of Monkey Sperm, *J. Lipid Res. 39*, 1404–1411.

16. Lindenthal, B., Aldaghlas, T.A., Kelleher, J.K., Henkel, S.M., Tolba, R., Haidl, G., and von Bergmann, K. (2001) Neutral Sterols of Rat Epididymis: High Concentrations of Dehydrocholesterols in Rat Caput Epididymis, *J. Lipid Res. 42*, 1089–1095.

17. Popjak, G., Meenan, A., Parish, E.J., and Nes, W.D. (1989) Inhibition of Cholesterol Synthesis and Cell Growth by 24 (R,S), 25-Iminolanosterol and Triparanol in Cultured Rat Hepatoma Cells, *J. Biol. Chem. 264*, 6230–6238.

18. Lange, Y., Echevarria, F., and Steck, T.L.(1991) Movement of Zymosterol, a Precursor of Cholesterol, Among Three Membranes in Human Fibroblasts, *J. Biol. Chem. 266*, 21439–21443.

19. Roberts, K.D. (1987) Sterol Sulfates in the Epididymis: Synthesis and Possible Function in the Reproductive Process, *J. Steroid. Biochem. 27*, 337–341.

20. Kidroni, G., Har-Nir, R., Menczel, J., Frutkoff, I.W., Palti, Z., and Ron, M. (1983) Vitamin D3 Metabolites in Rat Epididymis: High 24,25-Dihydroxyvitamin D3 Levels in the Cauda Region, *Biochem. Biophys. Acta 113*, 982–989.

21. Walters, M.R., Hunziker, W., and Norman, A.W. (1982) 1,25-Dihydroxyvitamin D3 Receptors: Exchange Assay and Presence in Reproductive Tissues, in *Vitamin D, Chemical, Biochemical and Clinical Endocrinology of Calcium Metabolism*, Walter de Gruyter and Co., Berlin, pp. 91–93.

22. Moody, J.P., Humphries, C.A., Allan, S.M., and Paterson, C.R. (1990) Determination of 7-Dehydrocholesterol in Human Skin by High-Performance Liquid Chromatography, *J. Chromatogr. 530*, 19–27.

23. Burger, K., Gimpl, G., and Fahrenholz, F.(2000) Regulation of Receptor Function by Cholesterol, *Cell. Mol. Life Sci. 57*, 1577–1592.

24. Phillips, J.E., Rodrigueza, W.V., and Johnson, W.J. (1998) Basis for Rapid Efflux of Biosynthetic Desmosterol from Cells, *J. Lipid Res. 39*, 2459–2470.

25. Izumi, A., Pinkerton, F.D., Nelson, S.O., Pyrek, J.S., Neill, P.J., Smith, J.H., and Schroepfer, G.J. Jr. (1994) Inhibitors of Sterol Synthesis. Submicromolar 14 alpha-ethyl-5 alpha-cholest-7-ene-3 beta, 15 alpha-diol Causes a Major Modification of the Sterol Composition of CHO-K1 Cells and a Marked Change in Cell Morphology, *J. Lipid Res. 35*, 1251–1266.

26. Byskov, A. G., Andersen, C.Y., Leonardsen, L., and Baltsen, M. (1999) Meiosis Activating Sterols (MAS) and Fertility in Mammals and Man, *J. Exp. Zool. 285*, 237–242.

Chapter 11

Physiological and Biophysical Properties of Male Germ Cell Sulfogalactosylglycerolipid

Nongnuj Tanphaichitr[a,b,c,*], Maroun Bou Khalil[a,b], Wattana Weerachatyanukul[a], Morris Kates[b], Hongbin Xu[a,b], Euridice Carmona[a], Mayssa Attar[a,b], and Danielle Carrier[b]

[a]Hormones/Growth/Development Research Group, Ottawa Health Research Institute, Ottawa, Ontario, Canada
[b]Department of Biochemistry/Microbiology/Immunology, Faculty of Medicine, University of Ottawa, Ottawa, Ontario, Canada
[c]Department of Obstetrics and Gynecology, Faculty of Medicine, University of Ottawa, Ottawa, Ontario, Canada

Abstract

Sulfogalactosylglycerolipid (SGG) is present in high amounts in spermatogenic cells and sperm. It is synthesized via sulfation of galactosylglycerolipid in early primary spermatocytes, and once synthesized SGG is stable throughout spermatogenesis and sperm maturation and capacitation. Using affinity purified anti-SGG IgG antibody, we have shown by indirect immunofluorescence that SGG is localized in patches to the plasma membranes of spermatogenic cells including primary spermatocytes and round and elongated spermatids, as well as the mature sperm head, the site of zona pellucida binding. In fact, sperm SGG is involved in sperm-zona binding, as anti-SGG-treated sperm have decreased binding to the zona. Furthermore, SGG liposomes specifically bind to the zona. Our FTIR studies reveal that SGG forms lamellar crystalline bilayers that undergo transition to the liquid crystalline phase at a T_{m} of 45°C. SGG interacts with a saturated model phospholipid, dimyristoylglycerophosphorylcholine, as well as natural phospholipids isolated from ram testes, which contain an appreciable level of polyunsaturated fatty acyl chains. This interaction leads to an increase in T_{m} of the hydrocarbon chains melting of the mixed lipid bilayers, indicative of the membrane-stabilizing role of SGG. SGG also interacts with cholesterol and both lipids are components of capacitated sperm rafts, possessing zona-binding ability. Our results therefore demonstrate that SGG contributes to the process of gamete binding as an adhesive molecule and as an ordered lipid participating in the formation of sperm rafts, which may be the zona-binding microdomains on the sperm surface.

Introduction

Sulfogalactosylglycerolipid (SGG), also known as seminolipid, was first described in boar testes and sperm (1) and in rat testes (2) independently by two groups of investigators. TLC revealed a unique R_f of the lipid with positive staining for a sugar moiety. The lipid was also eluted from silicic acid column chromatography with the same solvent used for other glycolipids (1). It reacted with Azure A (1) and rhodizonate (2), which is typical of a sulfatide, and infrared spectroscopy confirmed the presence of a sulfate group of the lipid (1). In a later publication, Kornblatt *et al.* (3) also showed that ^{35}S radiolabel was incorporated into seminolipid following injection of $Na_2{}^{35}SO_4$ into the testis of an adult rat. All of these results indicate that seminolipid is a sulfoglycolipid. Infrared spectroscopy and NMR also demonstrated the presence of a sulfate ester at the equatorial hydroxy-group and the β-anomeric configuration of hexopyranoside (1). Analyses of chemically degraded products of seminolipid revealed that the lipid was composed of an alkylether alcohol, mainly chimyl alcohol (*i.e.,* 1-*O*-hexadecyl glycerol); a fatty acyl chain, mainly 16:0; a galactose residue; and a sulfate residue, in equimolar stoichiometric ratio. Therefore, the chemical structure of seminolipid was concluded to be 1-*O*-alkyl-2-*O*-acyl[β-D-(3′-sulfatoxy)galactopyranosyl(1′-3)]-*sn*-glycerol (Fig.11.1A).

Later work employing gas chromatography, mass spectrometry, NMR and FTIR also revealed the same structure of seminolipid isolated from bovine testes (4) and ram testes (5,6). Simpler nomenclatures have also been used for the lipid, including SGG (our preferred term) or sulfotoxygalactosylalkylacylglycerol (Sulfo-GalAAG). SGG is structurally related to sulfogalactosylceramide (SGC) (or cerebroside sulfate, [β-D-(3′-sulfatoxy)galactopyranosyl]-(1′-1)]-*N*-tetracosanoylsphingosine) (Fig. 11.1B), the main sulfogalactolipid present in mammalian brain and kidney and in testis of lower vertebrates and invertebrates (7). Both lipids have a hydrophilic galactosyl sulfate head group with two hydrocarbon chains; only their backbones differ, SGG with a glycerol backbone and SGC with a sphingosine.

(A)

(B)

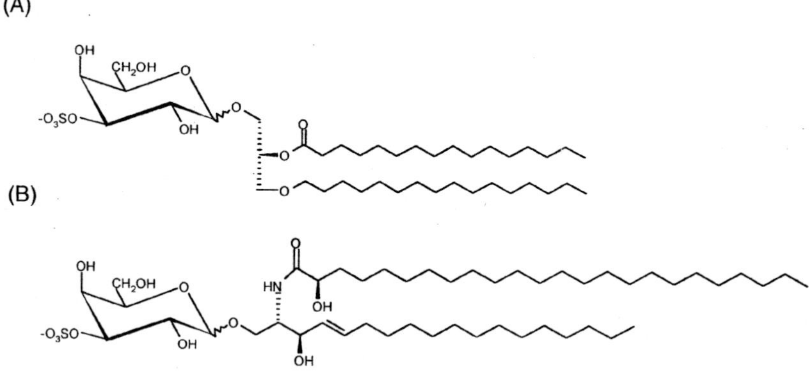

Fig. 11.1. (A) Chemical structure of 1-*O*-hexadecyl-2-*O*-hexadecanoyl-β-D-(3′-sulfatoxy)galactopyranosyl(1′-3)]-*sn*-glycerol (SGG) and (B) [β-D-(3′-sulfatoxy)galactopyranosyl]-1′-1-*N*-tetracosanoylsphingosine (SGC).

Metabolism of SGG: Biosynthesis, Cellular Localization, SGG Binding Protein, and Degradation

Accumulated evidence indicates that SGG is synthesized in spermatogenic cells during spermatogenesis (3,8), which occurs in the testicular seminiferous tubules and involves meiotic division and cell differentiation to form sperm. Temporal development of spermatogenic cells to sperm, *i.e.,* from spermatogonia to early and late primary spermatocytes, secondary spermatocytes, round spermatids, elongated spermatids, and, finally, testicular sperm, occurs with precise kinetics. In rodents, the first wave of spermatogenesis initiates right after birth. Therefore, the number of spermatogenic cells at more advanced developmental stages increases with the age of the neonatal animals. At days 15–20 after birth, the first wave of rat primary spermatocytes has been produced through mitotic division of spermatogonia, which already exist at birth. TLC of isolated testicular glycolipids from these 15–20-day-old rats indicated the first appearance of SGG, suggesting that SGG is synthesized in primary spermatocytes (3). This finding also holds true in adult rats. Intratesticular injection of [^{35}S]sulfate into adult rats results in radiolabeling newly synthesized SGG. Upon fractionation and isolation of early primary spermatocytes, late spermatocytes, and round spermatids from each other on an albumin gradient, early primary spermatocytes show a high degree of ^{35}S incorporation into SGG. ^{35}S is also present in SGG in late primary spermatocytes, although at a much lower level. In contrast, SGG in spermatids shows minimal incorporation of the radiolabel (8). This finding therefore indicates that SGG is preferentially synthesized in early primary spermatocytes and not in spermatids.

Galactosylglycerolipid (GG,β-D-galactopyranosyl-1′-3-sn-glycerol) is present in newborn rats at 15–20 days of age, although at a lower level than SGG, and its level declines dramatically on postnatal day 36 and is minimal in adult rats. In contrast, SGG level remains stable throughout mouse development and into adulthood (3). Intratesticular injection of [^{14}C]palmitate, [^{14}C]galactose, and [^{14}C]cetyl alcohol performed by Hsu *et al.* (9) revealed radioactivity in both GG and SGG, but the radioactivity peak of GG preceded that of SGG. These results suggested that SGG was synthesized from GG via sulfation. As in the sulfation reaction of galactosylceramide (GC, β-D-galactopyranosyl-1′-1-*N*-tetracosanoylsphingosine) to form SGC, catalyzed by a sulfotransferase, 3′-phosphoadenosine-5′-phosphosulfate (PAPS) has been shown to be a sulfate donor for GG sulfation. In fact, sulfotransferase isolated from testes (3,10–12) and other tissues (13,14) can sulfate both GG and GC when PAPS is present in the reaction mixture. Recent results (15) indicate that testicular GG sulfotransferase is encoded by the same gene as that of cerebroside sulfotransferase (CST) present in brain and kidney. *Cst*$^{-/-}$ mice genetically depleted of CST possess no SGC in brain and no SGG in testis. A buildup of GG in *Cst*$^{-/-}$ testes also confirms that GG is the precursor of SGG (15)

Subcellular fractionation of testis homogenate indicates enrichment of GG sulfotransferase in the Golgi apparatus, suggesting that GG sulfation to generate SGG occurs in this organelle (10). The activity of this enzyme is developmentally regulated and is highest at the onset of SGG synthesis (*i.e.,* at the early stage of primary spermatocytes). It then rapidly declines to a low level (9,16) due to the appearance of a small molecular weight inhibitor (17), identified as a glycosyl phosphoinositide (18). This report on the maximum GG sulfotransferase activities in primary spermatocytes corroborates the results described previously that SGG *de novo* synthesis is the highest in these cells.

In the metabolic radiolabeling experiments of Hsu *et al.* (9), a small amount of alkylacylglycerol (AAG) was detected, and therefore AAG was postulated to be galactosylated to form GG. UDP-galactose was presumed to be a galactose donor based on the discerned galactosylation reaction of ceramide to GC, which is catalyzed by ceramide galactosyltransferase (CGT) (19). Recently, *Cgt* null mice have been generated, and in these *Cgt$^{-/-}$* mice, GG is not present in brain nor in testis (20,21). Thus, this indicates that formation of GG from AAG is via the same enzyme responsible for GC formation, and UDP-galactose is also the galactose donor in the GG formation.

Once synthesized in primary spermatocytes, SGG remains stable throughout spermatogenesis (22). The *in vivo* ^{35}S radiolabeling studies indicate that SGG has a very slow turnover rate, with $t_{1/2}$ of 25 days, the same value as the half life of spermatogenic cell DNA radiolabeled with [^{3}H]thymidine. Therefore, this slow decrease of SGG reflects cell death rather than its degradation *per se* (22), and the results corroborate the fact that GG is usually present in a very low amount and that lysoSGG or lysoGG has not been found in testes or fertile adult animals (23). Furthermore, SGG remains stable during sperm transit through the epididymis (22) and is the only glycolipid of freshly ejaculated pig sperm (24). Epididymal mouse sperm with their SGG metabolically labeled with ^{35}S also do not show any SGG desulfation during the initial phase of *in vitro* capacitation in albumin-containing medium (25). The stability of SGG during spermatogenesis and early sperm capacitation suggests that the lipid may be involved in development of spermatogenic cells and egg binding, respectively. However, after a period of incubation in capacitating medium, at which time spontaneous acrosome reaction starts to occur, ~15% of SGG becomes desulfated (25). Physiologically, sperm undergo the acrosome reaction upon binding to the zona pellucida (ZP) (details discussed later), and it remains to be seen whether SGG becomes desulfated when sperm undergo the ZP-induced acrosome reaction.

Among various tissues of adult male rats, including the testis, epididymis, heart, intestine, kidney, liver, lung, spleen, and stomach, only the testis has the ability to synthesize SGG, as shown by the existence of ^{35}S in SGG following intraperitoneal injection of [^{35}S]-sulfate (26). However, a similar experiment performed later by Burkatt *et al.* (27) revealed that the brain also possesses an ability to synthesize SGG. Characterization of brain lipids also reveals the presence of SGG in a small amount (one third of the amount found in the testis as compared per gram wet weight and one fifteenth of the GC amount present in the brain) (23). Indirect immunofluorescence of frozen rat testis sections demonstrates the presence of SGG in pachytene spermatocytes and spermatids but not in spermatogonia and Sertoli cells (28). Similar results have been described by the same investigators with loose spermatogenic cells released from the minced testis. Interestingly, fluorescence staining of SGG is discontinuous, appearing as patches in these cells prefixed with an aldehyde. However, SGG staining was not observed in testicular or epididymal sperm, and this was explained as the antigen being masked (26). In a later publication, the same author described immunofluorescent staining of SGG in the epididymal sperm head but did not explain the discrepancy of the result from his earlier work (29).

We recently produced a polyclonal rabbit anti-SGG IgG antibody using the regimen originally described by Zalc (30), which required frequent and multiple intravenous injections of SGG liposomes without any adjuvant into the animal. By the TLC overlayering technique, we demonstrated that this antibody is monospecific to SGG and SGC, and it does not cross-react with cholesterol sulfate, phospholipids, or monogalactosyldiacylglycerol (31). Using this affinity-purified anti-SGG antibody to perform immunofluorescent studies, we demonstrated that live mouse spermatogenic cells, including primary spermatocytes and round spermatids, show positive staining for SGG with patchy patterns, similar to those described by Lingwood *et al.* (26), although these SGG patches are more separated in primary spermatocytes.

In contrast to Lingwood's previous results, elongating spermatids, testicular sperm, and epididymal sperm are also stained positively for SGG with patchy patterns that are very close to each other (Fig. 11.2A). Since an antibody cannot cross the plasma membrane, our results suggest that SGG is exposed on the plasma membrane of spermatogenic cells and sperm. Our observation also supports the previous finding describing SGG presence in isolated plasma membranes of spermatogenic cells (32). The patchy immunofluorescent staining patterns suggest that SGG molecules might exist in microdomains. In mature sperm, SGG is localized to the head plasma membrane overlying both the acrosomal ridge and the postacrosome (Fig. 11.2B). Notably, these two sperm head entities are the sites to which the ZP binds (33). During the course of these indirect immunofluorescence studies, we noticed that sperm that were left in the medium for a long time could lose reactivity to anti-SGG antibody. This suggests that SGG could be released from the sperm surface when the handling of the sperm suspension is prolonged, and this might explain why Lingwood did not see SGG staining in his first study (28).

At least 20 proteins have been shown to have affinity to SGG and SGC *in vitro* (7). Among these, sulfolipid immobilizing protein 1 (SLIP1) has been the most studied due to its coexistence with SGG in both spermatogenic cells and sperm (29,34). SLIP1 (68 kDa), SLIP2 (34 kDa), and SLIP3 (24 kDa) were first isolated from testis homogenates by SGG affinity column chromatography. Among these three SLIPs, SLIP1 is the major band. Purified SLIP1 has affinity to both SGG and ATP (35,36), and immunoblotting indicates that it is an evolutionarily conserved protein (35). We have shown for the first time that SLIP1 is involved in sperm-egg interaction. Sperm preincubated with anti-SLIP1 antibody have a decreased ability to bind to the egg ZP (37–39), and female mice inseminated with anti-SLIP1-coincubated sperm have a marked decrease in fertilization *in vivo* (40). Further, purified SLIP1 binds to ZP of

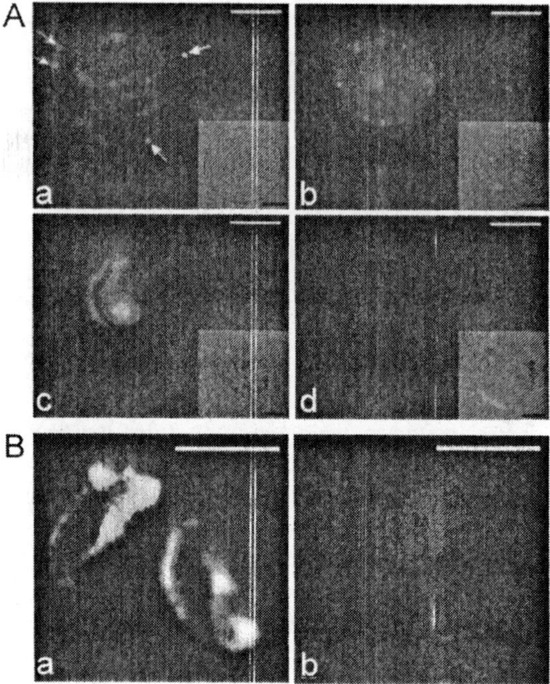

Fig. 11.2. Indirect immunofluorescence (IIF) of isolated primary spermatocytes, round spermatids, elongating spermatids, and caudal epididymal sperm with affinity purified anti-SGG antibody. (A) Primary spermatocytes (a), round spermatids (b) and elongating spermatids (c) were incubated with affinity-purified anti-SGG followed by Alexa-488-conjugated secondary antibody. Round spermatids incubated with pre-immune serum in place of anti-SGG antibody served as a negative control (d). Insets are the corresponding phase-contrast micrographs. Bar = 20 μm. (B) Caudal epididymal sperm were incubated with affinity-purified anti-SGG followed by Alexa-488-conjugated secondary antibody (a). Caudal epididymal sperm incubated with pre-immune serum in place of anti-SGG antibody served as a negative control (b). Bar = 10 μm.

intact eggs (37). SLIP1's physiological significance prompted us and Lingwood to discern its identity. Immunoblotting and tryptic peptide sequencing indicate that SLIP1 consists of three proteins, arylsulfatase A (AS-A), heat shock protein 70 (Hsp70), and albumin (41–43). Both AS-A and Hsp70 have been confirmed in their specific binding to SGG (43–45), but the binding of albumin to SGG may be nonspecific. Albumin also does not have any affinity to ZP. Therefore, attention has been focused mainly on AS-A and Hsp70.

Our accumulated work has conclusively shown that AS-A exists on the sperm surface and is the ZP binding component of SLIP1 (46–48). Preincubation of sperm with antiAS-A IgG/Fab inhibits sperm binding to the ZP in a dose-dependent manner.

Purified AS-A (formerly referred to as P68) at 10 nM could inhibit sperm-ZP binding to the minimal level. In contrast, whereas purified recombinant Hsp70 can also competitively inhibit sperm-ZP binding, it is effective at a high concentration (>50 μM), and the highest inhibition is only 50% of the control values (our unpublished results). Presently, it is unclear what the function of Hsp70 is in fertilization. Recently we showed that AS-A on the sperm surface originates from the epididymal fluid. Testicular sperm do not possess AS-A on their surface, although the enzyme is present in the acrosome. Principal cells, the major epididymal epithelial cells, synthesize AS-A, which is then secreted into the epididymal fluid. The AS-A in the fluid deposits onto the sperm surface via its high affinity to SGG (our unpublished data). Hsp70 is also present in the epididymal fluid (49) and presumably deposits onto the sperm surface, as shown by immunogold labeling studies (43), via the same mechanism. In essence, SGG may function in capturing proteins that are beneficial to sperm fertilizing ability, and thus its presence on the sperm surface may be crucial to the epididymal sperm maturation process.

Functions of SGG in Spermatogenesis and Fertilization

Several lines of evidence indicate the involvement of glycolipids in cell-cell adhesion (50,51), and SGG may also be involved in this event, particularly in gamete interaction, which occurs in a stepwise manner. Acrosome intact sperm first bind to the ZP, the egg extracellular matrix, via receptor-ligand interaction mechanisms. Whereas only one or two ZP sulfoglycoproteins are involved in sperm binding (52,53), a number of ZP-binding molecules have been described on the sperm surface (54–56). It is possible that these molecules may act together or in sequence in ZP binding and they can be backups for each other to an extent (57). Following their initial binding to the ZP, sperm are induced to acrosome react by the ZP sulfoglycoprotein. This is initiated by fusion between the plasma membrane overlying the acrosome and the outer acrosomal membrane, leading to a release of the acrosomal contents, which mainly consist of hydrolases. These soluble enzymes can digest the ZP and create a path for sperm to migrate through the ZP layer into the perivitelline space. Finally, acrosome reacted sperm bind to the egg plasma membrane and one is incorporated into the egg proper, signifying that fertilization has occurred (58,59).

As described above, SGG is localized to the convex ridge and postacrosome on the mouse sperm head plasma membrane, the sites engaged in ZP binding (33). This prompted us to investigate the role of SGG in sperm-ZP binding. Pretreatment of both mouse and human capacitated sperm with various concentrations of anti-SGG IgG or Fab resulted in a dose-dependent decrease in ZP binding (31,60) (Fig. 11.3A). Furthermore, inclusion of SGG liposomes in the sperm-egg coincubates reduced sperm binding to the ZP. When liposomes of 3-*sn*-glycerolphosphorylserine (PS) (negatively charged like SGG) or GG liposomes were used in place of SGG liposomes for gamete coincubation, there was no inhibition of sperm-egg binding, which indicated the specificity of SGG in this binding event (Fig. 11.3B). Finally, SGG lipo-

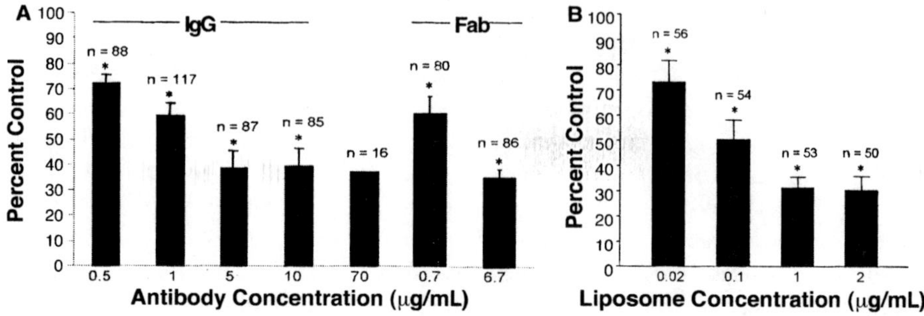

Fig. 11.3. Inhibition of mouse sperm-ZP binding by pretreatment of sperm with affinity-purified anti-SGG IgG or Fab (A) and by exogenous SGG liposomes (B). Except for data regarding the 70 μg/mL anti-SGG IgG sample, all data are expressed as mean ± SD of percentage control of averages from three or more experiments. Sperm-ZP coincubates (in a 60μL droplet) treated with PS liposomes (2 μg) served as a control. All liposomes used were unilamellar (diameter, 200 nm). n = Total number of eggs analyzed for each sample; * significant difference, as compared with controls. Taken with permission from White *et al.* (31).

somes, fluorescently labeled by including a small amount of *N*-rhodamine-conjugated 3-*sn*-glycerolphosphorylethanolamine (*N*-Rh-PE) during preparation showed direct binding to ZP of intact eggs and to isolated ZP, whereas PS and GG liposomes bound minimally to the ZP (Fig. 11.4). These results indicate that the sulfate group of the galactosyl moiety of SGG is essential for its binding to ZP, although this binding is not merely dependent on electrostatic interaction. All of our observations described herein indicate that SGG on the sperm surface plays an important role in ZP binding. This binding is specific to unfertilized eggs; once the eggs are fertilized, SGG no longer binds to their ZP (31).

At the present time, it is not clear how SGG interacts with the ZP sulfoglycoprotein(s). Having high affinity to AS-A, which is also involved in ZP binding, SGG and AS-A may act together as complexes in this binding event. These complexes as stated above would comprise a high molar ratio of SGG to AS-A. As discussed in the section below, these SGG/AS-A complexes are components of sperm raft membranes, being in a liquid ordered state due to the presence of cholesterol, which interacts with SGG and saturated phospholipids. This liquid-ordered property on the sperm raft domains might be beneficial for the interaction with ZP, and capacitated sperm rafts in fact have ZP binding ability (61). Being a peripheral plasma membrane sulfatase, AS-A may first bind to the sulfated sugar residues present in the distal part of the ZP glycans (the moieties that are involved in sperm binding). This will capture the ZP glycans next to the sperm surface, allowing carbohydrate-carbohydrate interaction between the glycans and the galactosyl sulfate moieties of SGG that extend only a short distance above the sperm plasma membrane bilayers. Although this carbohy-

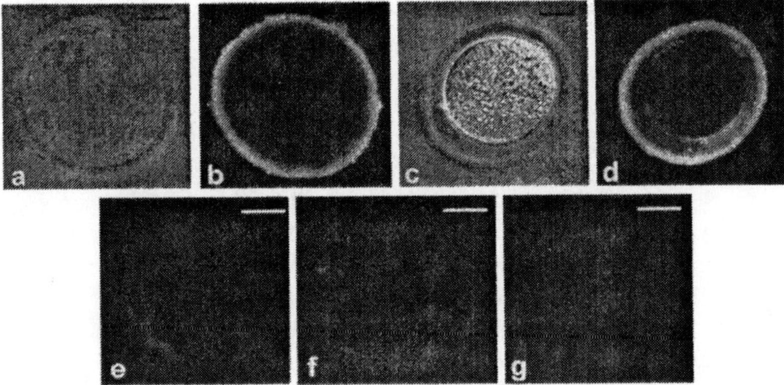

Fig. 11.4. Fluorescent staining of isolated ovarian ZP, unfertilized zona-intact eggs by fluorescently labeled SGG liposomes. The ZP (panels a and b) and unfertilized zona-intact eggs (panels c and d) were incubated with SGG/*N*-Rh-PE liposomes; unfertilized zona-intact eggs were incubated with PS/*N*-Rh-PE (panel e) liposomes, GG/*N*-Rh-PE (panel f,) or SGG/*N*-Rh-PE with SGG/PE (200x concentration of SGG/*N*-Rh-PE) (panel g). All panels are fluorescent micrographs, except for panels a and c, which are corresponding phase-contrast micrographs of panels b and d, respectively. Note fluorescent staining of the isolated ZP and the ZP and plasma membrane of unfertilized eggs exposed to SGG/*N*-Rh-PE (panels b and d), whereas eggs incubated with other liposomes did not show fluorescent staining. Bar = 20 μm. Taken with permission from White *et al.* (31).

drate-carbohydrate interaction is not very strong, it is stabilized by the multiplicity of SGG molecules. This postulated function of SGG in cell-cell adhesion is analogous to the involvement of gangliosides in cell adhesion events, including interaction between trout sperm and egg (50,51,62).

In acrosome reacted sperm, SGG is localized mainly to the plasma membrane overlying the postacrosomal region (our unpublished results). The plasma membrane at the beginning of the postacrosomal region is known to be involved in binding to and fusing with the egg plasma membrane (58). Sperm treated with anti-SGG IgG/Fab have reduced ability to bind to the plasma membrane of zona-free eggs, suggesting the importance of SGG in this sperm-egg plasma membrane binding event (63). The mechanism of sperm surface SGG-egg plasma membrane binding is different from that of SGG-ZP interaction. Immunofluorescence of live zona-free eggs reveals the presence of AS-A (*i.e.*, SLIP1, an SGG binding protein) on the egg plasma membrane (63). SGG on the sperm postacrosomal surface would bind to the egg plasma membrane AS-A because of their mutual high affinity (44). This postulation is supported by the finding that zona-free eggs pretreated with anti-SLIP1 have minimal ability to bind to sperm (63).

SGG may also be involved in cell signaling events in sperm. ZP sulfoglycoprotein induces the acrosome reaction following its initial binding to its receptors on the sperm surface (58). The currently accepted concept states that this induction is via ZP receptor aggregation due to the multivalency of sperm binding moieties of the ZP glycans (64). This aggregation leads to activation of sperm signaling events via Gi_α protein. Finally, calcium influx occurs, thus initiating the membrane fusion events of the acrosome reaction. Since there exists a number of ZP receptors, this aggregation-induced acrosome reaction has to be demonstrated using a ZP mimetic, *i.e.,* a specific binding ligand of the receptor that is also multivalent. AS-A, the SGG binding protein, is a dimer at physiological pH (47,65,66). Therefore, it is an ideal surrogate for the sperm receptor, ZP sulfoglycoprotein. Purified AS-A, when added to mature mouse sperm, binds to the sperm head exactly at the same sites where SGG is present, and the binding does not occur when sperm are pretreated with anti-SGG (44). The results suggest that purified AS-A binds to sperm via its affinity to SGG present on the sperm surface. Interestingly, treatment of both mouse and human sperm with purified AS-A at the amount equal to that existing on the sperm surface induces the acrosome reaction, and this results in drastic decreases in sperm binding to the ZP as well as fertilization *in vivo* (44). This treatment causes neither SGG desulfation nor changes sperm lipid composition. Therefore, the acrosome reaction induction is not via AS-A's enzymatic activity. On the other hand, this may be due to the tight binding of the AS-A dimers to SGG molecules, existing in multiplicity on the sperm surface (48). The binding would then lead to SGG sequestration and activation of signal transduction. SGG relocalization on the sperm plasma membrane has in fact been previously described (67,68).

Our results indicating the significance of SGG in fertilization corroborate previous findings that development of anti-SGG antibody in women is a cause of infertility (69) and that SGG and SGC are engaged in cell-cell adhesion. For the latter aspect, SGG has been described to have direct binding to gp120, the surface glycoprotein of HIV-1 (70,71,72), as well as infertility-induced mycoplasmas (73). The interactions of sperm surface SGG with these pathogenic microbials and viruses (46) may be a basis for the spread of sexually transmitted diseases (STD). Thus, our observations on tight binding of exogenous AS-A to SGG, leading to premature acrosome reaction and inhibition of gamete binding, may have promising application in contraception and STD prevention. AS-A or its mimicry may be used as a vaginal nonhormonal contraceptive that can also prevent the spread of STD. SGG and SGC have also been shown to bind *in vitro* to several extracellular proteins involved in cell adhesion, including L-selectin, laminin, thrombospondin, von Willebrand factor, and circumsporozoite proteins, the major surface proteins of malaria sporozoites (74–76). However, the physiological relevance of these interactions, particularly to male reproduction, is still unclear.

SGG is also important for development of spermatogenic cells into sperm. Spermatogenic cells organize themselves in the seminiferous tubules in a precise manner. Spermatogonia are localized above the basal membrane underneath the tight junctions of Sertoli cells, which span from the basal membrane to the lumen. Developing spermatogenic cells are in the adluminal compartment of Sertoli cells, above the tight junctions, with the more advanced stages closer to the lumen. In fact, elongated spermatids impregnate their heads into the Sertoli cell cytoplasm at the apical membrane region. Once the germ cells are fully developed into testicular sperm, they are then ejected from Sertoli cells into the lumen. Apparently, interactions among male germ cells themselves and between them and Sertoli cells are important during spermatogenesis (77).

As described above, both $Cgt^{-/-}$ and $Cst^{-/-}$ mice show complete absence of SGG in their testes. Both of these knockout male mice are infertile with clear evidence of spermatogenesis disruption; development of spermatogenic cells is arrested in the pachytene stage. Apoptosis occurs in these arrested spermatocytes, although spermatogonia and Sertoli cells appear to be normal (15,20). A higher amount of GG accumulated in the testes of $Cst^{-/-}$ mice, as compared to wild type mice, does not rescue this spermatogenesis arrest. All of these results indicate the high significance of SGG on the spermatogenic cell surface in spermatogenesis. The mechanism of SGG involvement in this process is still not clear. SGG may interact with cell surface proteins of spermatogenic and Sertoli cells, and this interaction may be essential for the development of spermatogenic cells beyond the primary spermatocyte stage. Perhaps, these proteins could be testicular SLIPs that Lingwood (34) has described previously.

Biophysical Properties of SGG

The involvement of glycolipids as cell surface recognition sites and as membrane structural elements has been documented (50,78). General functions of glycolipids in membranes include stabilization, shape determination, and recognition, as well as ion binding by the negatively charged glycolipids (79,80). Being commercially available, GC and its sulfate ester, SGC, have been extensively studied (81–85) and have served as structural analogs of SGG, the major sulfoglycolipid of the mammalian male germ cell. Like other glycolipids, SGG is expected to contribute to the biophysical properties of the male germ cell, and knowledge of its conformational properties and dynamics may provide a better understanding of the ZP adhesion function of SGG. Therefore, we have employed FTIR spectroscopy to elucidate the biophysical properties of SGG and its structural analogs, SGC and GC. The use of FTIR spectroscopy is advantageous because it gives detailed information on the molecular vibrations of individual structural groups of biological molecules without any need for an external probe (86,87).

The structural properties of GC, SGG's analog, were first explored by x-ray crystallography, revealing that the galactose head group of GC is oriented parallel to the bilayer plane. This conformation involves extensive lateral interactions via hydrogen bonding between the amide groups of the ceramide backbone of GC and its galactosyl hydroxyl groups, thus imparting greater bilayer stability (88). Pascher and colleagues (88,89) suggested that the α-hydroxy fatty acid in GC increases hydrogen bonding and gives rise to a locked/shovel conformation of the GC molecule with respect to the hydrocarbon chain axis (88,89,90). No crystal structures of SGC have been reported to date, but differential scanning calorimetry (DSC) indicates that the α-hydroxy fatty acid of SGC increases the phase transition temperature of the glycolipid, suggesting that it contributes to bilayer stability by participating in interfacial hydrogen bonding (91), a concept that was consolidated by our pressure tuning FTIR spectroscopic studies revealing extensive hydrogen bonding networks of SGC (81).

Like SGC, SGG is also well endowed with galactosyl hydroxyl groups, and these groups are expected to engage in hydrogen bonding, bringing stability to lipid bilayers. Moreover, the acyl and alkyl moieties of SGG isolated from different mammalian testes are predominantly 16:0 (4–6). Thus, the saturated character of SGG would allow tight packing of the hydrocarbon chains in the bilayer matrix. The phase behavior of SGG, SGC, and GC was investigated by pressure tuning and temperature dependent FTIR spectroscopy. Our results reveal that the hydrocarbon chains of hydrated SGG/SGC bilayers are interdigitated (5), a phenomenon that was also observed for crystalline SGC (83) and GC (90). This interdigitation would result in the formation of dense, near crystalline bilayers of SGG and SGC. Temperature dependent FTIR experiments also indicate that SGG (Fig. 11.5A), like SGC and GC, exhibits a relatively high T_m in aqueous dispersions, as well as engages in strong inter-molecular hydrogen bonding, which results in an increased stability of the bilayers (5,6,81,84,85). This high interfacial hydrogen bonding decreases the rotational disorder of both SGG (6) and SGC/GC (85), thereby promoting the formation of ordered, lamellar crystalline bilayers. Spectral changes indicated that the formation of the lamellar crystalline structures of SGG, SGC, and GC was accompanied by partial dehydration and by rearrangements of the hydrogen bonding network and bilayer packing modes (85).

The negatively charged sulfate group of SGG has the potential to bind cations on the sperm surface, and this binding may be of importance in the sequential events leading to fertilization. Ca^{2+} has been shown to be present on the sperm surface (92). Among numerous divalent cations present in the female reproductive tract fluid, Ca^{2+} appears to be necessary for various activities of mammalian sperm. These include (i) capacitation, which involves biochemical modification of the sperm plasma membrane in preparation for egg binding and the acrosome reaction (93,94); (ii) acquisition of hyperactivated motility patterns of capacitated sperm (58,95); (iii) sperm acrosome reaction, which results in the release of the hydrolytic enzymes of the acrosome, essential for sperm penetration through the egg extracellular matrix (96,97); (iv) sperm binding to the zona pellucida, the egg extracellular matrix of sulfoglycoproteins (98); and (v) sperm-egg membrane fusion (58,99).

Sulfoglycolipids, such as SGG and SGC, have been proposed to participate in cation transport (100,101). This proposal was further strengthened by our pressure tuning FTIR spectroscopic studies, revealing that the divalent cation Ca^{2+} binds to the sulfate moiety of SGC (81) and SGG (5), most likely cross-linking neighboring sulfo-glyoclipid molecules. Moreover, the presence of Ca^{2+} ions abolishes the interdigitated state of SGG bilayers, thus increasing the orientational disorder of the hydrocarbon

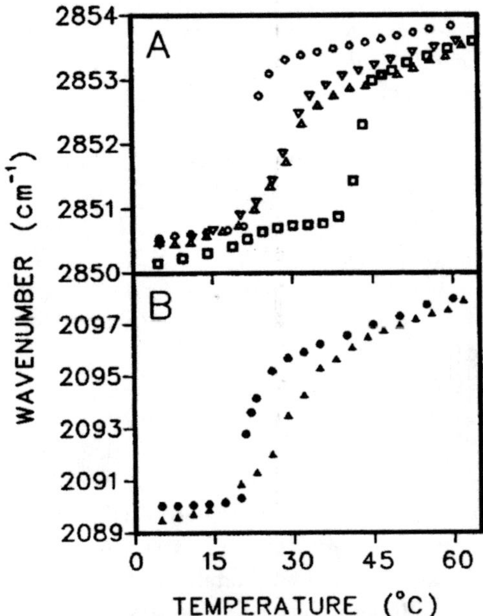

Fig. 11.5. (A) FTIR temperature profiles of DMPC (○), SGG (□), and mixed bilayers containing DMPC + SGG (molar ratio 3:2) (▽) or DMPC$_{d54}$ + SGG (molar ratio 3:2) (△) in the CH$_2$ (2850–2854 cm^{-1}) symmetric stretching region. (B) FTIR temperature profile of DMPC$_{d54}$ (●) and mixed DMPC$_{d54}$ + SGG (molar ratio 3:2) (▲) in the CD$_2$ (2089-2099 cm^{-1}) symmetric stretching region. The wave numbers of the CH$_2$ and CD$_2$ symmetric stretching vibrations were recorded as a function of temperature, and their frequencies were obtained after Fourier derivation of the original FTIR spectra with a power of 3 and a breakpoint of 0.3. Modified from Attar *et al.* (6).

chains of SGG. Such a phenomenon may result in increased bilayer fluidity, as previously proven relevant to fertilization-related events, *e.g.*, capacitation and acrosome reaction (102).

For a better understanding of the contribution of SGG to the biophysical properties of the mammalian male germ cell, the interaction of SGG with dimyristoylglycerophosphorylcholine (DMPC, 1,2-ditetradecanoyl-*sn*-glycerophosphorylcholine) model membranes was investigated by FTIR spectroscopy (6). The CH$_2$ symmetric stretching vibration was monitored as a function of temperature. The hydrocarbon chains are in the *trans* conformation in the gel phase and shift to higher frequencies when lipid bilayers undergo a transition from the gel phase into the relatively disordered/fluid liquid-crystalline phase (103). FTIR spectroscopic analysis showed that the gel to liquid-crystalline phase transition of DMPC and mixed DMPC + SGG bilayers (molar ratio 3:2) were 24 and 28°C, respectively (Fig. 11.5A). The higher T_m of the mixed bilayers implies that the mixed DMPC + SGG bilayers are more conformationally ordered than corresponding DMPC bilayers. These results indicated that SGG increased the stability of DMPC model membranes. This was further confirmed in an analogous set of FTIR spectroscopic experiments, in which perdeuterated DMPC ($DMPC_{d54}$) was used in mixtures with SGG. The temperature dependence of the frequency of the methylene symmetric C-H (~ 2850 cm^{-1}) and C-D (~ 2090 cm^{-1}) stretching vibration bands allows us to monitor the conformation of the lipid hydrocarbon chains of SGG and $DMPC_{d54}$ specifically in the mixed liposomes. In the mixed $DMPC_{d54}$ + SGG bilayers (molar ratio 3:2) the T_m of $DMPC_{d54}$ and SGG were both 29°C, between that of $DMPC_{d54}$ (21°C) and SGG (45°C) (Fig. 11.5). This confirmed that the hydrocarbon chains of SGG truly contributed to the observed T_m of 28°C in the mixed DMPC + SGG bilayers (Fig. 11.5A), and strengthened our findings that SGG directly imparts stability to DMPC model membranes. The saturated hydrocarbon chains of SGG (16:0) and DMPC favor the formation of tightly packed bilayers due to the strong van der Waals interaction among them. Moreover, the galactosylsulfate moiety of SGG might play an important role at the interfacial region, engaging in hydrogen bonding (5) and thus bringing further stability to DMPC bilayers.

Besides possessing SGG, mammalian male germ cells are noted for their content of polyunsaturated fatty acid containing phospholipids (46,104,105,106,107). Although our results reveal the membrane stabilizing role of SGG in DMPC bilayers, the coexistence of SGG with testicular/sperm phospholipids, containing polyunsaturated fatty acyl chains, raises the question of whether this stabilizing effect of SGG still prevails in highly fluid phospholipid bilayers. Therefore, we employed FTIR spectroscopy to elucidate the contribution of SGG to the conformational properties of ram testicular phospholipids. While the temperature profile of testicular total phospholipids showed a gel to liquid crystalline phase transition at 20°C, that of total testicular lipids displayed a T_m near 26°C (Fig. 11.6). This was reflective of the higher order status of testicular total lipids compared to total phospholipids. Since SGC and SGG form intermolecular hydrogen bonding (5,81) and increase the stability of DMPC model membranes (6,84), the increased order of testicular total lipids, compared to testicular phospholipids, may be attributable to SGG. In fact, mixed total testicular phospholipids + SGG bilayers showed an increase in T_m compared to total testicular phospholipids. At 10 mole percent SGG, the mixed bilayers displayed a broad phase transition with a T_m near 26°C, similar to that of the total testicular lipids (Fig.11.6). As was found for the mixed DMPC + SGG bilayers (Fig. 11.5), the present results demonstrate that SGG stabilizes testicular phospholipid bilayers and increases the ordering of the hydrocarbon chains, despite their appreciable content of unsaturated fatty acyl chains. This was revealed by the observed increase in T_m and by the lower frequencies of the CH_2 symmetric stretching band of the SGG containing bilayers, compared to testicular total phospholipids alone (Fig. 11.6).

Cholesterol is an important membrane component of animal cells, including male germ cells (108,109). In an attempt to mimic the nature of the mammalian male germ cell plasma membrane, we generated mixed testicular phospholipids + SGG + cholesterol bilayers (molar ratio 6.8:1:2.2) using the molar ratio determined from our quanti-

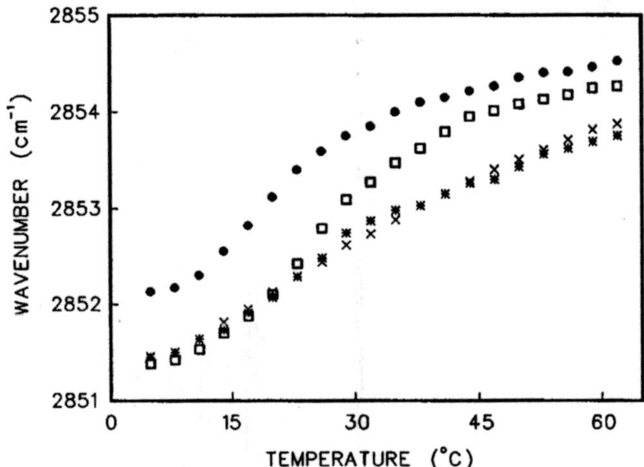

Fig. 11.6. FTIR temperature profiles of total testicular phospholipids (●), isolated total testicular lipids (*), and mixed bilayers containing testicular phospholipids + SGG (molar ratio 9:1) (□) and phospholipids + SGG + cholesterol bilayers (molar ratio 6.8:1: 2.2) (×). The wave number of the CH_2 symmetric stretching vibration was recorded as a function of temperature, and its frequency was obtained after Fourier derivation of the original FTIR spectra with a power of 3 and a breakpoint of 0.3.

tative colorimetric or fluorometric analysis of phospholipids with SGG and cholesterol in the same testicular lipid extract. The mixed testicular phospholipids + SGG + cholesterol bilayers (molar ratio of 6.8:1:2.2) exhibit a phase transition near 26°C, a value higher than the T_m of total testicular phospholipids (20°C) but similar to that of aqueous dispersions of isolated total testicular lipids (Fig. 11.6). These model membranes, consisting of isolated testicular phospholipids, SGG, and cholesterol, are physiologically relevant and reveal that SGG imparts stability to testicular phospholipids enriched in unsaturated fatty acids. Significantly, the T_m of ram testicular total lipids reported here (26°C) is similar to that previously reported for mammalian whole sperm, isolated sperm plasma membrane, and reconstituted sperm lipid bilayers (109,110), which suggests that lipids govern the phase behavior of male germ cells. Therefore, our findings revealing the stabilizing effects of SGG on isolated testicular phospholipids (containing appreciable levels of polyunsaturated fatty acids) should hold true for plasma membranes of male germ cells.

Accumulated evidence from studies employing cell biological and biophysical approaches suggests that there is selective segregation of lipids and proteins in discrete regions of the membrane, termed rafts (111,112). Initially, Simons and colleagues (113,114) showed that glycosphingolipid-rich patches exist in the Golgi and that apical membrane proteins (*e.g.*, glycosylphosphatidylinositol (GPI)-linked proteins) associate with the lipids for packaging into vesicles for transport to the apical plasma membrane. Independently, cholesterol- and glycosphingolipid-rich detergent resistant membranes (DRM) containing GPI-linked proteins were isolated from mammalian cells as a low density, light scattering band following discontinuous sucrose gradient ultracentrifugation (111). These findings support the model proposed by Simons and colleagues (113,114) and reveal the correlation between the formation of rafts in situ and DRM. Since glycosphingolipids play important roles in cell adhesion and signaling (78,115), rafts have been proposed to engage in these events. This was further supported by the discovery that rafts are enriched in cell adhesion and signaling molecules (50,116).

Simons and Ikonen (112) proposed that cholesterol is recruited to rafts due to its ability to fill gaps in the bilayer created by the discrepancy in size between the large glycosphingolipid headgroups and their acyl chains. Raft lipids have been proposed to exist in a separate phase from the rest of the bilayer, in a state similar to the liquid-ordered, cholesterol-enriched phase described in model membranes (117,118). In the liquid-ordered phase, the acyl chains of lipids are extended and tightly packed with cholesterol, similar to those in the gel phase but nevertheless laterally diffuse in the plane of the membrane (119). Thus, lipid structural features (such as acyl chains) that enhance formation of the gel phase can also enhance formation of the liquid-ordered phase when mixed with cholesterol (118). The saturated character of SGG and its extensive hydrogen-bonding network among themselves and with cholesterol may promote phase separation and formation of liquid-ordered domains in the presence of testicular phospholipids (enriched in unsaturated fatty acids). Significantly, our indirect immunofluorescence experiments reveal that SGG exists in clusters on the sperm head (Fig. 11.2). SGC (SGG's analog) was also shown to be enriched in sea urchin sperm rafts (120), and these rafts bind to egg rafts via carbohydrate-carbohydrate mediated interactions (121). Being a structural analog of SGC, SGG may also exist in mammalian sperm rafts. Our preliminary results support this postulation (61). We have shown that SGG and cholesterol are integral components of mammalian sperm rafts isolated as low density Triton X-100 insoluble domains, and our FTIR spectroscopic data revealed a strong interaction between SGG and cholesterol. SGG and its binding protein, AS-A, coexist in mammalian sperm rafts, which have ZP binding ability (61). Therefore, SGG may contribute to fertilization both by participating in the formation of mammalian sperm rafts through its strong interaction with cholesterol, an integral raft component, and by acting as a ZP adhesion molecule in these rafts

Acknowledgments

The authors wish to thank Ms. Terri van Gulik for her assistance in manuscript preparation. This work is supported by grants from CIHR (MT 10366) and from NSERC (183958) to Nongnuj Tanphaichitr. Maroun Bou Khalil is a recipient of Ontario Graduate Studentship in Science and Technology (OGSST) and Ontario Graduate Scholarship (OGS), respectively. Wattana Weerachatyanukul was a recipient of a graduate study fellowship from National Science and Technology Development Agency of Thailand.

References

1. Ishizuka, I., Suzuki, M., and Yamakawa, T. (1973) Isolation and Characterization of a Novel Sulfoglycolipid, Seminolipid, from Boar Testis and Spermatozoa, *J. Biochem. 73*, 77–87.

2. Kornblatt, M.J., Schachter, H., and Murray, R.K. (1972) Partial Characterization of a Novel Glycerogalactolipid from Rat Testis, *Biochem. Biophys. Res. Commun. 48*, 1489–1494.

3. Kornblatt, M.J., Knapp, A., Levine, M., Schachter, H., and Murray, R.K. (1974) Studies on the Structure and Formation during Spermatogenesis of the Sulfoglycerogalactolipid of Rat Testis, *Can. J. Biochem. 52*, 689–697.

4. Alvarez, J.G., Storey, B.T., Hemling, M.L., and Grob, R.L. (1990) High-Resolution Proton Nuclear Magnetic Resonance Characterization of Seminolipid from Bovine Spermatozoa, *J. Lipid Res. 31*, 1073–1081.

5. Tupper, S., Wong, P.T.T., Kates, M., and Tanphaichitr, N. (1994) Interaction of Divalent Cations with Germ Cell Specific Sulfogalactosylglycerolipid and the Effects on Lipid Chain Dynamics, *Biochemistry 33*, 13250–13258.

6. Attar, M., Kates, M., Bou Khalil, M., Carrier, D., Wong, P.T.T., and Tanphaichitr, N. (2000) A Fourier-Transform Infrared Study of the Interaction Between Germ-Cell Specific Sulfogalactosylglycerolipid and Dimyristoylglycerophosphocholine, *Chem. Phys. Lipids 106*, 101–114.

7. Vos, J.P., Lopes-Cardozo, M.G., and Gadella, B.M. (1994) Metabolic and Functional Aspects of Sulfogalactolipids, *Biochim. Biophys. Acta 1211*, 125–149.

8. Letts, P.J., Hunt, R.C., Shirley, M.A., Pinteric, L., and Schachter, H. (1978) Late Spermatocytes from Immature Rat Testis: Isolation, Electron Microscopy, Lectin Agglutinability, and Capacity for Glycoprotein and Sulfogalactoglycerolipid Biosynthesis, *Biochim. Biophys. Acta 541*, 59–75.

9. Hsu, L.H., Narasimhan, R., and Levine, M. (1983) Studies of the Biosynthesis and Metabolism of Rat Testicular Galactoglycerolipids, *Can. J. Biochem. Cell Biol. 61*, 1272–1281.

10. Knapp, A., Kornblatt, M.J., Schachter, H., and Murray, R.K. (1973) Studies on the Biosynthesis of Testicular Sulfoglycerogalactolipid: Demonstration of a Golgi-Associated Sulfotransferase Activity, *Biochem. Biophys. Res. Commun. 55*, 179–186.

11. Handa, S., Yamoto, K., Ishizuka, I., Suzuki, A., and Yamakawa, T. (1974) Biosynthesis of Seminolipid: Sulfation *in Vivo* and *in Vitro*, *J. Biochem. 75*, 77–83.

12. Sakac, D., Zachos, M., and Lingwood, C.A. (1992) Purification of the Testicular Galactolipid: 3′-Phosphoadenoisine 5′-Phosphosulfate Sulfotransferase, *J. Biol. Chem. 267*, 1655–1659.

13. Honke, K., Yamane, M., Ishii, A., Kobayashi, T., and Makita, A. (1996) Purification and Characterization of 3′-Phosphoadenosine-5′-Phosphosulfate:GalCer Sulfotransferase from Human Renal Cancer Cells, *J. Biochem. 119*, 421–427.

14. Honke, K., Tsuda, M., Hirahara, Y., Ishii, A., Makita, A., and Wada, Y. (1997) Molecular Cloning and Expression of cDNA Encoding Human 3′-Phosphoadenyl-ylsulfate:Galactosylceramide 3′-Sulfotransferase, *J. Biol. Chem. 272*, 4864–4868.

15. Honke, K., Hirahara, Y., Dupree, J., Suzuki, K., Popko, B., Fukushima, K., Fukushima, J., Nagasawa, T., Yoshida, N., Wada, Y., and Taniguchi, N. (2002) Paranodal Junction Formation and Spermatogenesis Require Sulfoglycolipids, *Proc. Natl. Acad. Sci. U.S.A. 99*, 4227–4232.

16. Lingwood, C.A. (1985) Developmental Regulation of Galactoglycerolipid and Galactosphingolipid Sulphation during Mammalian Spermatogenesis: Evidence for a Substrate-Selective Inhibitor of Testicular Sulphotransferase Activity in the Rat, *Biochem. J. 231*, 393–400.

17. Lingwood, C.A. (1985) Timing of Sulphogalactolipid Biosynthesis in the Rat Testis Studied by Tissue Autoradiography, *J. Cell Sci. 75*, 329–338.

18. Lingwood, C., Sakac, K., and Saltiel, A. (1994) Developmentally Regulated Testicular Galactolipid Sulfotransferase Inhibitor is a Phosphoinositol Glycerolipid and Insulin-Mimetic, *Mol. Reprod. Dev. 37*, 462–466.

19. Morell, P., and Radin, N.S. (1969) Synthesis of Cerebroside by Brain from Uridine Diphosphate Galactose and Ceramide Containing Hydroxy Fatty Acid, *Biochemistry 8*, 506–512.

20. Fujimoto, H., Tadano-Aritomi, K., Tokumasu, A., Ito, K., Hikita, T., Suzuki, K., and Ishizuka, I. (2000) Requirement of Seminolipid in Spermatogenesis Revealed by UDP-Galactose:Ceramide Galactosyltransferase-Deficient Mice, *J. Biol. Chem. 275*, 22623–22626.

21. Coetzee, T., Fujita, N., Dupree, J., Shi, R., Blight, A., Suzuki, K., and Popko, B. (1996) Myelination in the Absence of Galactorcerebroside and Sulfatide: Normal Structure with Abnormal Function and Regional Instability, *Cell 86*, 209–219.

22. Kornblatt, M.J. (1979) Synthesis and Turnover of Sulfogalactoglycerolipid, a Membrane Lipid, during Spermatogenesis, *Can. J. Biochem. 57*, 255–258.

23. Murray, R.K., and Narasimhan, R. (1990) Glycoglycerolipids of Animal Tissues, in *Glycolipids, Phosphoglycolipids, and Sulfoglycolipids*, Kates, M. (Ed.), Plenum Press, New York, pp. 321–361.

24. Gadella, B.M., Colenbrander, B., Van Golde, L.M.G., and Lopes-Cardozo, M. (1993) Boar Seminal Vesicles Secrete Arylsulfatases into Seminal Plasma: Evidence that Desulfation of Seminolipid Occurs only after Ejaculation, *Biol. Reprod. 48*, 483–489.

25. Tanphaichitr, N., Smith, J., and Kates, M. (1990) Levels of Sulfogalactosylglycerolipid in Capacitated Motile and Immotile Mouse Sperm, *Biochem. Cell Biol. 68*, 528–535.

26. Lingwood, C.A., Hay, G., and Schachter, H. (1981) Tissue Distribution of Sulfolipids in the Rat. Restricted Location of Sulfatoxygalactosylacylalkylglycerol, *Can. J. Biochem. 59*, 556–563.

27. Burkart, T., Caimi, L., Herschkowitz, N.N., and Wiesmann, U.N. (1983) Metabolism of Sulfogalactosyl Glycerolipids in the Myelinating Mouse Brain, *Dev. Biol. 98*, 182–186.

28. Lingwood, C.A. (1981) Localization of Sulfatoxygalactosylacylalkylglycerol at the Surface of Rat Testicular Germinal Cells by Immunocytochemical Techniques: pH Dependence of a Nonimmunological Reaction Between Immunoglobulin and Germinal Cells, *J. Cell Biol. 89*, 621–630.

29. Lingwood, C.A. (1986) Colocalization of Sulfogalactosylacylalkylglycerol (SGG) and Its Binding Protein During Spermatogenesis and Sperm Maturation. Topology of SGG Defines a New Testicular Germ Cell Membrane Domain, *Biochem. Cell Biol. 64*, 984–992.

30. Zalc, B., Jacque, C., Radin, N.S., and Dupouey, P. (1977) Immunogenicity of Sulfatide, *Immunochem. 14*, 775–779.

31. White, D., Weerachatyanukul, W., Gadella, B., Kamolvarin, N., Attar, M., and Tanphaichitr, N. (2000) Role of Sperm Sulfogalactosylglycerolipid in Mouse Sperm-Zona Pellucida Binding, *Biol. Reprod. 63*, 147–155.

32. Shirley, M.A., and Schachter, H. (1980) Enrichment of Sulfogalactosylalkylacylglycerol in a Plasma Membrane Fraction from Adult Rat Testis, *Can. J. Biochem. 58*, 1230–1239.

33. Kerr, C.L., Hanna, W.F., Shaper, J.H., and Wright, W.W. (2002) Characterization of Zona Pellucida Glycoprotein 3 (ZP3) and ZP2 Binding Sites on Acrosome-Intact Mouse Sperm, *Biol. Reprod. 66(6)*, 1585–1595.

34. Lingwood, C.A. (1985) Protein-Glycolipid Interactions during Spermatogenesis. Binding of Specific Germ Cell Proteins to Sulfatoxygalactosylacylalkylglycerol, the Major Glycolipid of Mammalian Male Germ Cells, *Can. J. Biochem. Cell Biol. 63*, 1077–1085.

35. Law, H., Itkonnen, O., and Lingwood, C.A. (1988) Sulfogalactolipid Binding Protein SLIP1: A Conserved Function for a Conserved Protein, *J. Cell. Physiol. 137*, 462–468.

36. Lingwood, C.A., and Nutikka, A. (1991) Studies on the Spermatogenic Sulfogalactolipid Binding Protein SLIP1, *J. Cell. Physiol. 146*, 258–263.

37. Tanphaichitr, N., Smith, J., Mongkolsirikieart, S., Gradil, C., and Lingwood, C. (1993) Role of a Gamete Specific Sulfoglycolipid-Immobilizing Protein on Mouse Sperm-Egg Binding, *Dev. Biol. 156*, 164–175.

38. Moase, C.E., Kamolvarin, N., Kan, F.W.K., and Tanphaichitr, N. (1997) Localization and Role of Sulfoglycolipid Immobilizing Protein 1 on the Mouse Sperm Head, *Mol. Reprod. Dev. 48*, 1–11.

39. Rattanachaiyanont, M., Weerachatyanukul, W., Leveille, M.-C., Taylor, T., D'Amours, D., Rivers, D., Leader, A., and Tanphaichitr, N. (2001) Anti-SLIP1-Reactive Proteins Exist on Human Sperm and Are Involved in Zona Pellucida Binding, *Mol. Human Reprod. 7*, 633–640.

40. Tanphaichitr, N., Tayabali, A., Gradil, C., Juneja, S., Leveille, M.C., and Lingwood, C. (1992) Role of Germ Cell-Specific Sulfolipidimmobilizing Protein (SLIP1) in Mouse *in Vivo* Fertilization, *Mol. Reprod. Dev. 32*, 17–22.

41. Tanphaichitr, N., Moase, C., Taylor, T., Surewicz, K., Hansen, C., Namking, M., Bérubé, B., Kamolvarin, N., Lingwood, C.A., Sullivan, R., Rattanachaiyanont, M., and White, D. (1998) Isolation of Anti-SLIP1-Reactive Boar Sperm P68/62 and Its Binding to Mammalian Zona Pellucida, *Mol. Reprod. Dev. 49*, 203–216.

42. Tanphaichitr, N., White, D., Taylor, T., Attar, M., Rattanachaiyanont, M., and Kates, M. (1999) Role of Male Germ-Cell Specific Sulfogalactosylglycerolipid (SGG) and Its Binding Protein, SLIP1, in Mammalian Sperm-Egg Interaction, in *The Male Gamete: From Basic Knowledge to Clinical Applications*, Gagnon, C., Cache Press, Vienna, IL, pp. 227–235.

43. Boulanger, J., Faulds, D., Eddy, E.M., and Lingwood, C.A. (1995) Members of the 70 kDa Heat Shock Protein Family Specifically Recognize Sulfoglycolipids: Role in Gamete Recognition and Mycoplasma-Related Infertility, *J. Cell. Physiol. 165*, 7–17.

44. Carmona, E., Weerachatyanukul, W., Xu, H., Fluharty, A.L., Anupriwan, A., Shoushtarian, A., Chakrabandhu, K., and Tanphaichitr, N. (2002) Binding of Arylsulfatase A to Mouse Sperm Inhibits Gamete Interaction and Induces the Acrosome Reaction, *Biol. Reprod. 66*, 1820–1827.

45. Mamelak, D., and Lingwood, C. (2001) The ATPase Domain of hsp70 Possesses a Unique Binding Specificity for 3'-Sulfogalactolipids, *J. Biol. Chem. 276*, 449–456.

46. Flesch, F.M., and Gadella, B.M. (2000) Dynamics of the Mammalian Sperm Plasma Membrane in the Process of Fertilization, *Biochim. Biophys. Acta 1469*, 197–235.

47. Carmona, E., Weerachatyanukul, W., Soboloff, T., Fluhary, A.L., White, D., Promdee, L., Ekker, M., Berger, T., Buhr, M., and Tanphaichitr, N. (2002) Arylsulfatase A is Present on the Pig Sperm Surface and Is Involved in Sperm-Zona Pellucida Binding, *Dev. Biol. 247*, 182–196.

48. Tantibhedhyangkul, J., Weerachatyanukul, W., Carmona, E., Xu, H., Anupriwan, A., Michaud, D., and Tanphaichitr, N. (2002) Role of Sperm Sufrace Arylsulfatase A in Mouse Sperm-Zona Pellucida Binding, *Biol. Reprod. 67*, 212–219.

49. Miller, D., Brough, S., and al-Harbi, O. (1992) Characterization and Cellular Distribution of Human Spermatozoal Heat Shock Proteins, *Hum. Reprod. 7*, 637–645.

50. Hakomori, S. (2000) Cell Adhesion/Recognition and Signal Transduction Through Glycosphingolipid Microdomain, *Glycoconj. J. 17*, 143–151.

51. Hakomori, S. (2000) Traveling for the Glycosphingolipid Path, *Glycoconj. J. 17*, 627–647.

52. Dunbar, B.S., Timmons, T.M., Skinner, S.M., and Prasad, S.V. (2001) Molecular Analysis of a Carbohydrate Antigen Involved in the Structure and Function of Zona Pellucida Glycoproteins, *Biol. Reprod. 65*, 951–960.

53. Prasad, S.V., Skinner, S.M., Carino, C., Wang, N., Cartwright, J., and Dunbar, B.S. (2000) Structure and Function of the Proteins of the Mammalian Zona Pellucida, *Cells Tissues Organs 166*, 148–164.

54. Dell, A., Morris, H.R., Easton, R.L., Patankar, M., and Clark, G.F. (1999) The Glycobiology of Gametes and Fertilization, *Biochim. Biophys. Acta 1473*, 196–205.

55. Wassarman, P.M. (1999) Mammalian Fertilization: Molecular Aspects of Gamete Adhesion, Exocytosis, and Fusion, *Cell 96*, 175–183.

56. Wassarman, P.M., and Litscher, E.S. (2001) Towards the Molecular Basis of Sperm and Egg Interaction during Mammalian Fertilization, *Cells Tissues Organs 168*, 36–45.

57. Jansen, S., Ekhlassi-Hundrieser, M., and Topfer-Petersen, E. (2001) Sperm Adhesion Molecules: Structure and Function, *Cells Tissues Organs 168*, 82–92.

58. Yanagimachi, R. (1994) Mammalian Fertilization, in *The Physiology of Reproduction*, Knobil, E., and Neill, J.E., Raven Press Ltd., New York,, pp. 189–317.

59. Primakoff, P., and Myles, D.G. (2002) Penetration, Adhesion, and Fusion in Mammalian Sperm-Egg Interaction, *Science 296*, 2183–2185.

60. Weerachatyanukul, W., Rattanachaiyanont, M., Carmona, E., Furimsky, A., Mai, A., Shoushtarian, A., Sirichotiyakul, S., Ballakier, H., Leader, A., and Tanphaichitr, N. (2001) Sulfogalactosylglycerolipid Is Involved in Human Gamete Interaction, *Mol. Reprod. Dev. 60(4)*, 569–578.

61. Bou Khalil, M., Chakrabandhu, K., Carmona, E., Xu, H., Vuong, N., Kamarasathan, P., da Silva, S., Carrier, D., Wong, P., and Tanphaichitr, N. (2002) Pig Sperm Raft Membranes Have Zona Pellucida Binding Ability and Contain Male Germ Cell Specific Sulfogalactosylglycerolipid (SGG) and Arylsulfatase A (AS-A), *Biol. Reprod. 66 Suppl 1*, 72 Abstract 432.

62. Yu, S., Kojima, N., Hakomori, S.I., Kudo, S., Inoue, S., and Inoue, Y. (2002) Binding of Rainbow Trout Sperm to Egg Is Mediated by Strong Carbohydrate-to-Carbohydrate Interaction Between (KDN) GM3 (deaminated neuraminyl ganglioside) and Gg3-like Epitope, *Proc. Natl. Acad. Sci. U.S.A. 99*, 2854–2859.

63. Ahnonkitpanit, V., White, D., Suwajanakorn, S., Kan, F., Namking, M., Wells, G., and Tanphaichitr, N. (1999) Role of Egg Sulfolipidimmobilizing Protein 1 (SLIP1) on Sperm-Egg Plasma Membrane Binding, *Biol. Reprod. 61*, 749–756.

64. Leyton, L., and Saling, P. (1989) Evidence that Aggregation of Mouse Sperm Receptors by ZP3 Triggers the Acrosome Reaction, *J. Cell Biol. 108*, 2163–2168.

65. Lukatela, G., Krauss, N., Theis, K., Selmer, T., Gieselmann, V., von Figura, K., and Saenger, W. (1998) Crystal Structure of Human Arylsulfatase A: The Aldehyde Function and the Metal Ion at the Active Site Suggest a Novel Mechanism for Sulfate Ester Hydrolysis, *Biochemistry 37*, 3654–3664.

66. Rahi, H., and Srivastava, P.N. (1983) Isolation and Characterization of the Pig Endometrial Arylsulphatase A, *Biochem. J. 211*, 649–659.

67. Gadella, B.M., Gadella, T.W.J., Colenbrander, B., Van Golde, L.M., and Lopes-Cardozo, M. (1994) Visualization and Quantification of Glycolipid Polarity Dynamics in the Plasma Membrane of the Mammalian Spermatozoon, *J. Cell Sci. 107*, 2151–2163.

68. Gadella, B.M., Lopes-Cardoza, M., van Golde, L.M.G., Colenbrander, B., and Gadella, T.W.J.J. (1995) Glycolipid Migration from the Apical to the Equatorial Subdomains of the Sperm Head Plasma Membrane Precedes the Acrosome Reaction, *J. Cell Sci. 108*, 935–945.

69. Tsuji, Y., Fukuda, H., Iuchi, A., Ishizuka, I., and Isojima, S. (1992) Sperm Immobilizing Antibodies React to the 3-*O*-Sulfated Galactose Residue of Seminolipid on Human Sperm, *J. Reprod. Immunol. 22*, 225–236.

70. Harouse, J.M., Bhat, S., Spitalnik, S.L., Laughlin, M., Stefano, K., Silberberg, D.H., and Gonzalez-Scarano, F. (1991) Inhibition of Entry of HIV-1 in Neural Cell Lines by Antibodies Against Galactosyl Ceramide, *Science 253*, 320–323.

71. Gadella, B.M., Hammache, D., Pieroni, G., Colenbrander, B., van Golde, L.M.G., and Fantini, J. (1998) Glycolipids as Potential Binding Sites for HIV: Topology in the Sperm Plasma Membrane in Relation to the Regulation of Membrane Fusion, *J. Reprod. Immunol. 41*, 233–253.

72. Piomboni, P., and Baccetti, B. (2000) Spermatozoon as a Vehicle for HIV-1 and Other Viruses: A Review, *Mol. Reprod. Dev. 56 Suppl 2*, 238–242.

73. Lingwood, C., Schramayr, S., and Quinn, P. (1990) Male Germ Cell Specific Sulfogalactoglycerolipid is Recognized and Degraded by Mycoplasmas Associated with Male Infertility, *J. Cell. Physiol. 142*, 170–176.

74. Suzuki, Y., Toda, Y., Tamatani, T., Watanabe, T., Suzuki, T., Nakao, T., Murase, K., Kiso, M., Hasegawa, A., Tadano-Aritomi, K., Ishizuka, I., and Miyasaka, M. (1993) Sulfated Glycolipids Are Ligands for a Lymphocyte Homing Receptor, L-selectin (LECAM-1), Binding Epitope in Sulfated Sugar Chain, *Biochem. Biophys. Res. Commun. 190*, 426–434.

75. Roberts, D.D., and Ginsburg, V. (1988) Sulfated Glycolipids and Cell Adhesion, *Arch. Biochem. Biophys. 267*, 405–415.

76. Pancake, S.J., Holt, G.D., Mellouk, S., and Hoffman, S.L. (1993) Malaria Sporozoites and Circumsporozoite Protein Bind Sulfated Glycans: Carbohydrate Binding Properties Predicted from Sequence Homologies with Other Lectins, *Parassitologia 35*, 77–80.

77. Sharpe, R.M. (1994) Regulation of Spermatogenesis, in *The Physiology of Reproduction*, Knobil, E., and Neill, J.D., Raven Press Ltd., New York,, pp. 1363–1434.

78. Hakomori, S. (1990) Bifunctional Role of Glycosphingolipids, *J. Biol. Chem. 265*, 18713–18716.

79. Curatolo, W. (1987) Glycolipid Function, *Biochim. Biophys. Acta 906*, 137–160.

80. Curatolo, W. (1987) The Physical Properties of Glycolipids, *Biochim. Biophys. Acta 906*, 111–136.

81. Tupper, S., Wong, P.T.T., and Tanphaichitr, N. (1992) Binding of Ca^{2+} to Sulfogalactosylceramide and the Sequential Effects on the Lipid Dynamics, *Biochemistry 31*, 11902–11907.

82. Haas, N.S., and Shipley, G.G. (1995) Structure and Properties of *N*-Palmitoleoylgalacto-sylsphingosine (Cerebroside), *Biochim. Biophys. Acta 1240*, 133–141.

83. Nabet, A., Boggs, J.M., and Pézolet, M. (1996) Study by Infrared Spectroscopy of the Interdigitation of C26:0 Cerebroside Sulfate into Phosphatidylcholine Bilayers, *Biochemistry 35*, 6674–6683.

84. Attar, M., Wong, P.T.T., Kates, M., Carrier, D., Jaklis, P., and Tanphaichitr, N. (1998) Interaction Between Sulfogalactosylceramide and Dimyristoylphosphatidylcholine Increases the Orientational Fluctuations of the Lipid Hydrocarbon Chains, *Chem. Phys. Lipids 94*, 228–238.

85. Bou Khalil, M., Carrier, D., Wong, P.T.T., and Tanphaichitr, N. (2001) Polymorphic Phases of Galactocerebrosides: Spectroscopic Evidence of Lamellar Crystalline Structures, *Biochim. Biophys. Acta 1512*, 158–170.

86. Wong, P.T.T., Siminovitch, D.J., and Mantsch, H.H. (1988) Structure and Properties of Model Membranes: New Knowledge from High-Pressure Vibrational Spectroscopy, *Biochim. Biophys. Acta 947*, 139–171.

87. Lewis, R.N.A.H., and McElhaney, R.N. (1990) Subgel Phases of *n*-Saturated Diacylphosphatidylcholines: A Fourier-Transform Infrared Spectroscopic Study, *Biochemistry 29*, 7946–7953.

88. Pascher, I., and Sundell, S. (1977) Molecular Arrangements in Sphingolipids. The Crystal Structure of Cerebroside, *Chem. Phys. Lipids 20*, 175–191.

89. Nyholm, P., Pascher, I., and Sundell, S. (1990) The Effect of Hydrogen Bonds on the Conformation of Glycosphingolipids. Methylated and Unmethylated Cerebroside Studied by X-ray Single Crystal Analysis and Model Calculations, *Chem. Phys. Lipids 52*, 1–10.

90. Bunow, M.R., and Levin, I.W. (1980) Molecular Conformations of Cerebrosides in Bilayers Determined by Raman Spectroscopy, *Biophys. J. 32*, 1007–1022.

91. Boggs, J.M., Koshy, K.M., and Rangaraj, G. (1988) Influence of Structural Modifications on the Phase Behavior of Semi-Synthetic Cerebroside Sulfate, *Biochim. Biophys. Acta 938*, 361–372.

92. Ruknudin, A. (1989) Cytochemical Study of Intracellular Calcium in Hamster Spermatozoa during the Acrosome Reaction, *Gamete Res. 22*, 375–384.

93. Kaul, G., Singh, S., Gandhi, K.K., and Anand, S.R. (1997) Calcium Requirement and Time Course of Capacitation of Goat Spermatozoa Assessed by Chlortetracycline Assay, *Andrologia 29*, 243–251.

94. Fraser, L.R. (1998) Sperm Capacitation and Acrosome Reaction, *Hum. Reprod. 13 Suppl 1*, 9–19.

95. Suarez, S., Varosi, S.M., and Dai, X. (1993) Intracellular Calcium Increases with Hyperactivation in Intact, Moving Hamster Sperm and Oscillates with the Flagellar Beat Cycle, *Cell Biol. 90*, 4660–4664.

96. Fraser, L.R. (1993) Calcium Channels Play a Pivotal Role in the Sequence of Ionic Changes Involved in Initiation of Mouse Sperm Acrosomal Exocytosis, *Mol. Reprod. Dev. 36*, 368–376.

97. Tomes, C.N., Michaut, M., De Blas, G., Visconti, P., Matti, U., and Mayorga, L.S. (2002) SNARE Complex Assembly Is Required for Human Sperm Acrosome Reaction, *Dev. Biol. 243*, 326–338.

98. Saling, P.M., Wolf, D.P., and Storey, B.T. (1978) Calcium-Dependent Binding of Mouse Epididymal Spermatozoa to the Zona Pellucida, *Dev. Biol. 65*, 515–525.

99. Fraser, L.R. (1987) Minimum and Maximum Extracellular Ca^{2+} Requirements during Mouse Sperm Capacitation and Fertilization *in Vitro, J. Reprod. Fertil. 81*, 77–89.

100. Hakomori, S.I. (1981) Glycosphingolipids in Cellular Interaction, Differentiation, and Oncogenesis, *Ann. Rev. Biochem. 50*, 733–764.

101. Karlsson, K.A., Samuelsson, B.E., and Steen, G.O. (1974) The Lipid Composition and Na^+/K^+-Dependent Adenosine-Triphosphatase Activity of the Salt (Nasal) Gland of Eider Duck and Herring Gull: A Role for Sulphatides in Sodium-Ion Transport, *Eur. J. Biochem. 46*, 243–258.

102. Wolf, D., Hagopian, S., and Ishijima, S. (1986) Changes in Sperm Plasma Membrane Lipid Diffusibility after Hyperactivation during *in Vitro* Capacitation in the Mouse, *J. Cell Biol. 102*, 1372–1377.

103. Mantsch, H.H., and McElhaney, R.N. (1991) Phospholipid Phase Transitions in Model and Biological Membranes as Studied by Infrared Spectroscopy, *Chem. Phys. Lipids 57*, 213–226.

104. Beckman, J.K., Gray, M.E., and Coniglio, J.G. (1978) The Lipid Composition of Isolated Rat Spermatids and Spermatocytes, *Biochim. Biophys. Acta 530*, 367–374.

105. Grogan, W.M., Franham, W.F., and Szopiak, B.A. (1981) Long-Chain Polyenoic Acid Levels in Viably Sorted, Highly Enriched Mouse Testis Cells, *Lipids 16*, 401–410.

106. Grogan, W.M., and Huth, E.G. (1983) Biosynthesis of Long-Chain Polyenoic Acids from Arachidonic Acid in Cultures of Enriched Spermatocytes and Spermatids from Mouse Testis, *Lipids 18*, 275–284.

107. Cooper, T.G., and Yeung, C.-H. (1997) Physiology of Sperm Maturation and Fertilization, in *Andrology: Male Reproductive Health and Dysfunction*, Nieschlag, E., and Behre, H.M., Springer-Verlag, Berlin Heidelberg, pp. 61–78.

108. Nikolopoulou, M., Soucek, D., and Vary, J. (1985) Changes in the Lipid Content of Boar Sperm Plasma Membranes during Epididymal Maturation, *Biochim. Biophys. Acta 815*, 486–498.

109. Parks, J.E., and Lynch, D.V. (1992) Lipid Composition and Thermotropic Phase Behavior of Boar, Bull, Stallion, and Rooster Sperm Membranes, *Cryobiology 29*, 255–266.

110. Wolf, D.E., Maynard, V.M., McKinnon, C.A., and Melchior, D.L. (1990) Lipid Domains in the Ram Sperm Plasma Membrane Demonstrated by Differential Scanning Calorimetry, *Proc. Natl. Acad. Sci. U.S.A. 87*, 6893–6896.

111. Brown, D.A., and Rose, J.K. (1992) Sorting of GPI-Anchored Proteins to Glycolipid-Enriched Membrane Subdomains during Transport to the Apical Cell Surface, *Cell 68*, 533–544.

112. Simons, K., and Ikonen, E. (1997) Functional Rafts in Cell Membranes, *Nature 387*, 569–572.

113. Simons, K., and van Meer, G. (1988) Lipid Sorting in Epithelial Cells, *Biochemistry 1988*, 27.

114. Van Meer, G., Stelzer, E.H.K., Wijnaendts-van-Resandt, R.W., and Simons, K. (1987) Sorting of Sphingolipids in Epithelial (Mardin-Darby Canine Kidney) Cells, *J. Cell Biol. 105*, 1623–1635.

115. Hakomori, S.-I., Yamamura, S., and Handa, K. (1998) Signal Transduction Through Glyco(sphingo)lipids, *Ann. NY Acad. Sci. 845*, 1–10.

116. Iwabuchi, K., Yamamura, S., Prinetti, A., Handa, K., and Hakomori, S. (1998) GM3-Enriched Microdomain Involved in Cell Adhesion and Signal Transduction through Carbohydrate-Carbohydrate Interaction in Mouse Melanoma B16 Cells, *J. Biol. Chem. 273*, 9130–9138.

117. Brown, D.A., and London, E. (1998) Structure and Origin of Ordered Lipid Domains in Biological Membranes, *J. Membrane Biol. 164*, 103–114.

118. Schroeder, R., London, E., and Brown, D. (1994) Interactions Between Saturated Acyl Chains Confer Detergent Resistance On Lipids and Glycosylphosphatidylinositol (GPI)-Anchored Proteins: GPI-Anchored Proteins in Liposomes and Cells Show Similar Behavior, *Proc. Natl. Acad. Sci. U.S.A. 91*, 12130–12134.

119. Sankaram, M.B., and Thompson, T.E. (1990) Modulation of Phospholipid Acyl Chain Order by Cholesterol. A Solid-State ^{2}H Nuclear Magnetic Resonance Study, *Biochemistry 29*, 10676–10684.

120. Ohta, K., Sato, C., Matsuda, T., Toriyama, M., Lennarz, W., and Kitajima, K. (1999) Isolation and Characterization of Low-Density Detergent-Insoluble Membrane (LD-DIM) Fraction from Sea Urchin Sperm, *Biochem. Biophys. Res. Commun. 258*, 616–623.

121. Ohta, K., Sato, C., Matsuda, T., Norohashi, N., Lennarz, W.J., and Kitajima, K. (1999) Egg Receptor for Sperm Binds to Gangliosides in the Low-Density Detergent-Insoluble Membrane (LD-DIM) Domain of the Sperm Surface. Possible Involvement of the LD-DIM in Sperm-Egg Binding Coupled with Signal Transduction during Fertilization, *Glycoconj. J. 16*, S63 Abstract.

Chapter 12

Regulation of Oxytocinase Activity in the Testis by Dietary Lipids

M.J. Ramírez-Expósito, M.J. García-López, M.D. Mayas, M.P. Carrera, and J.M. Martínez-Martos

Department of Health Sciences, Physiology Laboratory, University of Jaén, Spain

Abstract

The nonapeptide hormone oxytocin (OTX) is locally synthesized in the testis, where it may act as autocrine/paracrine factor regulating the metabolism of androgens and, consequently, take a part in the regulatory mechanisms of male fertility. Oxytocinase (cystinyl aminopeptidase) activity hydrolyzes and inactivates OTX, reflecting the functional status of its substrate. It has been proposed that dietary lipids affect fertility in mammals. Previous studies have demonstrated that cholesterol, sex steroids, and the type and amount of fatty acids used in the diet affect several aminopeptidase activities in serum and several tissues. In the present work, we describe the influence of several polyunsaturated and saturated oils and cholesterol in the diet on oxytocinase activity in the soluble and membrane-bound fractions of testis in mice. The results demonstrated higher levels of oxytocinase activity in mice fed the diet supplemented with polyunsaturated oils than in those that were fed diets containing saturated oils. Higher levels of oxytocinase activity were also found in mice fed the cholesterol-enriched diet. Thus, the type and amount of dietary lipids modifies oxytocinase activity in the testis, probably through the action of their fatty acid content but also through their influence on cholesterol metabolism. These changes on oxytocinase activity modify the OTX degradation rate and, therefore, alter the testicular functions in which OTX is involved.

Introduction

Classically, it has been described that the nonapeptide hormone oxytocin (OTX) is synthesized in the hypothalamus and secreted by the posterior pituitary, its functions being related to parturition and lactation. However, we now recognize that OTX exerts a wide spectrum of central and peripheral effects. Thus, the actions of OTX range from the modulation of neuroendocrine reflexes to the establishment of complex social and bonding behaviors related to the reproduction and care of offspring. Overall, OTX and its structurally related peptides facilitate the reproduction in all vertebrates at several levels (1). In this way, it is now well established that OTX is locally synthesized in the testis, where it may act as autocrine/paracrine factor regulating the metabolism of androgens and, consequently, take a part in the regulatory mechanisms of male fertility (2,3). The balance between OTX synthesis and its degradation determines the availability of this bioactive peptide (4). Oxytocinase (also called cystinyl aminopeptidase, EC 3.4.11.3), hydrolyzes and inactivates OTX (5). Therefore, the study of this enzymatic activity may reflect the functional status of its substrate.

It has been proposed that dietary fatty acid composition affects fertility in mammals (6,7). However, the mechanisms that underlie this effect remain unclear. Some studies have suggested that the use of n-3 polyunsaturated fatty acids in the diet may improve male and female fertility in mammals (6). In contrast, low levels of n-3 together with the simultaneous high levels of n-6 polyunsaturated fatty acids in sperm could be involved in male infertility (8). Previous studies have demonstrated that cholesterol, sex steroids (9), and the type and amount of fatty acids used in the diet (10–12) affect several aminopeptidase activities in serum and several tissues. In the present work, we describe the effects of the use of several polyunsaturated (olive oil and fish oil) and saturated oils (lard and coconut oils) in the diet on oxytocinase activity in the soluble and membrane-bound fractions of testis of mice. Cholesterol can modulate OTX receptor function by changing both membrane fluidity and direct binding effects (13); therefore, the effect of a high cholesterol diet was also investigated. The modifications found on oxytocinase activity clearly indicate a role in testicular function.

Material and Methods

Experiment 1

Twelve male Balb/C mice (13 days old) were used in this experiment. Six animals were fed a high-fat diet containing 20% virgin olive oil (20% protein, 49.58% carbohydrates, 5% non-nutritive bulk, and 20% olive oil), whereas the other six animals were fed a low-fat diet (14.6% protein, 48.4% carbohydrates, 18.6% non-nutritive bulk, and 2.4% unspecified oil) (10). All animals were fed for ten weeks and were allowed access to water and food *ad libitum*. After this time, the animals were perfused with saline through the left cardiac ventricle under equithensin anaesthesia, and samples from the right testis (interstitial area and seminiferous tubules) were quickly removed and processed as described below.

Experiment 2

Male Balb/C mice, 1–2 weeks old and weighing 11–14 g at the start of the study, were used. Three groups of animals were fed with isocaloric diets containing 2.4% of the respective experimental oil: fish oil (*n* = 10), lard (*n* = 10), and coconut oil (*n* = 9) (12). All mice were fed during 10 weeks and were allowed free access to water and food. After the feeding period, the animals were perfused with saline through the left cardiac ventricle under equithensin anaesthesia and samples from the right testis (interstitial area and seminiferous tubules) were quickly removed and processed as described below.

Experiment 3

Twenty adult male Balb/C mice were used in this study. Ten animals with a body weight of 26.8 g (SEM 1.01) were fed a standard diet containing 15.6% of protein, 2.8% of fat, and 55% of carbohydrate (control groups). Ten other animals, 27.1 g (SEM 0.93) body weight, were fed the same diet enriched with cholesterol 1% and cholic acid 0.5% (cholesterol group). All animals were fed during 15 days and allowed access to water and food *ad libitum*. After this time, the animals were perfused with saline through the left cardiac ventricle under equithensin anaesthesia and samples from the right testis (interstitial area and seminiferous tubules) were quickly removed and processed as described below.

In all the experiments, the mice were housed at constant temperature (25°C) with a constant light/dark cycle of 12 h/12 h. The experimental procedures for animal use and care were in accordance with the European Community Council Directive (86/609/EEC).

Sample Preparation

To obtain the soluble fraction, tissue samples were homogenized in 10 volumes of 10 mM HCl-Tris buffer (pH 7.4) and ultracentrifuged at $100,000 \times g$ for 30 min (4°C). The resulting supernatants were used to measure soluble enzymatic activity and protein content, assayed in triplicate. To solubilize membrane proteins, the pellets were rehomogenized in HCl-Tris buffer (pH 7.4) plus 1% Triton X-100. After centrifugation ($100,000 \times g$, 30 min, 4°C) the supernatants were used to measure solubilized membrane-bound activity and proteins, also in triplicate. To ensure complete recovery of activity, the detergent was removed from the medium by adding adsorbent polymeric Biobeads SM-2 (100 mg/ml) (Bio-Rad, Richmond, CA) to the samples and shaking for 2 h at 4°C.

Oxytocinase Activity Assay

Oxytocinase activity was measured fluorimetrically using cystinyl-β-naphthylamide (CysNNap) as the substrate as previously described (14). Briefly, 10 μL of each supernatant were incubated for 30 min at 37°C with 1 mL of the substrate solution containing 100 μM CysNNap, 1.5 mM bovine serum albumin (BSA), and 0.65 mM dithiothreitol (DTT) in 50 mM of phosphate buffer, pH 7.4. The reactions were stopped by adding 1 mL of 0.1 M acetate buffer, pH 4.2. The amount of β-naphthylamine released as a result of the enzymatic activity was measured fluorimetrically at 412 nm emission wavelength with an excitation wavelength of 345 nm. Proteins were quantified in triplicate by the method of Bradford using BSA as a standard. Specific soluble and membrane-bound oxytocinase activities were expressed as nmol of CysNNap hydrolyzed per min per mg of protein by using a standard curve prepared with the latter compound under corresponding assay conditions. The fluorogenic assay was linear with respect to time of hydrolysis and protein content.

Results

In experiment 1, specific soluble oxytocinase activity was significantly increased in the testis ($P < 0.01$), whereas membrane-bound oxytocinase activity did not differ between the two groups (Fig. 12.1). It is interesting to note that serum total cholesterol concentration was significantly higher (by 13.4%; $P < 0.05$) in the olive oil group than in control mice.

For experiment 2, specific soluble and membrane-bound oxytocinase activities in the testis of mice fed the different diets are shown in Figure 12.2. Soluble oxytocinase activity progressively decreased ($P < 0.001$) depending on the degree of saturation of the fatty acid used in the diet. The order of activities were fish oil > lard oil > coconut oil.

In experiment 3, specific soluble and membrane-bound oxytocinase activities in the testis of mice fed a high cholesterol diet are shown in Figure 3. Both soluble and membrane-bound oxytocinase activity increased significantly ($P < 0.05$ and $P < 0.001$, respectively) in the cholesterol-fed group. Serum total cholesterol levels increased by 44% ($P < 0.001$) in the cholesterol-fed group.

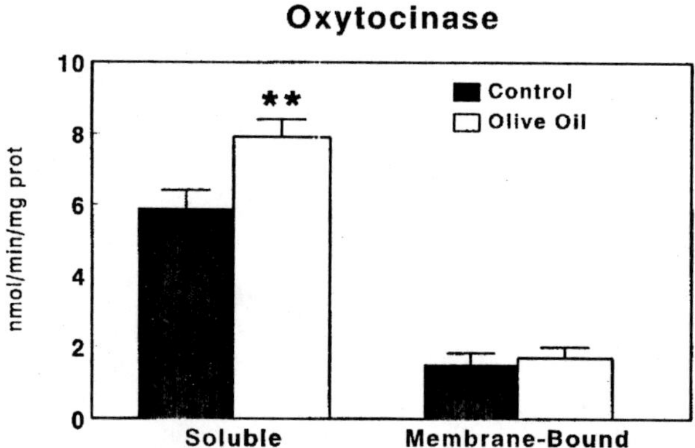

Fig. 12.1. Specific soluble and membrane-bound oxytocinase activities in testis of control and olive oil fed animals. Results are expressed as nmol of cystinyl-ß-naphthylamide hydrolyzed per min and per mg of proteins (mean with SEM error bars; $n = 6$; **$P < 0.01$).

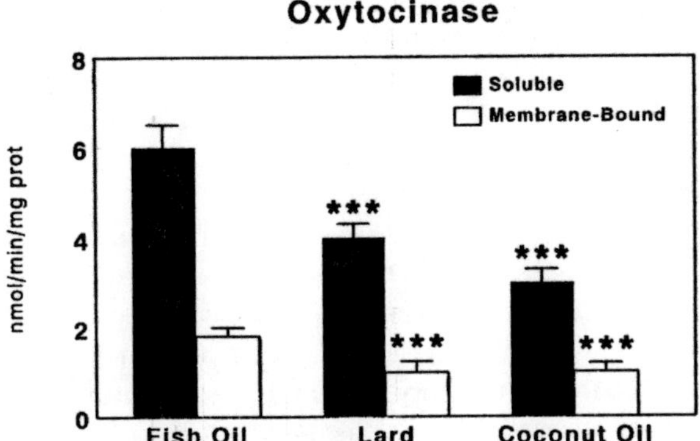

Fig. 12.2. Specific soluble and membrane-bound oxytocinase activities in testis of mice fed a diet containing fish oil, lard, or coconut oil. Groups are ordered from left to right according to the degree of saturation of the fat used in the diet. Oxytocinase activities are expressed as nmol of cystinyl-ß-naphthylamide hydrolyzed per min and per mg of protein (mean with SEM error bars; $n = 9$–10; ***$P < 0.001$).

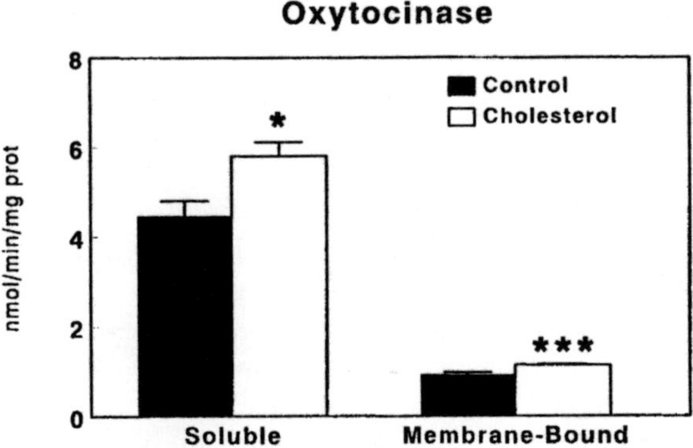

Fig. 12.3. Specific soluble and membrane-bound oxytocinase activities in testis of control and cholesterol-fed animals. Results are expressed as nmol of cystinyl-ß-naphthylamide hydrolyzed per min and per mg of protein (mean with SEM error bars; $n = 10$; *$P < 0.05$; ***$P < 0.001$).

Discussion

In male mammals, clear effects of dietary n-3 polyunsaturated fatty acids on both sperm membrane phospholipid composition and fertilizing ability have been demonstrated (6). It has been described that sperm phospholipids and their fatty acid composition are altered in infertile men (8). The levels of phosphatidylethanolamine and n–3 polyunsaturated fatty acids (eicosopentaenoic and docosahexaenoic) were dramatically lower, whereas the levels of some n-6 polyunsaturated fatty acids (linoleic and docosatretaenoic) were higher. There was a positive correlation between docosahexaenoic acid and sperm motility and a negative correlation between linolenic acid and sperm motility (8).

The role of OTX on male fertility remains controversial. Primarily two functions have been ascribed to testicular OTX, namely, the regulation of seminiferous tubule contractility and the modulation of steroidogenesis. In the testis, the seminiferous tubules are surrounded by smooth muscle-like cells, the myoid cells. OTX has been shown to enhance the contractility of the tubules; therefore, the responsiveness to OTX was higher at a certain stage of the spermatogenic cycle, around the time when the sperm are shed into the lumen (15). OTX promotes the spermiation and the subsequent transport of the immotile spermatozoa to the epididymis. Because Sertoli cells exhibit the components of a local OTX system under some circumstances, they may also be involved in the contractile activity of seminiferous tubules. OTX receptors have also been identified in the interstitial spaces in the rat testis consistent with binding to Leydig cells (16). The Leydig cells drive spermatogenesis via the secretion of testosteron, which acts on the Sertoli and/or peritubular cells to create an environment that enables normal progression of germ cells through the spermatogenic cycle. Daily subcutaneous injections of OTX led to an increase in the plasma and testicular levels of testosteron. In contrast, continuous administration of the peptide into the testis, either by implants or in the transgenic mouse, which overexpresses the bovine OTX gene in its testes, produced a decrease in testosteron but an increase in dihydrotestosteron concentrations (17,18) Although the predominant androgen in the testis is testosteron, elsewhere in the male reproductive tract testosteron acts as a prohormone and is converted to its active metabolite dihydrotestosteron by the enzyme 5α-reductase. OTX was shown to increase the activity of 5α-reductase in both testis and epididymis and may thus have an autocrine/paracrine role modulating steroid metabolism in these tissues (19). The results presented here clearly show that oxytocinase activity is increased after high olive oil and cholesterol administration, and mice fed a diet containing fish oil exhibited remarkably higher levels of oxytocinase activity in the testis when compared with animals fed diets containing lard or coconut oil. Increased oxytocinase activity would probably imply a higher catabolic rate of OTX and a decrease of its half-life. Therefore, the testicular functions in which OTX is involved may be attenuated. According to this, the metabolism of testosteron to 5α-dihydrotestosteron may be reduced, which could have repercussions in male reproductive function. Furthermore, OTX receptors require at least two essential components for high affinity OTX binding: divalent cations and cholesterol. The interaction of cholesterol with both soluble and membrane-bound OTX receptors is of high specificity and is not due to changes of membrane fluidity (20), appearing a direct and cooperative molecular interaction of cholesterol with OTX receptors. Cholesterol acts as an allosteric modulator and stabilizes the OTX receptor in a high-affinity state for agonists and antagonists. It has been suggested that high-affinity state OTX receptors are preferentially localized in cholesterol-rich subdomains of the plasma membrane. Therefore, cholesterol may be involved in the regulation of OTX-mediated signaling functions, particularly in reproductive tissues, where the cholesterol concentrations may be highly dynamic. Thus, changes in cell membrane lipid composition induced by cholesterol must be also taken into account.

To conclude, we can summarize that the type and amount of dietary lipids modifies oxytocinase activity in the testis, probably through the action of their fatty acids content but also through their influence on cholesterol metabolism. These changes on oxytocinase activity modify OTX degradation rate and, therefore, alter the testicular functions in which OTX is involved.

References

1. Gimpl, G., and Fahrenholz, F. (2001) The Oxytocin Receptor System: Structure, Function, and Regulation, *Physiol. Rev. 81*, 629–683.
2. Adashi, E.Y., and Huseh, A.J. (1981) Direct Inhibition of Testicular Androgen Biosynthesis by Arginine-Vasopressin: Mediation through Pressor-Selective Testicular Recognition Sites, *Endocrinology 109*, 1793–1795.
3. Inaba, T., Nakayama, Y., Tani, H., Tamada, H., Kawate, N., and Sawada, T. (1999) Oxytocin Gene Expression and Action in Goat Testis, *Theriogenology 52*, 425–434.
4. Knights, E.B., Baylin, S.B., and Foster, G.V. (1973) Control of Polypeptide Hormones by Enzymatic Degradation, *Lancet 2*, 719–723.
5. Itoh, C., and Nagamatsu, A. (1995) An Aminopeptidase Activity from Porcine Kidney that Hydrolyzes Oxytocin and Vasopressin: Purification and Partial Characterization, *Biochim. Biphys. Acta 1243*, 203–208.
6. Abayasekara, D.R., and Wathes, D.C. (1999) Effects of Altering Dietary Fatty Acid Composition on Prostaglandin Synthesis and Fertility, *Prostaglandins Leukot. Essent. Fatty Acids 61*, 275–287.
7. Sebokova, E., Garg, M.L., Wierzbicki, A., Thomson, A.B., and Clandinin, M.T. (1990). Alteration of the Lipid Composition of Rat Testicular Plasma Membranes by Dietary (n-3) Fatty Acids Changes the Responsiveness of Leydig Cells and Testosterone Synthesis, *J. Nutr. 120*, 610–618.
8. Gulaya, N.M., Margitich, V.M., Govseeva, N.M., Klimashevsky, V.M., Gorpynchenko, I.I., and Boyko, M.I. (2001) Phospholipid Composition of Human Sperm and Seminal Plasma in Relation to Sperm Fertility, *Arch. Androl. 46*, 169–175.
9. Martínez-Martos, J.M., Ramírez-Expósito, M.J., Prieto, I., Alba, F., and Ramírez, M. (1998) Sex Differences and *in Vitro* Effects of Steroids on Serum Aminopeptidase Activities, *Peptides 19*, 1637–1640.
10. Ramírez-Expósito, M.J., Martínez-Martos, J.M., Prieto, I., Alba, F., and Ramírez, M. (1998) Dietary Supplementation with Olive Oil Influences Aminopeptidase Activities in Mice, *Nutr. Res. 18*, 99–107.
11. Arechaga, G, Martínez-Martos, J.M., Prieto, I., Ramírez-Expósito, M.J., Sánchez, M.J. Alba, F., De Gasparo, M., and Ramírez, M. (2001) Serum Aminopeptidase Activity of Mice Is Related to Dietary Fat Saturation, *J. Nutr. 131*, 1177–1179.

12. Segarra, A.B., Arechaga, G., Prieto, I., Ramírez-Expósito, M.J., Martínez-Martos, J.M., Alba, F., Ruiz-Larrea, B., Ruiz-Sanz, J.I., and Ramírez, M. (2002) Effects of Dietary Supplementation with Fish Oil, Lard, or Coconut Oil on Oxytocinase Activity in the Testis of Mice, *Arch. Androl. 48*, 233–236.

13. Gimpl, G., Burger, K., and Fahrenholz, F. (1997) Cholesterol as Modulator of Receptor Function, *Biochemistry 36*, 10959–10974.

14. Ramírez-Expósito, M.J., Mayas, M.D., García, M.J., Ramírez, M., and Martínez-Martos, J.M. (2001) Pituitary Aminopeptidase Activities Involved in Blood Pressure Regulation Are Modified by Dietary Cholesterol. Sex Differences, *Regul. Pep.102*, 87–82.

15. Okuda, K., Uenoyama, Y., Fujita, Y., Iga, K., Sakamoto, K., and Kimura, T. (1997) Functional Oxytocin Receptors in Bovine Granulosa Cells, *Biol. Reprod. 56*, 625–631.

16. Bathgate, R.A., and Sernia, C. (1994) Characterization and Localization of Oxytocin Receptors in the Rat Testis, *J. Endocrinol. 141*, 343–352.

17. Ang, H.L., Ivell, R, Walther, N., Nicholson, H, Hngerfroren, H., Millar, M., Carter, D., and Murphy, D. (1994) Over-Expression of Oxytocin in the Testes of a Transgenic Mouse Model, *J. Endocrinol 140*, 53–62.

18. Nicholson, H.D., Guldenaar, S.E., Boer, G.J., and Pickering B.T. (1991) Testicular Oxytocin: Effects of Intratesticular Oxytocin in the Rat, *J. Endocrinol. 130*, 231–238.

19. Nicholson, H.D., and Jenkin, L. (1995) Oxytocin and Prostatic Function, *Adv. Exp. Med. Biol. 395*, 529–538.

20. Gimpl, G., Burger, K., Politowska, E., Clarkowski, J., and Fahrenholz, F. (2000) Oxytocin Receptors and Cholesterol: Interaction and Regulation, *Exp. Physiol. 85*, 41–50.

Chapter 13

Significance of Oxidative Stress and Sperm Chromatin Damage in Male Infertility

Ashok Agarwal

Director, Andrology Laboratory and Sperm Bank, and Director, Center for Advanced Research in Human Reproduction, Infertility, and Sexual Function, Urological Institute and Department of Obstetrics-Gynecology, Cleveland Clinic Foundation, Cleveland, OH 44195

Abstract

Researchers studying the causes of male infertility have recently focused on the role played by reactive oxygen species (ROS)—a highly reactive oxidizing agent belonging to the class of free radicals. ROS are produced by a variety of semen components, and antioxidants in the seminal fluid keep their levels in check. Small amounts of ROS help spermatozoa acquire their necessary fertilizing capabilities. However, when ROS production exceeds the scavenging capacity of the antioxidants—a state referred to as oxidative stress (OS)—ROS become toxic to sperm. Research suggests that ROS attack the integrity of DNA in the sperm nucleus by causing base modification, DNA strand breaks, and chromatin cross-linking. DNA damage induced by excessive levels of ROS may accelerate the process of germ cell apoptosis, leading to the decline in sperm counts associated with male infertility. This chapter will discuss in more detail the cellular origins of ROS in human semen, how ROS damages sperm nuclear DNA, and how such DNA damage contributes to male infertility. Research highlights from the Cleveland Clinic, including the novel ROS-TAC (ROS total antioxidant capacity) score for assessing OS, will also be presented.

Introduction

Defective sperm function is the most prevalent cause of male infertility and is difficult to treat (1). The mechanisms underlying abnormal sperm function are still poorly understood. This may be due to a lack of basic knowledge about biochemical and physiological processes involved in spermatogenesis (2).

One possible mechanism that is currently being studied is the generation of reactive oxygen species (ROS) in the male reproductive tract. ROS are highly reactive oxidizing agents that belong to the class of free radicals. A free radical is defined as "any atom or molecule that possesses one or more unpaired electrons" (3). When produced in large amounts, ROS have potentially toxic effects on sperm quality and function. Recent reports have indicated that high levels of ROS are detected in semen samples of 25 to 40% of infertile men (4,5). However, a strong body of evidence suggests that small amounts of ROS are necessary for spermatozoa to acquire fertilizing capabilities (6).

Spermatozoa, like all cells living under aerobic conditions, constantly face the oxygen (O_2) paradox, *i.e.*, O_2 is required to support life, but its metabolites, such as ROS, can modify cell functions, endanger cell survival, or both (7). Hence, ROS must be continuously inactivated to keep only the small amount necessary to maintain normal cell function. It is not surprising that a battery of different types of antioxidants protect against oxidants (8). An antioxidant is defined as "any substance that, when present at low concentrations compared with those of an oxidizable substrate, significantly delays or prevents oxidative damage to that substrate." The term "oxidizable substrate" includes almost every molecule found in living cells, including proteins, lipids, carbohydrates, and DNA (9).

Spermatozoa are particularly susceptible to the damage induced by excessive ROS because their plasma membranes contain large quantities of polyunsaturated fatty acids (PUFA) (10), and their cytoplasm contains low concentrations of scavenging enzymes (7,11–13). In addition, the intracellular antioxidant enzymes cannot protect the plasma membrane that surround the acrosome and the tail, forcing spermatozoa to supplement their limited intrinsic antioxidant defenses by depending on the protection afforded by the seminal plasma, which bathes these cells (14,15). Excessive generation of ROS in the reproductive tract not only attacks the fluidity of the sperm plasma membrane but also the integrity of DNA in the sperm nucleus. DNA bases are susceptible to oxidative damage resulting in base modification, strand breaks, and chromatin cross-linking. There is strong evidence that DNA fragmentation commonly observed in spermatozoa of infertile men is mediated by high levels of ROS.

ROS and Sperm Physiology

Until recently, ROS were exclusively considered toxic to human spermatozoa. The idea that limited amounts of ROS can physiologically regulate some sperm functions was first evoked in a study by Aitken *et al.* (16). They observed that ROS, at low levels, enhanced the ability of human spermatozoa to bind zonae pellucida, an effect that was reversed by the addition of vitamin E. As a general rule, incubating spermatozoa with low concentrations of hydrogen peroxide (H_2O_2) stimulates sperm capacitation, hyperactivation, and the ability of the spermatozoa to undergo acrosome reaction and oocyte fusion (17–21). Reactive oxygen species other than H_2O_2, such as nitric oxide and superoxide anion ($O_2^{\bullet-}$), have also been shown to promote sperm capacitation and acrosome reaction (22,23).

Cellular Origin of ROS in Human Semen

A variety of semen components, including morphologically abnormal spermatozoa, precursor germ cells, and leukocytes, can generate ROS in semen. However, seminal leukocytes and morphologically abnormal spermatozoa are the main sources of ROS in human ejaculates (24,25).

ROS Production by Spermatozoa

Clear evidence suggests that human spermatozoa produce oxidants (26–28). Levels of ROS produced by pure sperm populations are negatively correlated with quality of sperm in the original semen (29). The link between poor semen quality and increased ROS generation lies in the presence of excess residual cytoplasm (cytoplasmic droplet). When spermatogenesis is impaired, the cytoplasmic extrusion mechanisms are defective, and spermatozoa are released from the germinal epithelium carrying surplus residual cytoplasm (Fig. 13.1). Under these circumstances, spermatozoa released during spermiation are thought to be immature and functionally defective (30). Retention of residual cytoplasm by spermatozoa is positively correlated with ROS generation via mechanisms that may be mediated by the cytostolic enzyme glucose-6-phosphate-dehydrogenase (G_6PD). This enzyme controls the rate of glucose flux through hexose monophosphate shunt, which in turn controls the intracellular availability of nicotinamide adenine dinucleotide phosphate (NADPH). Spermatozoa use NADPH as a source of electrons to fuel the generation of ROS by an enzyme system known as NADPH-oxidase (31,32).

Spermatozoa may generate ROS in two ways: (i) NADPH-oxidase system at the level of the sperm plasma membrane (26) and (ii) NADH-dependent oxido-reductase (diphorase) at the level of mitochondria (33). The mitochondrial system is the major source of ROS in spermatozoa from infertile men (34) (Fig. 13.1).

The primary ROS generated in human spermatozoa is the $O_2^{\bullet -}$. This one-electron reduction product of oxygen secondarily reacts with itself in a dismutation reaction, which is greatly accelerated by superoxide dismutase (SOD), to generate H_2O_2. In

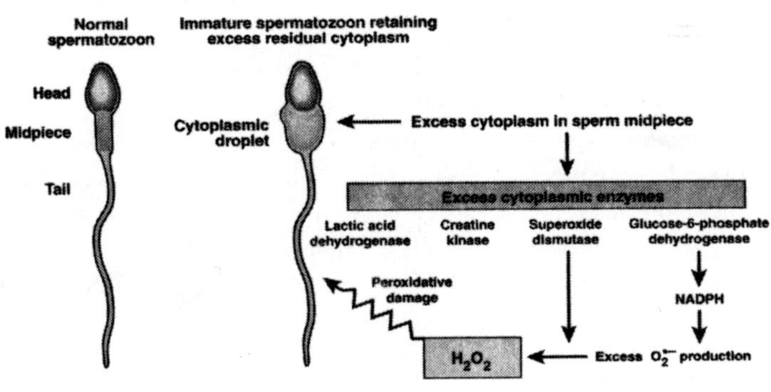

Fig. 13.1. Mechanism of increased production of reactive oxygen species (ROS) by abnormal spermatozoa.

addition to H_2O_2 and $O_2^{\cdot-}$, a variety of secondary cytotoxic radicals and oxidants are generated by human spermatozoa. In the presence of transition metals such as iron and copper, H_2O_2 and $O_2^{\cdot-}$ can interact in a Haber-Weiss reaction to generate the extremely pernicious hydroxyl radical ($OH^\cdot$) as in Equation 1.

$$O_2^{\cdot-} + H_2O_2 \rightarrow OH + OH^- + O_2 \qquad [1]$$

Alternatively, the hydroxyl radical can be produced from hydrogen peroxide by the Fenton reaction, which requires a reducing agent, such as ascorbate or ferrous ions (Eq. 2) (35).

$$H_2O_2 + Fe^{2+} \rightarrow Fe^{3+} + OH^\cdot + OH^- \qquad [2]$$

The hydroxyl radical, which is thought to be an extremely powerful initiator of the lipid peroxidation (LPO) cascade, can precipitate a loss of sperm function.

ROS Production by Leukocytes

With respect to all nonsperm cells, the majority of the so-called round cells consist of immature germ cells with fewer than 5% leukocytes under normal conditions (36). Peroxidase-positive leukocytes are the major source of ROS in semen (20,37,38). Peroxidase-positive leukocytes include polymorphonuclear (PMN) leukocytes, which represent 50 to 60% of all seminal leukocytes, and macrophages, which represent the remaining 40 to 50% of all seminal leukocytes (39–41). Peroxidase-positive leukocytes in semen are contributed largely by the prostate and the seminal vesicles (42). Sperm damage from ROS produced by leukocytes occurs if seminal leukocyte concentrations are abnormally high, *i.e.,* leukocytospermia (43), if the patient has epididymitis, or if seminal plasma was removed during sperm preparation for assisted reproduction (38). Seminal plasma contains large amounts of ROS scavengers but confers a very variable (10 to 100%) protection against ROS generated by leukocytes (44).

Activated leukocytes can produce 100-fold higher amounts of ROS than nonactivated leukocytes (34). Leukocytes may be activated in response to a variety of stimuli including inflammation and infection (45). Activated leukocytes increase the NADPH production via the hexose monophosphate shunt. The myeloperoxidase system of both PMN leukocytes and macrophages is also activated leading to respiratory burst with production of high levels of ROS (46,47). Such an oxidative burst is an early and effective defense mechanism in cases of infection for killing the microbes (48).

ROS Scavenging Strategies

Interestingly, the seminal plasma is well endowed with an array of antioxidant defense mechanisms to protect spermatozoa against oxidative insult (49). These mechanisms compensate for the deficiency in cytoplasmic enzymes in sperm (50). Seminal plasma contains enzymatic antioxidants, such as SOD (51), glutathione peroxidase/glutathione reductase (GPX/GRD) system (52), and catalase (53), as well as nonenzymatic antioxidants, such as ascorbate (54), urate (55), vitamin E (56,57), pyruvate (58), glutathione (59), taurine, and hypotaurine (60). Seminal plasma from fertile men has a higher total antioxidant capacity than that of infertile men (61). However, pathological levels of ROS detected in semen from infertile men are more likely due to increased ROS production rather than reduced antioxidant capacity of the seminal plasma (15). Antioxidant defense mechanisms include three levels of protection: prevention, interception, and repair.

Prevention

Prevention of ROS formation is the first line of defense against oxidative damage. An example is the binding of metal ions, iron and copper ions in particular, which prevents them from initiating a chain reaction (8). Chelation of transition metals is a major means of controlling LPO and DNA damage. When transition metals become loosely bound to biological molecules such as oxygen reduction products, they can produce secondary and more reactive oxidants, particularly OH• (9).

Interception

Free radicals have a tendency toward chain reaction, *i.e.,* a compound carrying an unpaired electron will react with another compound to generate an unpaired electron, "radical begets radical." Hence, the basic problem is to intercept a damaging species from further activity, which is the process of deactivation leading to the formation of nonradical end products (8). Vitamin E, a chain-breaking antioxidant, inhibits LPO in membranes by scavenging peroxyl (RO•) and alkoxyl (ROO•) radicals. The ability of α-tocopherol to maintain a steady-state rate of peroxyl radical reduction in the plasma membrane depends on the recycling of α-tocopherol by external reducing agents, such as ascorbate or thiols (62). In this way, α-tocopherol can function again as a free radical chain-breaking antioxidant, even though its concentration is low (63). A prerequisite for efficient interception is a relatively long half-life of the radical to be intercepted (8). The peroxyl radicals are major reaction partners because their half-life extends into the range of seconds (7 s). In contrast, the hydroxyl radical, with its high reactivity and extremely short half-life (10^{-9} s), cannot be intercepted with reasonable efficiency.

Repair

Protection from the effects of oxidants can also occur by repairing the damage once it has occurred. Unfortunately, spermatozoa are unable to repair the damage induced by ROS because they lack the cytoplasmic enzyme systems that are required to accomplish this repair. This is one of the features that make spermatozoa unique in their susceptibility to oxidative insult (16,51).

The Concept of Oxidative Stress (OS)

Oxidative stress (OS) is the term applied when oxidants outnumber antioxidants (8), when peroxidation products develop (64), and when these phenomena cause pathological effects. Oxidative stress has been implicated in numerous disease states such as cancer, arthritis, connective tissue disorders, aging, toxin exposure, physical injury, infection, inflammation, acquired immunodeficiency syndrome, and male infertility (12,20,26,65).

In the context of human reproduction, a balance is present between ROS generation and scavenging in the male reproductive tract. As a result, only a minimal amount of ROS remains, which is needed to regulate normal sperm functions, such as sperm capacitation, acrosome reaction, and sperm-oocyte fusion (66). Excessive ROS production, which is related to abnormalities of the male reproductive tract, can overwhelm all antioxidant defense strategies of spermatozoa and seminal plasma when it exceeds critical levels, causing an OS status (13,67,68).

Mechanisms of ROS Toxicity

Virtually every human ejaculate is contaminated with potential sources of OS, such as peroxidase-positive leukocytes and morphologically abnormal spermatozoa. It follows that some of the sperm cells will incur oxidative damage and a concomitant loss of function in every ejaculate. Thus, the impact of OS on male fertility is a question of degree rather than the presence or absence of the pathology (69). All cellular components, lipids, proteins, nucleic acids, and sugars are potential targets for ROS. The extent of damage caused by ROS depends not only on type and the amount of ROS involved but also on the moment and duration of ROS exposure and on extra-cellular factors such as temperature, oxygen tension, and the composition of the surrounding environment, including ions, proteins, and ROS scavengers.

Lipid Peroxidation

Lipid peroxidation can be broadly defined as "oxidative deterioration of PUFA," *i.e.,* fatty acids that contain more than two carbon-carbon double bonds (70). The LPO cascade occurs in two fundamental stages: initiation and propagation.

Initiation Stage

The hydroxyl radical (OH$^{\bullet}$) is a powerful initiator of LPO (12). Most membrane PUFA have unconjugated double bonds that are separated by methylene groups. The presence of a double bond adjacent to a methylene group makes the methylene C-H bonds weaker, and therefore hydrogen is more susceptible to abstraction. Once this abstraction has occurred, the radical that is produced is stabilized by the rearrangement of the double bonds, which forms a conjugated diene radical that can then be oxidized. This means that lipids, which contain many methylene-interrupted double bonds, are particularly susceptible to peroxidation (47). Conjugated dienes rapidly react with O_2 to form a lipid peroxyl radical (ROO$^{\bullet}$), which abstracts hydrogen atoms from other lipid molecules to form lipid hydroperoxides (ROOH). Thus, the chain reaction of LPO is continued (70).

Propagation Stage

Lipid hydroperoxides are stable under physiological conditions until they contact transition metals such as iron or copper salts. These metals or their complexes cause lipid hydroperoxides to generate alkoxyl and peroxyl radicals, which then continue the chain reaction within the membrane and propagate the damage throughout the cell (70). Lipid peroxidation propagation will depend upon the antioxidant strategies employed by spermatozoa. One of the by-products of lipid peroxide decomposition is malonaldehyde (MDA), which has been used as an end product in biochemical assays to monitor the degree of peroxidative damage sustained by spermatozoa (12,16). The results of such an assay exhibit an excellent correlation with the degree to which sperm function is impaired in terms of motility and the capacity for sperm-oocyte fusion (71,72).

Impairment of Sperm Motility

Increased production of ROS has been correlated with a reduction of sperm motility (14,16,73,74). The link between ROS and reduced motility may be due to a cascade of events that results in a decrease in axonemal protein phosphorylation and sperm immobilization, both of which are associated with a reduction in membrane fluidity that is necessary for sperm-oocyte fusion (7). Another hypothesis is that H_2O_2 can diffuse across the membranes into the cells and inhibit the activity of some enzymes, such as G_6PDH, leading to a decrease in the availability of NADPH and a concomitant accumulation of oxidized glutathione and reduced glutathione. This can cause a decrease in the antioxidant defenses of the spermatozoa, which ultimately leads to the peroxidation of membrane phospholipids (75).

Sperm Nuclear DNA Damage

Sperm DNA is organized in a specific manner to keep the chromatin in the nucleus compact and stable (76). In 1991, Ward and Coffey proposed four levels of organization for DNA packaging in the spermatozoon: (i) chromosomal anchoring, which refers to the attachment of the DNA to the nuclear annulus; (ii) formation of DNA loop domains as the DNA attaches to the newly added nuclear matrix; (iii) replacement of histones by protamines, which condense the DNA into compact doughnuts; and (iv) chromosomal positioning. Chromosomes become organized, with their centromeres located in the center of the nucleus and their telomeres at the nuclear periphery; active genes are localized to the nuclear center and the inactive genes to the periphery (Fig. 13.2).

This DNA organization not only permits the very tightly packaged genetic information to be transformed to the egg but also ensures that the DNA is delivered in a physical and chemical form that allows the developing embryo to access the genetic information (76).

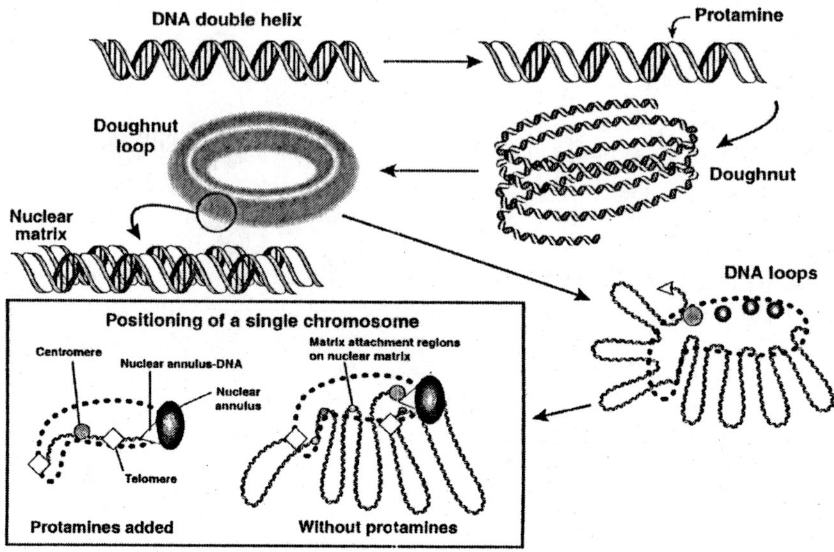

Organization of DNA in the human sperm nucleus (Sakkas et al., 1999).

Fig. 13.2. DNA packaging in human spermatozoa.

Origin Of DNA Damage in Spermatozoa

Defective Chromatin Packaging

Endogenous nicks in DNA occur most frequently during the transition from round to elongated spermatids in the testis. In rat and mouse spermatozoa, the nicks occur before protamination is completed (77). Protamination for chromatin packaging might require the formation and ligation of nicks through endogenous nuclease activity. Researchers have proposed that the endogenous nuclease, topoisomerase II (topo II), might play a role in both the creation and ligation of nicks during spermiogenesis. These nicks are thought to relieve stress due to torsion and to aid chromatin rearrangement as histones are replaced by protamines. Therefore, the presence of endogenous nicks in ejaculated spermatozoa indicates incomplete maturation during spermiogenesis (76). This hypothesis is supported by observations that the presence of DNA damage in mature spermatozoa is correlated with poor chromatin packaging due to under-protamination (78,79).

Apoptosis

Spermatogenesis is a dynamic process of germ cell proliferation and differentiation from stem spermatogonia to mature spermatozoa through a complex series of mitotic and meiotic divisions. Apoptosis, also described as programmed cell death, is a physiological phenomenon characterized by cellular morphological and biochemical alterations leading the cell to commit suicide (80). Apoptosis is genetically determined and takes place at specific moments during normal embryonic life to allow definitive forms of tissues to develop and during adult life to discard cells that have an altered function or no function at all (81). In the context of male reproductive function, apoptosis may be responsible for controlling overproduction of male gametes (76,82). Testicular germ cell apoptosis occurs normally and continuously throughout life.

One factor that is thought to play a role in sperm apoptosis is the cell surface protein Fas (83). Fas is a type I membrane protein that belongs to the tumor necrosis factor-nerve growth factor receptor family and mediates apoptosis (84). Binding of Fas-ligand (Fas-L) or agonistic anti-Fas antibody to Fas kills cells by apoptosis (85). In men with abnormal semen parameters, the percentage of Fas-positive spermatozoa can be as high as 50%. Samples with low sperm concentration are more likely to have a high proportion of Fas-positive spermatozoa (76). This evidence suggests that in subfertile men the correct clearance of spermatozoa via apoptosis is not occurring. The presence of spermatozoa that possess apoptotic markers, such as positive Fas and DNA damage, indicates that in men with abnormal semen parameters such as abnormal morphology, abnormal biochemical functions, and nuclear DNA damage, an "abortive apoptosis" has taken place (30,76).

Fas-positive spermatozoa may not be cleared due to dysfunction at one or more levels. First, apoptosis limits any excess in the number of developing germ cells so that the supportive capacity of Sertoli cells is not overloaded. Because Sertoli cells can limit their proliferation by producing Fas-L, the production of spermatozoa may not be enough to trigger apoptosis in cases with hypo-spermatogenesis. In these men, Fas-positive spermatogonia may escape the signal to undergo apoptosis. Second, Fas-positive spermatozoa may also exist because of problems in activating Fas-mediated apoptosis. These problems could be inherent to a particular patient or may be due to lack of synchronization between apoptosis and spermatogenesis. In the latter case, the spermatozoa will go through spermiogenesis and fail to complete apoptosis even though apoptosis has been initiated. This hypothesis may explain why patients with abnormal semen characteristics also possess a high percentage of spermatozoa containing DNA damage and abnormal spermatozoa that display markers of apoptosis (76).

Oxidative Stress-Induced DNA Damage

Two factors protect spermatozoal DNA from oxidative insult: the characteristic tight packaging of the sperm DNA and the antioxidants present in the seminal plasma (86). Exposing the sperm to artificially produced ROS causes DNA damage in the form of modification of all bases, production of base-free sites, deletions, frame shifts, DNA cross-links, and chromosomal rearrangements (87). Oxidative stress is also associated with high frequencies of single and double DNA strand breaks (86). This information has important clinical implications, particularly in the context of assisted reproductive techniques (ART). Spermatozoa selected for ART most likely originate from an environment experiencing OS, and a high percentage of these sperm may have damaged DNA (88,89). There is a substantial risk that spermatozoa carrying damaged DNA are being used clinically in this form of therapy (90). When intrauterine insemination (IUI) or *in vitro* fertilization (IVF) is used, such damage may not be a cause of concern because the collateral peroxidative damage to the sperm plasma membrane ensures that fertilization cannot occur with a DNA-damaged sperm. However, when intracytoplasmic sperm injection (ICSI) is used, this natural selection barrier is bypassed, and a spermatozoon with damaged DNA is directly injected into the oocyte (6,90).

Whether DNA-damaged spermatozoa used in ICSI can impair the process of fertilization and embryo development is not clear. On one hand, a recent study has indicated that spermatozoa with significantly damaged DNA still retain a residual capacity for fertilization. On the other hand, the percentage of sperm with DNA damage has been negatively correlated to the fertilization rate (91,92). In addition, a recent study has linked sperm DNA damage to increased rates of early embryo death (76). This is also supported by the results of Sanchez and colleagues who, in 1996, reported that miscarriage rates after ICSI were higher than that after conventional IVF.

Sperm preparation techniques involving repeated centrifugation may lead to high ROS production in sperm suspensions processed for ART (74). This may be important because exposing spermatozoa to high levels of ROS may increase the DNA fragmentation rate, which can have adverse consequences if they are used for ICSI (92). In 2000, Zini and colleagues reported that the improvement in sperm motility after Percoll processing is not associated with a similar improvement in sperm DNA integrity. The authors recommended that the current sperm preparation techniques be reexamined with the goal of minimizing sperm DNA damage. This can be accomplished by using more gentle sperm preparation methods such as the swim-up technique, which allows for good sperm recovery with minimal sperm dysfunction (93,94). In a recent study from our center, we found that recovery of sperm with intact nuclear DNA is significantly higher after the swim-up technique than the ISolate gradient technique (unpublished data).

Complications of Sperm Nuclear DNA Damage

Failure of Fertilization

When spermatozoa with DNA damage are selected for ICSI, the initiation or completion of de-condensation may be impeded, thereby preventing fertilization (76). Lopes *et al.* (92) have shown that men with a sperm population containing more than 25% of sperm with DNA damage are more likely to experience a fertilization rate of less than 20% after ICSI. However, Twigg *et al.* (90) found that the genetically damaged spermatozoa can achieve normal fertilization following ICSI.

Embryo Death

Several studies have indicated that damage to sperm DNA may be linked to an increase in early embryo death (76).

Childhood Cancer

Sperm nuclear DNA damage may have consequences for the health of the offspring, who show a particularly high incidence of childhood cancer (95). In a study from China, paternal smoking was associated with a four-fold overall increased risk of developing a childhood cancer (96). Smoking may induce a state of OS that is associated with free radical-mediated damage to sperm DNA. Furthermore, an independent epidemiological study in the United Kingdom concluded that 14% of all childhood cancers could be attributed directly to paternal smoking (97).

Infertility

Another possible consequence of free radical-mediated DNA damage in the male germ line is infertility in the offspring (6). This possibility relates specifically to forms of male infertility involving deletions on the long arm (q) of the Y chromosome. In this nonrecombining area of the Y chromosome (NRY), three regions have been identified that contain genes of importance to spermatogenesis; these loci have been designated AZF (azoospermia factor) a, b, and c (98). Deletions in each of these areas produce a particular testicular phenotype. Deletions in AZFa produce Sertoli cell only syndrome. Deletions in AZFb are associated with germ cell arrest at the pachytene stage and deletions in AZFc generate arrest at the spermatid stage of development (99). These deletions are not observed in fertile men or in the majority of fathers of affected patients. Therefore, the Y chromosome deletions leading to male infertility must arise *de novo* in the germ line of the patient's fathers (6).

Y chromosome deletions are found in approximately 15% of patients with azoospermia or severe oligozoospermia and in 10% of men with idiopathic infertility (98). Although these are not particularly high frequencies, it should be recognized that more than 90% of the human genome is noncoding and would not produce a phenotypic change on deletion. Moreover, for most of the genome, homologous recombination could provide a theoretical mechanism for repairing double-stranded DNA deletions on autosomes or on the X chromosome. However, since the Y chromosome does not possess a homologue, this repair mechanism cannot be invoked, and deletions on the nonrecombining region of this chromosome will persist. Thus, for Y chromosomal deletions to occur at the frequency observed, there must be an extremely high spontaneous rate of DNA fragmentation in the male germ line, most of which is either undetected or is repaired. However, deletions on the AZF on the NRY cannot be repaired and produce an extremely obvious phenotype (6).

Contributions of the Cleveland Clinic

The role of OS in male infertility has been the main focus of our research in the Cleveland Clinic Foundation during the last decade. Our research team has identified the critical role OS plays in male infertility. The main objective of our research was to transfer this important knowledge from the research bench to clinical practice. This objective was stated in a review article by Sharma and Agarwal (13), which described specific plans and strategies for future research in the area of OS. We designed studies with the aims of (i) understanding the exact mechanisms by which OS develops in semen, (ii) establishing assays for accurate assessment of OS status and running the quality control studies for this purpose, and (iii) identifying the clinical significance of seminal OS assessment in male infertility practice.

Mechanism of Seminal OS

We investigated the cellular origins of ROS in semen to track the source of OS and, accordingly, to create strategies to overcome the problem.

Role of Seminal Leukocytes

Shekarriz *et al.* (43) reported that peroxidase-positive leukocytes are the main source of ROS in semen and found that positive peroxidase staining is an accurate indicator of excessive ROS generation in semen. Recently, Sharma *et al.* (100) observed that seminal leukocytes may cause OS even at concentrations below the WHO cutoff value for leukocytospermia (concentrations greater than 1×10^6 peroxidase positive leukocytes/mL semen). Levels of ROS production by pure sperm suspensions were found to be significantly higher in infertile men with leukocytospermia than in infertile men without leukocytospermia and were strongly correlated with seminal leukocyte concentration (101) (Table 13.1). This new finding led us to postulate that seminal leukocytes play a potential role in enhancing sperm capacity for excessive ROS production either by direct sperm-leukocyte contact or by soluble products released by the leukocytes. This observation has significant implications for the fertility potential of sperm both *in vivo* and *in vitro*. Excessive production of ROS by sperm in the patients with leukocytospermia implies that both the free-radical generating sperm themselves and any normal sperm in the immediate vicinity are susceptible to oxidative damage. Furthermore, once the process of LPO is initiated, the self-propagating nature of this process ensures a progressive spread of the damage throughout the sperm population.

Role of Abnormal Spermatozoa

In addition to ROS production by seminal leukocytes, the production of ROS by human sperm was also the subject of extensive research by our group. Our data indicate that human sperm production of ROS was significantly increased by the repeated cycles of centrifugation involved in the conventional semen processing techniques

TABLE 13.1

Median (25 and 75% Interquartile Value) ROS Levels in Original Cell Suspension (Basal) in Leukocyte-Free Sperm Suspension (Pure Sperm); and ROS-TAC Score in Normal Donors, Nonleukocytospermic Patients, and Leukocytospermic Patients[a]

Variable	Donors ($n = 13$)	Non-Leukocytospermic ($n = 32$)	Leukocytospermic ($n = 16$)	A	B	C
Basal ROS ($\times 10^6$ cpm)	0.4 (0.1, 2.5)	2.7 (0.53, 12)	178 (32, 430)	0.06	0.0001	<0.0001
Pure sperm ROS ($\times 10^6$ cpm)	0.06 (0.01, 0.2)	0.31 (0.09, 1.2)	3.3 (0.5, 7.4)	0.05	0.001	0.002
ROS-TAC Score	54.5 (52, 60)	50.3 (42, 54.8)	27.8 (23.7, 35)	0.01	0.0003	0.0001

[a]A = *P* value of donors *versus* nonleukocytospermic; B = *P* value of donors *versus* leukocytospermic; and C = *P* value of nonleukocytospermic *versus* leukocytospermic. Wilcoxon rank-sum test was used for comparison and statistical significance was assessed at $P < 0.05$ level. ROS = reactive oxygen species; TAC = total antioxidant capacity.

(washing and resuspension) for ART (102). In addition, we have demonstrated that the duration of centrifugation is more important than the force of centrifugation for inducing ROS formation in semen (43). Based on these findings, we recommended the use of more gentle techniques for sperm preparation with shorter centrifugation periods to minimize the risk of OS-induced injury to the sperm.

Our group has also reported that ROS production by human sperm rises as sperm concentration increases and decreases with time (103). In addition, we emphasized the importance of adjusting sperm concentration for ROS measurements when comparing ROS levels between different specimens (104). Results from our most recent studies indicate that ROS production varies significantly in subsets of human spermatozoa at different stages of maturation (28,105). Following ISolate gradient fractionation of ejaculated sperm, ROS production was found to be highest in immature sperm with abnormal head morphology and cytoplasmic retention and lowest in mature sperm and immature germ cells. The relative proportion of ROS-producing immature sperm was directly correlated with nuclear DNA damage values in mature sperm and inversely correlated with the recovery of motile, mature sperm. These interesting findings led to the hypothesis that oxidative damage of mature sperm by ROS-producing immature sperm during their co-migration from seminiferous tubules to the epididymis may be an important cause of male infertility. This suggests that perhaps interventions directed to (i) increase antioxidant levels in immature germ cell membranes during spermatogenesis and (ii) isolate spermatozoa with intact DNA by *in vitro* separation techniques should be of particular benefit to these patients in which a defect in the normal regulation of spermiogenesis and spermiation leads to an abnormal increase in the production of ROS-producing immature sperm.

Assessment of OS Status

Extensive research in the field of male infertility has been conducted to develop adequate indices of OS that would help determine, with accuracy, if OS is a significant contributor in male infertility (106). Levels of OS vary greatly in infertile men (51). Because OS is an imbalance between levels of ROS production and antioxidant protection in semen, it is conceivable that any assessment of OS will rely on the measurement of ROS as well as total antioxidant capacity (TAC) of semen. Recently, a statistical formula described as the ROS-TAC score has been introduced for assessment of OS using principal component analysis (106).

Measurement of ROS

Levels of seminal ROS can be measured by a chemiluminescence assay (107) (Fig. 13.3). Liquefied semen is centrifuged at $300 \times g$ for 7 min, and the seminal plasma is separated and stored at $-80°C$ for measurement of TAC. The pellet is washed with phosphate buffered saline (PBS) and resuspended in the same media at a concentration of 20×10^6 sperm/mL. Levels of ROS are measured by a chemiluminescence assay using luminol (5-amino-2,3,-dihydro-1,4-phthalazinedione; Sigma Chemical Co., St. Louis, MO) as a probe. Four 100-µL aliquots of the resulting cell suspensions (containing sperm and leukocytes) are used for assessment of basal ROS levels. Eight microliters of horseradish peroxidase (HRP) (12.4 U of HRP Type VI, 310 U/mg; Sigma Chemical Co.) are added to sensitize the assay so that it can measure extracellular hydrogen peroxide. Ten microliters of luminol, prepared as 5-mM stock in dimethyl sulfoxide (DMSO), are added to the mixture. A negative control is prepared by adding 10 µL of 5-mM luminol to 400 µL of PBS. Levels of ROS are assessed by measuring the luminol-dependant chemiluminescence with a luminometer (model:

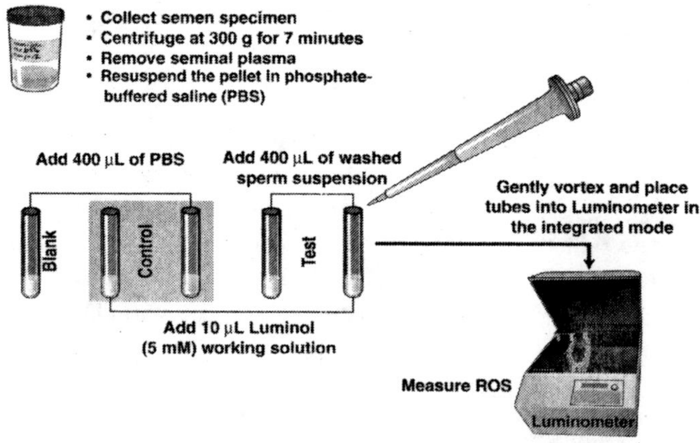

Fig. 13.3. Measurement of reactive oxygen species (ROS) in washed semen by chemiluminescence assay.

LKB 953; Wallac Inc., Gaithersburg, MD) in the integrated mode for 15 min. The results are expressed as $\times 10^4$ counted photons per minute (cpm) per 20×10^6 sperm. Normal ROS levels in washed semen range from 10 to 100×10^4 counted photons per minute (cpm) per 20×10^6 sperm.

Measurement of TAC

Total antioxidant capacity in the seminal plasma can be measured with an enhanced chemiluminescent assay (108). Frozen samples of seminal plasma are thawed at room temperature and immediately assessed for TAC. Seminal plasma is diluted 1:20 with deionized water (dH2O) and filtered through a 0.20-µ filter (Allegiance Healthcare Corporation, McGaw Park, IL). Signal reagent is prepared by adding 30 µL H_2O_2 (8.8 molar/L), 10 µL para-iodophenol stock solution (41.72 µM), and 110 µL of luminol stock solution (3.1 mM) to 10 mL of Tris Buffer (0.1 M, pH 8.0). Horseradish peroxidase working solution is prepared from the HRP stock solution by making a dilution of 1:1 of dH_2O to give a chemiluminescence output of 3×10^7 cpm. Trolox (6-hydroxyl-2,5,7,8-tetramethylchroman-2-carboxylic acid), a water-soluble tocopherol analogue, is prepared as a standard solution (25, 50, and 75 µM) for TAC calibration. With the luminometer in the kinetic mode, 100 µL of signal reagent and 100 µL of HRP working solution are added to 700 µL of dH_2O and mixed. The mixture is equilibrated to the desired level of chemiluminescent output (between 2.8 and 3.2×10^7 cpm) for 100 s. One hundred microliters of the prepared seminal plasma is immediately added to the mixture, and the chemiluminescence is measured. Suppression of luminescence and the time from the addition of seminal plasma to 10% recovery of the initial chemiluminescence are recorded. The same steps are repeated after the Trolox solutions are replaced with 100-µL aliquots of the prepared seminal plasma. The assay is conducted in a dark room because light affects the chemiluminescence. Plotting the three concentrations of Trolox solution versus 10% recovery time results in a linear equation (Fig. 13.4).

TAC Calculation

Seminal TAC levels are calculated using the following equation:

$$y = (Mx \pm C) \times d$$

In this equation, M refers to the slope increase in the value of Trolox equivalent for a one-second increase of the recovery time, whereas C accounts for the daily background variability. The results are multiplied by the dilution (d) factor and expressed as molar Trolox equivalents (106).

ROS-TAC Score: A New Development in the Field of OS

The fact that neither ROS alone nor TAC alone can adequately quantify seminal oxidative stress led us to the logical conclusion that combining these two variables may be a better index for diagnosis of the overall OS affecting spermatozoa. This con-

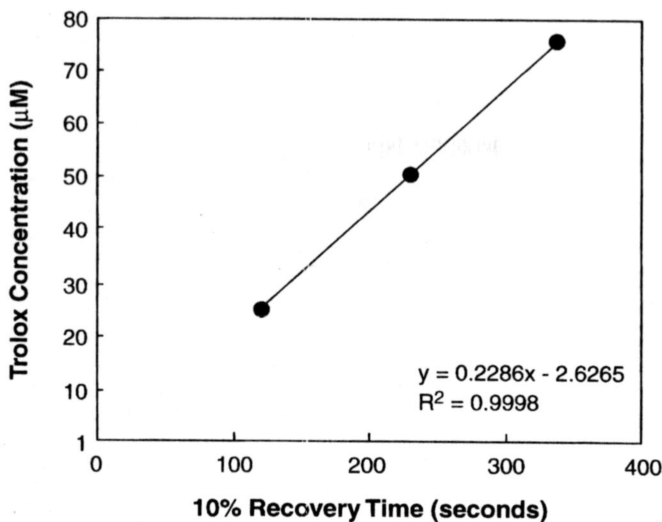

Fig. 13.4. Linear relationship between the concentrations of standard Trolox solution (µM) and 10% recovery time (sec.).

clusion was behind our landmark paper in which we introduced the ROS-TAC score as a new method for accurate assessment of OS status in infertile men (106). The new ROS-TAC score is derived from levels of ROS in washed semen and TAC in seminal plasma (106). The resulting score minimizes the variability present in the individual parameters of OS (ROS alone or TAC alone). In our study, the ROS-TAC score was calculated from a group of normal healthy fertile men who had very low levels of ROS. The composite ROS-TAC score calculated for these men was representative of the fertile population, and any scores significantly below levels in the fertile population were indicative of infertility. We found that individuals with ROS-TAC scores below 30, the lower limits of normal range, are at particular risk for prolonged inability to initiate pregnancies.

Quality Control of OS Indices (ROS and TAC)

It was of utmost importance to standardize the measures that we used as indices for OS, including measurement of ROS in washed semen and TAC in seminal plasma. We have demonstrated that the luminol-dependent chemiluminescence assay for ROS measurement in washed semen is both accurate and reliable when the sperm concentration is greater than 1×10^6/mL and the samples are analyzed within one hour after collection (108). Our results have also indicated that the enhanced chemiluminescence assay is both accurate and reliable for assessment of TAC in seminal plasma (109).

Clinical Significance of Assessment of Seminal OS

It was also of special interest to us to determine levels of seminal OS in different clinical settings (Table 13.2). We found a significant increase in levels of ROS in men with spinal cord injury, which was also associated with poor sperm motility and morphology (5). We also found elevated levels of ROS in infertile men with varicoceles (27). In a recent study, we demonstrated that varicocelectomy resulted in a significant increase in pregnancy and live birth rates for couples who underwent IUI, although standard semen parameters were not improved in all patients (110). We hypothesized that the improvement in pregnancy rates following varicocelectomy may be due to a functional factor not tested during standard semen analysis such as seminal OS or sperm DNA damage. Currently, studies are underway in our center to investigate this hypothesis. Patients with varicocele also had low levels of TAC in their seminal plasma. We speculated that these patients might benefit from antioxidant supplementation (27). A study on rats has indicated that free radical scavengers such as SOD can prevent free radical-mediated testicular damage (111).

Across all clinical diagnoses, the ROS-TAC score was a superior discriminator between fertile and infertile men to either ROS or TAC alone (106). Furthermore, analyses of male patients with a diagnosis of male-factor infertility indicated that those with partners who had subsequent successful pregnancies had an average ROS-TAC score in the normal range compared with significantly lower ROC-TAC scores in those men with partners who did not become pregnant. In addition, we found that the average ROS-TAC score for the fertile vasectomy reversal group was nearly identical to that of the controls (107). Infertile men with male-factor or idiopathic diagnoses had significantly lower ROS-TAC scores than the controls, and men with male-factor diagnoses that eventually were able to initiate a successful pregnancy had significantly higher ROS-TAC scores than those who failed (112). Also, infertile men with chronic prostatitis or prostatodynia have been shown to have lower ROS-TAC score than controls, and this was irrespective of their leukocytospermia status (113). Finally, male partners of couples who achieved pregnancy did not have significantly different ROS-TAC scores than controls. Therefore, the new ROS-TAC score may serve as an important measure in identifying those patients with a clinical diagnosis of male infertility who are likely to initiate a pregnancy over a period of time (45).

ROS in Neat (Raw) Semen: An Accurate and Reliable Test for OS

More recently, our group has introduced an additional test of OS in which ROS levels are measured directly in neat (raw) semen (114). The maximum ROS level observed in neat semen from normal healthy donors with a normal genital examination and normal standard semen parameters was 1.5×10^4 cpm/20 million sperm/mL. The test was subjected to all quality control studies and proved to be an accurate measure for seminal OS status. Using a cutoff value of 1.5×10^4 cpm/20 million sperm/mL, infertile men were reliably classified as either OS-positive (>1.5×10^4 cpm/20 million

TABLE 13.2

Mean and Standard Deviation (SD) between ROS, TAC, and ROS-TAC Score in Subgroups of Infertility Patients and Controls[a]

Diagnosis	ROS Log (ROS + 1)	P-value vs. controls[b]	TAC (Trolox Equivalent)	P-value vs. controls[b]	ROS-TAC score	P-value vs. controls[b]
Control (n = 24)	1.39 (SD 0.73)		1650.9 (SD 532.2)		50.00 (SD 10.00)	
Varicocele (n = 55)	2.10 (SD 1.21)	0.02	1100.1 (SD 410.3)	0.0002	34.87 (SD 13.54)	0.0001
Varicocele with prostatitis (n = 8)	3.25 (SD 0.89)	0.0002	1061.4 (SD 425.1)	0.03	22.39 (SD 13.48)	0.0001
Vasectomy reversal (infertile; n = 23)	2.65 (SD 1.01)	0.0004	1389.9 (SD 723.9)	0.30	33.22 (SD 15.24)	0.0002
Vasectomy reversal (fertile; n = 12)	1.76 (SD 0.86)	0.80	1876.9 (SD 750.8)	0.62	49.35 (SD 12.25)	1.00
Idiopathic infertility (n = 28)	2.29 (SD 1.20)	0.01	1052.0 (SD 380.9)	0.0003	32.25 (SD 14.40)	0.0001

[a]TAC = total antioxidant capacity; ROS = reactive oxygen species.
[b]Pairwise P-values from Student's t-test adjusted using Dunnett's method.

sperm/mL) or OS-negative ($\leq 1.5 \times 10^4$ cpm/20 million sperm/mL), irrespective of their clinical diagnosis or results of standard semen analysis.

We also found that assessing ROS directly in neat semen has diagnostic and prognostic capabilities identical to those obtained from the ROS-TAC score (Table 13.3). Levels of ROS in neat semen were strongly correlated with levels of ROS in washed semen and with ROS-TAC score (Fig. 13.5). A strong positive correlation was seen between ROS levels in neat semen and the extent of sperm chromatin damage (115). However, the difference in the extent of sperm DNA damage between OS-negative and OS-positive patients was not statistically significant, an indication that OS is associated with DNA damage or contributes to it in some way (or both) in some but not all infertility patients.

Strategies to Reduce Seminal OS

Long-term strategies must determine the cause of the enhanced generation of ROS by spermatozoa of infertile men. Reduced levels of OS will be beneficial in ART such as IUI and IVF. An insight into the molecular basis of these defects is vital in order to identify the underlying cause of the etiology of sperm pathologies. Such an understanding will help researchers develop appropriate therapeutic strategies in the treatment for male infertility. Determining the level and origin of ROS production in the ejaculate and precisely evaluating the scavenger system may be useful in treating patients. If the error in spermatogenesis that leads to such atypical activity (excessive ROS production) could be defined, it would provide an important lead in determining the etiology of male infertility, and a sensible basis for the design of effective therapies could be prepared.

The seminal leukocyte population should also be considered potentially detrimental and must be carefully monitored. It is important to minimize the interaction

TABLE 13.3

Median (25th and 75th Percentile) Values of Reactive Oxygen Species (ROS) in Neat Semen, ROS in Washed Semen, Total Antioxidant Capacity (TAC) in Seminal Plasma, and ROS-TAC Score in Donors and Oxidative Stress (OS)-Negative and OS-Positive Patients

Variable	Donors (n = 9)	OS-negative (n = 11)	OS-positive (n = 23)	A[a]	B[a]	C[a]
ROS-neat semen ($\times 10^4$ cpm)	0.3 (0.2, 0.9)	0.3 (0.2, 1)	19 (6, 143)	0.9	0.0001	0.0001
ROS-washed semen ($\times 10^4$ cpm)	10 (4, 17)	79 (13, 177)	1468 (514, 11496)	0.03	0.0003	0.0008
TAC (Trolox Equivalents)	908 (736, 1129)	797 (575, 966)	739 (627, 1047)	0.31	0.24	0.94
ROS-TAC score	53 (51, 55)	49 (47, 52)	36 (32, 44)	0.4	0.001	0.001

[a]A, donors *vs.* OS-negative patients; B, donors *vs.* OS-positive patients; C, OS-negative patients *vs.* OS-positive patients. Results were analyzed by Wilcoxon rank-sum test, $P < 0.05$ was significant.

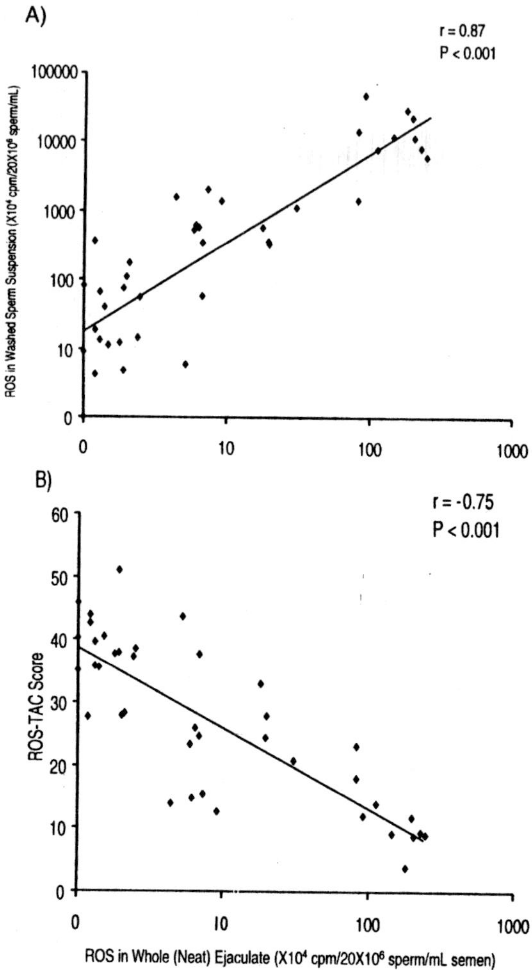

Fig. 13.5. Correlation of reactive oxygen species (ROS) levels in neat semen with (A) levels of reactive oxygen species in washed semen (r = 0.87, *P* < 0.001) and (B) reactive oxygen species – total antioxidant capacity (TAC) score (r = –0.75, *P* < 0.001).

between ROS-producing cells in semen, *e.g.*, PMN leukocytes, and spermatozoa that have a potential to fertilize. Differentiating between spermatozoa and leukocyte sources of ROS is important clinically because this will affect the strategies used to reduce OS on spermatozoa during the course of IVF therapy. It is important for the clinician also to know that sperm preparation techniques used for ART may induce damage to the spermatozoa by removing the seminal plasma with its powerful antioxidants and by inducing ROS generation by spermatozoa.

Future Directions

Future efforts should focus on elucidating why spermatozoa from some patients become over-reactive in the generation of ROS. It is also important to determine the period of sperm differentiation at which this self-destructive activity first appears. Further efforts are also required to identify sperm population at risk of collateral per-oxidative damage to the sperm membrane. An interesting area of future research is to investigate the oxidative damage to sperm DNA and its implication on male fertility potential and the outcome of assisted reproductive programs.

References

1. Aitken, R.J., and Clarkson, J.S. (1987) Cellular Basis of Defective Sperm Function and Its Association with the Genesis of Reactive Oxygen Species by Human Spermatozoa, *J. Reprod. Fertil. 81*, 459–469.
2. Purvis, K., and Christeansen, E. (1995) The Impact of Infection on Sperm Quality, *J. British Fertil. Soc. 1*, 31–41.
3. Warren, J.S., Johnson, K.J., and Ward, P.A. (1987) Oxygen Radicals in Cell Injury and Cell Death, *Pathol. Immunopathol. Res. 6*, 301–315.
4. de Lamirande, E., Leduc, B.E., Iwasaki, A., Hassouna, M., and Gagnon, C. (1995) Increased Reactive Oxygen Species Formation in Semen of Patients with Spinal Cord Injury, *Fertil. Steril. 64*, 637–642.
5. Padron, O.F., Brackett, N.L., Sharma, R.K., Kohn, S., Lynne, C.M., Thomas, A.J., Jr., and Agarwal, A. (1997) Seminal Reactive Oxygen Species, Sperm Motility, and Morphology in Men with Spinal Cord Injury, *Fertil. Steril, 67*, 1115–1120.
6. Aitken, R.J. (1999) The Amoroso Lecture. The Human Spermatozoon-a Cell in Crisis? *J. Reprod. Fertil. 115*, 1–7.
7. de Lamirande, E., and Gagnon, C. (1995) Impact of Reactive Oxygen Species on Spermatozoa: A Balancing Act between Beneficial and Detrimental Effects, *Hum. Reprod, 10*, 15–21.
8. Sies, H. (1993) Strategies of Antioxidant Defense, *Eur. J. Biochem. 215*, 213–219.
9. Halliwell, B. (1990) How to Characterize a Biological Antioxidant, *Free Radic. Res. Commun. 9*, 1–32.
10. Alvarez, J.G., and Storey, B.T. (1995) Differential Incorporation of Fatty Acids into and Peroxidative Loss of Fatty Acids from Phospholipids of Human Spermatozoa, *Mol. Reprod. Dev. 42*, 334–346.
11. Jones, R., Mann, T., and Sherins, R.J. (1979) Peroxidative Breakdown of Phospholipids in Human Spermatozoa: Spermicidal Effects of Fatty Acids Peroxidatives and Protective Action of Seminal Plasma, *Fertil. Steril. 31*, 531–537.
12. Aitken, R.J., and Fisher, H. (1994) Reactive Oxygen Species Generation and Human Spermatozoa: The Balance of Benefit and Risk, *Bioassays 16*, 259–267.
13. Sharma, R.K., and Agarwal, A. (1996) Role of Reactive Oxygen Species in Male Infertility (Review), *Urology 48*, 835–850.
14. Iwasaki, A., and Gagnon, C. (1992) Formation of Reactive Oxygen Species in Spermatozoa of Infertile Patients, *Fertil. Steril. 57*, 409–416.

15. Zini, A., de Lamirande, E., and Gagnon, C. (1993) Reactive Oxygen Species in the Semen of Infertile Patients: Levels of Superoxide Dismutase- and Catalase-like Activities in Seminal Plasma, *Int. J. Androl. 16*, 183–188.

16. Aitken, R.J., Clarkson, J.S., and Fishel, S. (1989) Generation of Reactive Oxygen Species, Lipid Peroxidation, and Human Sperm Function, *Biol. Reprod. 40*, 183–197.

17. de Lamirande, E., and Gagnon, C. (1993) Human Sperm Hyperactivation and Capacitation as Parts of an Oxidative Process, *Free Radic. Biol. Med. 14*, 255–265.

18. de Lamirande, E., Eiley, D., and Gagnon, C. (1993) Inverse Relationship between the Induction of Human Sperm Capacitation and Spontaneous Acrosome Reaction by Various Biological Fluids and the Superoxide Scavenging Capacity of these Fluids, *Int. J. Androl. 16*, 258–266.

19. Griveau, J.F., Renard, P., and Le Lannou, D. (1994) An in Vitro Promoting Role for Hydrogen Peroxide in Human Sperm Capacitation, *Int. J. Androl. 17*, 300–307.

20. Aitken, R.J., Paterson, M., Fisher, H., Buckingham, D.W., and Van Dubin, M. (1995) Redox Regulation of Tyrosine Phosphorylation in Human Spermatozoa is Involved in the Control of Human Sperm Function, *J. Cell Sci. 108*, 2017–2025.

21. Kodama, H., Kuribayashi, Y., and Gagnon, C. (1996) Effect of Sperm Lipid Peroxidation on Fertilization, *J. Androl. 16*, 151–157.

22. Griveau, J.F., Dumont, E., Renard, B., Callegari, J.P., and Lannou, D.L. (1995) Reactive Oxygen Species, Lipid Peroxidation and Enzymatic Defense Systems in Human Spermatozoa, *J. Reprod. Fertil. 103*, 17–26.

23. Zini, A., De Lamirande, E., and Gagnon, C. (1996) Low Levels of Nitric Oxide Promote Human Sperm Capacitation in Vitro, *J. Androl. 16*, 424–431.

24. Aitken, R.J., and West, K.M. (1990) Analysis of the Relationship Between Reactive Oxygen Species Production and Leukocyte Infiltration in Fractions of Human Semen Separated on Percoll Gradients, *Int. J. Androl. 3*, 433–451.

25. Kessopoulou, E., Tomlinson, M.J., Banat, C.L.R., Bolton, A.E., and Cooke, I.D. (1992) Origin of Reactive Oxygen Species in Human Semen-Spermatozoa or Leukocytes, *J. Reprod. Fertil. 94*, 463–470.

26. Aitken, R.J., Buckingham, D.W., and West, K.M. (1992) Reactive Oxygen Species and Human Spermatozoa: Analysis of the Cellular Mechanisms Involved in Luminol- and Lucigenin-Dependent Chemiluminescence, *J. Cell Physiol. 151*, 466–477.

27. Hendin, B., Kolettis, P., Sharma, R.K., Thomas, A.J., Jr., and Agarwal, A. (1999) Varicocele Is Associated with Elevated Spermatozoal Reactive Oxygen Species Production and Diminished Seminal Plasma Antioxidant Capacity, *J. Urol. 161*, 1831–1834.

28. Gil-Guzman, E., Ollero, M., Lopez, M.C., Sharma, R.K., Alvarez, J.G., Thomas, A.J., Jr., and Agarwal, A. (2001) Differential Production of Reactive Oxygen Species by Subsets of Human Spermatozoa at Different Stages of Maturation, *Hum. Reprod. 16*, 1922–1930.

29. Gomez, E., Irvine, D.S., and Aitken, R.J. (1998) Evaluation of a Spectrophotometric Assay for the Measurement of Malondialdehyde and 4-Hydroxyalkenals in Human Spermatozoa: Relationships with Semen Quality and Sperm Function, *Int. J. Androl. 21*, 81–94.

30. Huszar, G., Sbracia, M., Vigue, L., Miller, D.J., and Shur, B.D. (1997) Sperm Plasma Membrane Remodeling during Spermiogenic Maturation in Men: Relationship among Plasma Membrane Beta 1,4-Galactosyltransferase, Cytoplasmic Creatine Phosphokinase and Creatine Phosphokinase Isoform Ratios, *Biol. Reprod. 56*, 1020–1024.

31. Aitken, R.J., Fisher, H.M., Fulton, N., Gomez, E., Knox, W., Lewis, B., and Irvine, D.S. (1997) Reactive Oxygen Species Generation by Human Spermatozoa is Induced by

Exogenous NADPH and Inhibited by Flavoprotein Inhibitors Diphenylene Iodinium and Quinacrine, *Mol. Reprod. Dev. 47*, 468–482.

32. Richer, S., Whittington, K., and Ford, W.C.L. (1998) Confirmation of NADPH Oxidase Activity in Human Sperm, *J. Reprod. Fertil. Abstract series 21*, Abstract 118.

33. Gavella, M., and Lipovac, V. (1992) NADH-Dependent Oxido-Reductase (Diaphorase) Activity and Isozyme Pattern of Sperm in Infertile Men, *Arch. Androl. 28*, 135–141.

34. Plante, M., de Lamirande, E., and Gagnon, C. (1994) Reactive Oxygen Species Released by Activated Neutrophils, but not by Deficient Spermatozoa, Are Sufficient to Affect Normal Sperm Motility, *Fertil. Steril. 62*, 387–393.

35. Kwenang, A., Kroos, M.J., Koster, J.F., and Van Eijk, H.G. (1987) Iron, Ferritin, and Copper in Seminal Plasma, *Hum. Reprod. 2*, 387–388.

36. Eggert-Kruse, W., Bellman, A., Rohr, G., Tilgen, W., and Rumiebaum, B. (1992) Differentiation of Round Cells in Semen by Means of Monoclonal Antibodies and Relationship with Male Infertility, *Fertil. Steril. 58*, 1046–1055.

37. Tomlinson, M.J., Barrat, G.L.R., and Cooke, I.D. (1993) Prospective Study of Leukocytes and Leukocyte Subpopulations in Semen Suggests that They Are not a Cause of Male Infertility, *Fertil. Steril. 60*, 1069–1075.

38. Ochsendorf, F.R. (1999) Infections in the Male Genital Tract and Reactive Oxygen Species, *Hum. Reprod. 5*, 399–420.

39. Wolff, H., and Anderson, D.J. (1988) Immunohistologic Characterization and Quantitation of Leukocyte Subpopulation in Human Semen, *Fertil. Steril. 49*, 497–503.

40. Fedder, J., Askjaer, S.A., and Hjort, T. (1993) Nonspermatozoal Cells in Semen: Relationship to Other Semen Parameters and Fertility Status of the Couple, *Arch. Androl. 31*, 95–103.

41. Thomas, J., Fishel, S.B., Hall, J.A., Green, S., Newton, T.A., and Thornton, S.J. (1997) Increased Polymorphonuclear Granulocytes in Seminal Plasma in Relation to Sperm Morphology, *Hum. Reprod. 12*, 2418–2421.

42. Wolff, H. (1995) The Biologic Significance of White Blood Cells in Semen, *Fertil. Steril. 63*, 1143–1157.

43. Shekarriz, M., Sharma, R.K., Thomas, A.J., Jr., and Agarwal, A. (1995) Positive Myeloperoxidase Staining (Endtz Test) as an Indicator of Excessive Reactive Oxygen Species Formation in Semen, *J. Assist. Reprod. Genet. 12*, 70–74.

44. Kovalski, N.N., de Lamirande, E., and Gagnon, C. (1992) Reactive Oxygen Species Generated by Human Neutrophils Inhibit Sperm Motility: Protective Effects of Seminal Plasma and Scavengers, *Fertil. Steril. 58*, 809–816.

45. Pasqualotto, F.F., Sharma, R.K., Nelson, D.R., Thomas, A.J., Jr., and Agarwal, A. (2000) Relationship between Oxidative Stress, Semen Characteristics, and Clinical Diagnosis in Men Undergoing Fertility Investigation, *Fertil. Steril. 73*, 459–464.

46. Green, M.R., Allen, H., Hill, O., Okolowzubkowska, M.J., and Segal, A.W. (1979) The Production of OH and O_2^- by Stimulated Human Neutrophils-Measurement by Electron Paramagnetic Resonance Spectroscopy, *FEBS Lett. 100*, 23–26.

47. Blake, D.R., Allen, R.E., and Lunec, J. (1987) Free Radical in Biological Systems—A Review Oriented to Inflammatory Processes, *Br. Med. Bulletin 43*, 371–385.

48. Saran, M., Beck-Speier, I., Fellerhoff, B., and Bauer, G. (1999) Phagocytic Killing of Microorganisms by Radical Processes: Consequences of the Reaction of Hydroxyl Radicals with Chloride Yielding Chlorine Atoms, *Free Rad. Biol. Med. 26*, 482–490.

49. Smith, R., Vantman, D., Escobar, J., and Lissi, E. (1996) Total Antioxidant Capacity of Human Seminal Plasma, *Hum. Reprod. 11*, 1655–1660.

50. Donnelly, E.T., McClure, N., and Lewis, S. (1999) Antioxidant Supplementation *in Vitro* does not Improve Human Sperm Motility, *Fertil. Steril. 72,* 484–495.

51. Alvarez, J.G., Touchstone, J.C., Blasco, L., and Storey, B.T. (1987) Spontaneous Lipid Peroxidation and Production of Hydrogen Peroxide and Superoxide in Human Spermatozoa: Superoxide Dismutaseas Major Enzyme Protectant Against Oxygen Toxicity, *J. Androl. 8,* 336–348.

52. Chaudiere, J., Wilhelmsen, E.C., and Tappel, A.L. (1984) Mechanism of Selenium-Glutathione Peroxidase and its Inhibition by Mercaptocarboxylic Acids and other Mercaptans, *J. Biol. Chem. 259,* 1043–1050.

53. Jeulin, C., Soufir, J.C., Weber, P., Laval-Martin, D., and Calvayrac, R. (1989) Catalase Activity in Human Spermatozoa and Seminal Plasma, *Gam. Res. 24,* 185–196.

54. Fraga, G.G., Motchnik, P.A., Shigenaga, M.K., Helbrock, J.H., Jacob, R.A., and Ames, B. (1991) Ascorbic Acid Protects Against Endogenous Oxidative DNA Damage in Human Sperm, *Proc. Natl. Acad. Sci. USA. 88,* 11003–11006.

55. Thiele, J.J., Freisleben, H.J., Fuchs, J., and Oschendorf, F.R. (1995) Ascorbic Acid and Urate in Human Seminal Plasma: Determination and Interrelationship with Chemiluminescence in Washed Semen, *Hum. Reprod. 10,* 110–115.

56. Aitken, R.J., and Clarkson, J.S. (1988) Significance of Reactive Oxygen Species and Antioxidants in Defining the Efficacy of Sperm Preparation Techniques, *J. Androl. 9,* 367–376.

57. Moilanen, J., Hovatta, O., and Lindroth, L. (1993) Vitamin E Levels in Seminal Plasma can be Elevated by Oral Administration of Vitamin E in Infertile Men, *Int. J. Androl. 16,* 165–166.

58. de Lamirande, E., and Gagnon, C. (1992) Reactive Oxygen Species and Human Spermatozoa. II. Depletion of Adenosine Triphosphate (ATP) Plays an Important Role in the Inhibition of Sperm Motility, *J. Androl. 13,* 379–386.

59. Lenzi, A., Picardo, M., Gandini, L., Lombardo, F., Terminali, O., Passi, S., and Dondero, F. (1994) Glutathione Treatment of Dyspermia: Effect on the Lipoperoxidation Process, *Hum. Reprod. 9,* 2044–2050.

60. Alvarez, J.G., and Storey, B.T. (1983) Taurine, Hypotaurine, Epinephrine and Albumin Inhibit Lipid Peroxidation in Rabbit Spermatozoa and Protect Against Loss of Motility, *Biol. Reprod. 29,* 548–555.

61. Lewis, S.E.M., Boyle, P.M., McKinney, K.A., Young, I.S., and Thompson, W. (1995) Total Antioxidant Capacity of Seminal Plasma is Different in Fertile and Infertile Men, *Fertil. Steril. 64,* 868–870.

62. Wefers, H., and Sies, H. (1988) The Protection by Ascorbate and Glutathione Against Microsomal Lipid Peroxidation is Dependent on Vitamin E, *Eur. J. Biochem. 174,* 353–357.

63. Buettner, G.R. (1993) The Pecking Order of Free Radicals and Antioxidants, Lipid Peroxidation, Alpha-Tocopherol and Ascorbate, *Arch. Biochem. Biophys. 300,* 535–543.

64. Spitteler, G. (1993) Review: On the Chemistry of Oxidative Stress, *J. Lipid Mediators 7,* 77–82.

65. Clark, I.A., Hunt, N.H., and Cowden, W.B. (1986) Oxygen-Derived Free Radicals in the Pathogenesis of Parasitic Disease, *Adv. Parasitol. 25,* 1–44.

66. Griveau, J.F., and Le Lannou, D. (1997) Reactive Oxygen Species and Human Spermatozoa, *Int. J. Androl. 20,* 61–69.

67. Sikka, S.C., Rajasekaran, M., and Hellstrom, W.J.G. (1995) Role of Oxidative Stress and Antioxidants in Male Infertility, *J. Androl. 16,* 464–468.

68. Sikka, S.C. (2001) Relative Impact of Oxidative Stress on Male Reproductive Function, *Cur. Med. Chem. 8*, 851–862.

69. Aitken, R.J. (1995) Free Radicals, Lipid Peroxidation, and Sperm Function, *Reprod. Fertil. Dev. 7*, 659–668.

70. Halliwell, B. (1984) Tell Me about Free Radicals, Doctor: A Review, *J. Roy. Soc. Med. 82*, 747–752.

71. Aitken, R.J., Harkiss, D., and Buckingham, D. (1993) Relationship Between Iron-Catalyzed Lipid Peroxidation Potential and Human Sperm Function, *J. Reprod. Fertil. 98*, 257–265.

72. Sidhu, R.S., Sharma, R.K., Thomas, A.J., Jr., and Agarwal, A. (1998) Relationship Between Creatine Kinase Activity and Semen Characteristics in Sub-Fertile Men, *Int. J. Fertil. Women's Med. 43*, 192–197.

73. Lenzi, A., Cualosso, F., Gandini, L., Lombardo, F., and Dondero, F. (1993) Placebo-Controlled, Double-Blind, Cross-Over Trial of Glutathione Therapy, in Male Infertility, *Hum. Reprod. 9*, 2044–2050.

74. Agarwal, A., Ikemoto, I., and Loughlin, K.R. (1994) Levels of Reactive Oxygen Species before and after Sperm Preparation: Comparison of Swim-Up and L4 Filtration Methods, *Arch. Androl. 32*, 169–174.

75. Griveau, J.F., Renard, P., and Le Lannou, D. (1995) Superoxide Anion Production by Human Spermatozoa as a Part of the Ionophore-Induced Acrosome Reaction *in Vitro*, *Int. J. Androl. 18*, 67–74.

76. Sakkas, D., Mariethoz, E., Manicardi, G., Bizzaro, D., Bianchi, P., and Bianchi, U. (1999) Origin of DNA Damage in Ejaculated Human Spermatozoa, *Rev. Reprod. 4*, 31–37.

77. McPherson, S.M.G., and Longo, F.J. (1992) Localization of DNase I-Hypersensitive Regions during Rat Spermatogenesis: Stage-Dependent Patterns and Unique Sensitivity of Elongating Spermatids, *Mol. Reprod. Dev. 31*, 268–279.

78. Manicardi, G.C., Bianchi, P.G., Pantano, S., Azzoni, P., Bizzaro, D., Bianchi, U., and Sakkas, D. (1995) Presence of Endogenous Nicks in DNA of Ejaculated Human Spermatozoa and Its Relationship to Chromomycin A_3 Accessibility, *Biol. Reprod. 52*, 864–867.

79. Sailer, B.L., Jost, L.K., and Evenson, D.P. (1995) Mammalian Sperm DNA Susceptibility to *in Situ* Denaturation Associated with the Presence of DNA Strand Breaks as Measured by the Terminal Deoxynucleotidyl Transferase Assay, *J. Androl. 16*, 80–87.

80. Nagata, S. (1997) Apoptosis by Death Factor, *Cell 88*, 355–365.

81. Vaux, D.L., and Korsmeyer, S.J. (1999) Cell Death in Development, *Cell 96*, 245–254.

82. Sinha, H.A.P., and Swerdloff, R.S. (1999) Hormonal and Genetic Control of Germ Cell Apoptosis in the Testis, *Rev. Reprod. 4*, 38–47.

83. Lee, J., Richburg, J.H., Younkin, S.C., and Boekelheide, K. (1997) The Fas System is a Key Regulator of Germ Cell Apoptosis in the Testis, *Endocrinol. 138*, 2081–2088.

84. Krammer, P.H., Behrmann, I., Daniel, P., Dhein, J., and Debatin, K.M. (1994) Regulation of Apoptosis in the Immune System, *Current Opinions Immunol. 6*, 279–289.

85. Suda, T., Takahashi, T., Golstein, P., and Nagata, S. (1993) Molecular Cloning and Expression of Fas Ligand, a Novel Member of the Tumor Necrosis Factor Family, *Cell 75*, 1169–1178.

86. Twigg. J., Irvine, D.S., Houston, P., Fulton, N., Michael, L., and Aitken, R.J. (1998) Iatrogenic DNA Damage Induced in Human Spermatozoa during Sperm Preparation: Protective Significance of Seminal Plasma, *Mol. Hum. Reprod. 4*, 439–445.

87. Duru, N.K., Morshedi, M., and Oehninger, S. (2000) Effects of Hydrogen Peroxide on DNA and Plasma Membrane Integrity of Human Spermatozoa. *Fertil. Steril. 74*, 1200–1207.

88. Kodama, H., Yamaguchi, R., Fukuda, J., Kasai, H., and Tanaka, T. (1997) Increased Oxidative Deoxyribonucleic Acid Damage in the Spermatozoa of Infertile Male Patients, *Fertil. Steril. 65*, 519–524.

89. Lopes, S., Jurisicova, A., Sun, J., and Casper, R.F. (1998) Reactive Oxygen Species: A Potential Cause for DNA Fragmentation in Human Spermatozoa, *Hum. Reprod. 13*, 896–900.

90. Twigg. J., Irvine, D.S., and Aitken, R.J. (1998) Oxidative Damage to DNA in Human Spermatozoa does not Preclude Pronucleus Formation at Intracytoplasmic Sperm Injection, *Hum. Reprod. 13*, 1864–1871.

91. Sun, J.G., Jurisicova, A., and Casper, R.F. (1997) Deletion of Deoxyribonucleic Acid Fragmentation in Human Sperm: Correlation with Fertilization *in Vitro, Biol. Reprod. 56*, 602–607.

92. Lopes, S., Sun, J., Jurisicova, A., Meriano, J., and Casper, R.F. (1998) Semen Deoxyribonucleic Acid Fragmentation is Increased in Poor Quality Semen Samples and Correlates with Failed Fertilization in Intracytoplasmic Sperm Injection, *Fertil. Steril. 69*, 528–532.

93. Morales, P., Vantman, D., Darros, C., and Vigil, P. (1991) Human Spermatozoa Selected by Percoll Gradient or Swim-Up Are Equally Capable of Binding to the Human Zona Pellucida and Undergoing Acrosome Reaction, *Hum. Reprod. 6*, 401–404.

94. Ng, F.L., Liu, D.Y., and Baker, H.W. (1992) Comparison of Percoll, Mini-Percoll, and Swim-Up Methods for Sperm Preparation from Abnormal Semen Samples, *Hum. Reprod. 7*, 261–266.

95. Fraga, G.G., Motchnik, P., Wyrobek, A.J., Rempel, D.M., and Ames, B. (1996) Smoking and Low Antioxidant Levels Increase Oxidative Damage to Sperm DNA, *Mut. Res. 351*, 199–203.

96. Ji, B.T., Shu, X.O., Linet, M.S., Zheng, W., Milne, P.A., and Aitken, R.J. (1997) Paternal Cigarette Smoking and the Risk of Childhood Cancer Among Offspring of Nonsmoking Mothers, *J. Natl. Cancer Inst. 89*, 238–244.

97. Sorahan, T., Lancashire, R.J., Hulten, M.A., Peck, I., and Stewart, A.M. (1997) Childhood Cancer and Parental Use of Tobacco: Deaths from 1953 to 1955, *British J. Cancer 75*, 134–138.

98. Roberts, K.P. (1998) Y Chromosome Deletions and Male Infertility: State of the Art and Clinical Applications, *J. Androl. 19*, 255–259.

99. Vogt, P., Chandley, A.C., Hargreave, T.B., Keil, R., Ma, K., and Sharkey, A. (1992) Microdeletions in Interval 6 of Y Chromosome of Males with Idiopathic Sterility Point to Disruption of AZF, a Human Spermatogenesis Gene, *Hum. Genet. 89*, 491–496.

100. Sharma, R., Pasqualotto, F.F., Nelson, D.R., Thomas, A.J., Jr., and Agarwal, A. (2001) Relationship between Seminal White Blood Cell Counts and Oxidative Stress in Men Treated at an Infertility Clinic, *J. Androl. 22*, 575–583.

101. Saleh, R.A., Agarwal, A., Kandirali, E., Sharma, R.K., Thomas, A.J., Jr., Nada, E.A., Evenson, D.P., and Alvarez, J.G. (2002) Leukocytospermia is Associated with Increased Reactive Oxygen Species Production by Human Spermatozoa, *Fertil. Steril. 78*, 1215–1224.

102. Agarwal, A., Ikemoto, I. and Loughlin, K.R. (1994) Effect of Sperm Washing on Reactive Oxygen Species Level in Semen, *Arch. Androl. 33*, 157–162.

103. Shekarriz, M., Thomas, A.J., Jr., and Agarwal, A. (1995a) A Method of Human Semen Centrifugation to Minimize the Iatrogenic Sperm Injuries Caused by Reactive Oxygen Species, *Eur. Urol. 28*, 31–35.
104. Shekarriz, M., Thomas, A.J., Jr., and Agarwal, A. (1995) Incidence and Level of Seminal Reactive Oxygen Species in Normal Men, *Urology 45*, 103–107.
105. Ollero, M., Gil-Guzman, E., Lopez, M.C., Sharma, R.K., Agarwal, A., Larson, K.L., Evenson, D.K., Thomas, A.J., Jr., and Alvarez, J.G. (2001) Characterization of Subsets of Human Spermatozoa at Different Stages of Maturation: Implications in the Diagnosis and Treatment of Male Infertility, *Hum. Reprod. 16*, 1912–1921.
106. Sharma, R.K., Pasqualotto, F.F., Nelson, D.R., Thomas, A.J., Jr., and Agarwal, A. (1999) The Reactive Oxygen Species–Total Antioxidant Capacity Score is a New Measure of Oxidative Stress to Predict Male Infertility, *Hum. Reprod. 14*, 2801–2807.
107. Kobayashi, H., Gil-Guzman, E., Mahran, A.M., Sharma, R.K., Nelson, D.R., Thomas, A.J., Jr., and Agarwal, A. (2000) Quality Control of Reactive Oxygen Species Measurement by Luminol-Dependent Chemiluminescence Assay, *J. Androl. 22*, 568–574.
108. Kolettis, P., Sharma, R.K., Pasqualotto, F.F., Nelson, D.R., Thomas, A.J., Jr., and Agarwal, A. (1999) The Effects of Seminal Oxidative Stress on Fertility after Vasectomy Reversal, *Fertil. Steril. 71*, 249–255.
109. Saleh, R.A., Kobayashi, H., Ranganathan, P., Sharma, R.K., Nelson, D.R., Thomas, A.J., Jr., and Agarwal, A. (2001) Quality Control of Total Nonenzymatic Seminal Antioxidant Capacity by an Enhanced Chemiluminescence Assay, 7th International Congress of Andrology, Montreal, Canada, June 15–20.
110. Daitch, J.A., Bedaiway, M.A., Pasqualotto, F.F., Hendin, B., Hallak, J., Falcone, T., Thomas, A.J., Jr., Nelson, D.R., and Agarwal, A. (2001) Varicocelectomy Improves Intrauterine Insemination Success Rates among Men with Varicocele, *J. Urol. 165*, 1510–1513.
111. Agarwal, A., Ikemoto, I., and Loughlin, K.R. (1997) Prevention of Testicular Damage by Free-Radical Scavengers, *Urology 50*, 759–763.
112. Pasqualotto, F.F., Sharma, R.K., Kobayashi, H., Nelson, D.R., Thomas, A.J., Jr., and Agarwal, A. (2001) Oxidative Stress in Normospermic Men Undergoing Infertility Evaluation, *J. Androl. 73*, 459–464.
113. Pasqualotto, F.F., Sharma, R.K., Agarwal, A., Nelson, D.R., Thomas, A.J., Jr., and Potts, J.M. (2000) Seminal Oxidative Stress in Chronic Prostatitis Patients, *Urology 55*, 881–885.
114. Saleh, R.A., Esfandiari, N., Al-Dujaily, S., Sharma, R.K., Thomas, A.J., Jr., and Agarwal, A. (2001) An Accurate and Reliable Method for the Diagnosis of Seminal Oxidative Stress in Infertile Men, 57th Annual Meeting of the American Society for Reproductive Medicine, Orlando, Florida, October 20–25.
115. Saleh, R.A., Larson, K.L., Sharma, R.K., Thomas, A.J., Jr., Evenson, D.P., and Agarwal, A. (2001) Correlation of Reactive Oxygen Species in Neat Semen with Sperm Chromatin Structure Assay-Defined Sperm DNA Damage, 57th Annual Meeting of the American Society for Reproductive Medicine, Orlando, Florida, October 20–25.

Chapter 14

Scavenger Systems and Related Therapies Against Lipoperoxidation Damage of Polyunsaturated Fatty Acids in Spermatozoa

Andrea Lenzia[a], Loredana Gandini[a], Federica Tramer[c], Vittoria Maresca[b], Francesco Lombardo[a], Gabriella Sandri[c], Mauro Picardo[b], Enrico Panfili[c]

[a]Department of Medical Physiopathology, Laboratory of Seminology and Immunology of Reproduction, University of Rome "La Sapienza", Rome, Italy
[b]Laboratory of Physiopathology, IRCCS "S. Gallicano", Rome, Italy
[c]Department of Biochemistry, Biophysics and Macromolecular Chemistry, University of Trieste, Italy

Abstract

One of the principal energy sources in sperm cells comes from the metabolism of lipids. This is of great importance for the cell structure. The membrane double leaflets do not consist of a passive lipid film but are a highly complex and specialized structure. The sperm cell membrane requires various testicular lipid biosynthetic processes and passage through the epididymis for its full maturation. We describe the compositions of sperm and immature germ cell membranes with particular attention to their phospholipids rich in polyunsaturated fatty aicds (PUFA). Both testis germ cells and spermatozoa undergoing epididymal maturation have various enzymatic and nonenzymatic scavenger systems to prevent damage from lipoperoxidation. These include catalase, superoxide dismutase, and GSH-dependent oxidoreductases, present in different amounts depending on the stage of development. Discussed in depth are phospholipid hydroperoxide GSH peroxidase (PHGPx) activity and alpha tocopherol of rat epididymal spermatozoa and their distribution and roles in caput and cauda epididymal sperm cells. They are also considered with respect to aging. A highly specialized scavenger system is present in seminal plasma. This protects the sperm membrane from lipoperoxidation, and it is regulated by the degree of PUFA unsaturation. A disequilibrium of anti- and pro-oxidants may be the result of a systemic predisposition or one of various pathologies. GSH or other scavengers can restore the cell membrane's physiological PUFA constitution and so are useful for treating this imbalance. The results of a study using GSH therapy, as an example of scavenger therapy, are presented and discussed.

Physiological Role of Phospholipids in the Sperm Plasma Membrane

Sperm fertilization capacity and sperm-oocyte communication are greatly influenced by the sperm membrane. Its biochemical constitution is therefore one of the principal areas under investigation in the study of sperm physiology and pathology.

Spermatozoa are polarized cells consisting of structurally and functionally distinct domains. Sensitivity to capacitation stimuli is found in the two leaflets in the membrane of the cap region, which overlies the acrosomal vesicle (1). An increase in fluidity of the cap region is induced by the various capacitation steps. This leads to a fusogenic process, which possesses already the structural premise, which kicks off between this and the outer acrosomal vesicle membrane. Finally, pore formation allows the acrosomal enzymes acrosine and hyaluronidase to disperse. Intensification of the fusion process leads to the formation of mixed pseudovesicles comprising both the plasma and the outer acrosomal membrane. Demonstrated in animal models, although only partly confirmed in humans, is the penetration of the zona pellucida by the spermatozoa toward the end of this process. Current membrane fusion theories hold that membrane fluidity is paramount for normal cell function and that cell membrane fluidity and flexibility are largely related to the membranes lipid constitution.

Early pioneer sperm lipid analyses performed to investigate this area demonstrated the presence of neutral fatty acids, cholesterol, phospholipids (mainly lecithin, cephalin, and sphingomielin), and glycolipids (2–6) in mammalian and nonmammalian spermatozoa. It was also shown that the oxidative metabolism of endogenous fatty acids of up to two-carbon acyl fragments was particularly active in the epididymis as a result of the high concentration of carnitine and acetylcarnitine facilitating fatty acid passage into mitochondria, the site of beta-oxidation.

Also widely studied in recent years is the role of cholesterol in fusogenic events leading to capacitation. Cholesterol can inhibit protein insertion into plasma membrane phospholipids (7). It has also been shown to reduce lateral motility of proteic receptors, affecting their activity and altering their conformation (8). Conversely, cholesterol removal leads to membrane destabilization and allows protein migration, the basis of capacitation and the acrosome reaction (1).

During *in vitro* capacitation, cholesterol concentration is lowered mainly in the acrosomal cap plasma membrane (1,8). Albumin, one of the most well-studied sterol acceptors promoting cholesterol outflow from the sperm plasma membrane, is considered one of the main capacitating substances (9). The resulting higher membrane fluidity allows receptor migration to the equatorial region. This migration, or removal of glycolipoproteic components of the acrosomal membrane, has been demonstrated in guinea pigs (10,11). It has recently been suggested for human spermatozoa, with antisperm antibodies acting as probes of membrane antigenic change during capacitation events (12,13). Finally, the molecular signals that activate acrosome reactions are initiated, involving many second messenger pathways.

Analysis of lipid composition in sperm cell membranes has shown that phospholipids represent the main fraction, in particular, phosphatidylcholine and phosphatidylethanolamine (14,15). Plasmalogen forms a significant proportion of the phospholipids in sperm membranes. This is a distinct group of aldehydogenic phosphatidyl lipids, containing one fatty acid esterified with glycerol and a long carbon chain (C20; C24) unsaturated ester. Its hydrolysis yields a fatty aldehyde and a fatty acid. The exact role of these lipids is not yet fully understood. However, a similar membrane lipid constitution has been described in nervous system cells (16), that is, in other cells in which membrane transduction signals and cell-to-cell interaction are fundamental for their physiological function. On a related theme, free radicals have been recently suggested as second messengers, conducting signals from the outer to the inner leaflet of the membrane (17).

Analysis of fatty acids in membrane phospholipids and plasmalogen has revealed the presence of polyunsaturated fatty acids (PUFA) in significant quantities. Their contribution to membrane fluidity and flexibility is already known (18–20). The fatty acid composition of cell membranes controls the activity of various lipid-dependent membrane-bound enzymes, again including the second messenger systems, and affects the membrane resistance to chemical and physical stress.

In the membrane of spermatozoa from rams, an asymmetric transversal distribution of phospholipids has been demonstrated. Aminophospholipids are preferentially located in the inner and choline-containing phospholipids in the outer leaflet. The presence of an aminophospholipid translocase in the membrane, together with results from fluorescence studies, suggests a transbilayer phospholipid movement and points to the importance of their transversal segregation in the fusion process during fertilization (1,21).

The three PUFA classes are classified by the distance from the first double bond to the methyl terminal, *i.e.,* n-3, n-6, and n-9. α-Linolenic acid (18:3n-3), linoleic acid (18:2n-6), and oleic acid (18:1n-9) are the parent fatty acids of the three groups. Long-chain PUFA in cell membrane phospholipids are derived from the metabolism of the essential fatty acids linoleic acid (18:2n-6) and α-linolenic acid (18:3n-3). These parent essential fatty acids, after ingestion through normal diet, are converted into their long-chain derivatives by a series of elongations and desaturations.

Metabolism takes place mainly in the liver as desaturase activity is almost exclusively limited to this organ. Delta-6-desaturase is considered the rate-limiting enzyme and is probably regulated by vitamin E and selenium, thought to be its co-factors (22), and the lipid composition of hepatic microsomes. PUFA are also precursors of prostaglandins and leukotrienes, which are important factors in both sperm motility and inflammatory processes. Prostaglandin E and 19-OH PGE have both been shown to be related to sperm motility.

Epididymal maturation leads to the definitive lipid pattern of ejaculated spermatozoa. This was first demonstrated in rams, where different lipid patterns were seen in testicular and ejaculated sperm (23,24). In rats (1,27,28), guinea pigs (10,26), and rams (25) the sperm membrane undergoes a complete transformation of its preexisting protein and lipid structures during passage through the epididymis. In humans, too, biomembrane fluidity and degree of unsaturation (associated with the fatty acyl component of phospholipids) may increase proportionately as sperm pass from the caput to the cauda of the epididymis. This would indicate active lipid sperm metabolism.

Using combined gas chromatography–mass spectrometry (29) we studied the PUFA membrane composition in human ejaculated spermatozoa, examined after washing. Higher PUFA levels were detected in sperm than in blood serum phospholipids. This difference has already been noted in both humans (30,31) and mammalian spermatozoa (15) but without a proposed relationship to sperm fertilizing capability. However, both diet and, in animals, the season have been found to significantly affect this percentage. This suggests active fatty acid metabolism and desaturation during either spermatogenesis or epididymal sperm maturation.

To further investigate this, we studied sperm populations and immature germ cells (IGC) present in semen from the same subjects using an ad hoc modified Percoll gradient (32). In whole spermatozoa we found around 50% saturated fatty acids, with greatest levels of palmitic (16:0) and stearic acids (18:0). Oleic acid (18:1n-9) was the main monounsaturated fatty acid and the essential fatty acids linoleic (18:2n-6) and α-linolenic acid (18:3n-3) were both present, although in lower concentrations than oleic acid.

The following metabolites resulting from desaturase activity were found: 20:3n-6, 20:4n-6, 22:4n-6, 20:5n-3, and 22:6n-3. Total PUFA concentration was around 30%, with about 1/3 n-6 and 2/3 n-3 PUFA. Docosahexaenoic acid (DHA, 22:6n-3) was the PUFA found at the highest concentration.

Significant differences were found in fatty acid concentration in sperm populations and IGC separated on Percoll gradient. In sperm populations, there was no great change in the levels of saturated fatty acids, whereas for the unsaturated fatty acids a significant rearrangement was seen. Linoleic acid and α-linolenic acid decreased from lower to higher Percoll fractions. The 20:3n-6 level was relatively stable. 20:4n-6 progressively decreased, and this was associated with an increase in 22:4n-6. Conversely, the desaturase metabolites 20:5n-3 and 22:6n-3 progressively increased in the higher Percoll-concentrated layers. A significant inverse correlation of 18:2n-6 and 18:3n-3 with the Percoll gradient concentrations was found. In contrast, a direct linear correlation was found between DHA increase and higher Percoll gradients.

The high 22:6n-3 level correlates well with spermatozoa morphology. In fact, an inverse relationship was seen between the percentage of atypical forms scored in each layer and the 22:6n-3 levels evaluated in the same layers. The best morphological pattern is seen with the highest 22:6n-3 concentration.

Results for IGC isolated by the second Percoll gradient were quite different. As for sperm cells, saturated fatty acids were present mainly as 16:0 and 18:0, but their concentration in relation to total fatty acids present was significantly higher. Monounsaturated fatty acids consisted of 16:1n-7 and 18:1n-9. 18:2n-6 and 18:3n-3 concentrations were significantly higher than in mature sperm cells. In contrast, the desaturase metabolites n-6 PUFA and n-3 PUFA were significantly lower than seen in mature sperm cells. Di-homo gamma-linolenic acid (20:3n-6), arachidonic acid (20:4n-6), and docosahexanoic acid (22:6n-3) were the PUFA present in the greatest concentrations but were less concentrated than in mature sperm cells.

These results demonstrate the human germ cell active lipid metabolism, which causes changes to fatty acid concentration and elongation and saturation of essential fatty acids during spermatogenesis and possibly also during the sperm maturation process (33).

The high PUFA concentration in the membrane of mature and morphologically normal sperm suggests that spermatozoa are extremely sensitive to external stimuli. Their fertilizing function may explain why this cell is provided with a fragile, but very active membrane that is easily destabilized and activated. The high PUFA concentration may also give biochemical confirmation of the sperm plasma membrane's essential role in the fertilization process. It is notable that similar PUFA concentrations, particularly 22:6n-3, are detectable in membranes of nerve cells or cells derived from the neural crest, such as melanocytes (34).

Interestingly, rats fed with a diet deficient in essential fatty acids have shown, in addition to decreased PUFA levels in both red blood cells and serum, degeneration of the seminiferous tubules, progressive decrease in germ cells, and absence of spermatozoa in the lumina of the seminiferous tubules and epididymis (35). These alterations and the rats' consequent infertility are related to the marked reduction in the level of arachidonic acid as a proportion of total fatty acids present in the testis.

An alteration in PUFA constitution of the plasma membrane is a possible explanation of several andrological diseases (varicocele, germ-free genital tract inflammation) and may be the cause of the membrane's increased vulnerability after exposure to reproductive toxic compounds. PUFA are in fact one of the main victims of free radical damage, and an inverse relationship between sperm motility and lipid peroxides has been clearly demonstrated (36) both *in vivo* and *in vitro*.

Enzymatic and Nonenzymatic Scavenger Systems and Sperm Lipoperoxidation

Reactive oxygen species (ROS) are chemical species endowed with an unpaired electron that react promptly with both other free radicals and nonradical molecules, thus triggering a cascade of radical reactions (37). Figure 14.1 summarizes the glutathione-dependent enzymatic scavenger mechanism active on peroxidated fatty acids (LOOH). This system is founded on at least five different GSH peroxidases (GPx). One of these (PHGPx) specifically reduces *in situ* the membrane phospholipid hydroperoxides. The link with GR is compulsory for the correct turnover of the GSSG/GSH couple. A recent review by Ochsendorf (38) illustrates exhaustively the state of the art on the ROS and the male genital tract.

The single electron reduction, with the consequent generation of the superoxide anion radical, hydrogen peroxide, and the hydroxyl radical, is more frequent than the two-electron reduction, owing to the parallel electron spin arrangements in the latter

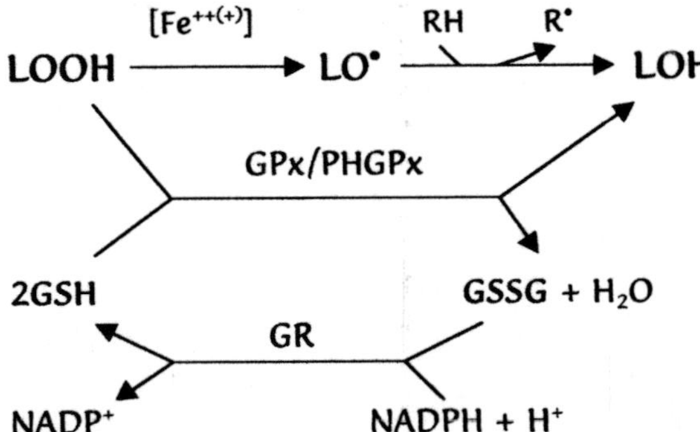

Fig. 14.1. Glutathione peroxidases system. LOOH: Hydroperoxide (PLOOH: phospholipid hydroperoxide for PHGPx); LO•: alkoxyl radical; LOH: hydroxylated fatty acid; RH: e.g. PUFA, α-tocopherol; R•: a radical; GPx: glutathione peroxidase; PHGPx: phospholipid hydroperoxide glutathione peroxidase; GR: glutathione reductase; GSH/GSSG: reduced /oxidated glutathione.

case. ROS are very unstable in biological material; they are highly reactive, and the hydroxyl radical is considered the most powerful. It can cause effective biological damage only if generated in close proximity to a potential target molecule or directly at the critical cellular target site. The hydroperoxyl radical, which is a more powerful oxidant, may be the predominant form of superoxide anion in phospholipid membranes. This is capable of peroxidizing PUFA and thus initiating a chain reaction.

It should be pointed out, however, that there is a growing body of evidence indicating that low ROS levels are responsible for the physiological control of some sperm functions (39,40).

The levels of peroxidable substances, such as PUFA, and free radical scavenger system activity and levels generally regulate cellular homeostasis. An oxidative stress can therefore be defined as any disturbance of the balance between pro- and antioxidants, where pro-oxidants are predominant. Studies of the processes resulting from the action of these two competing systems are therefore fundamental for the understanding of the complex sequence of events leading from spermatogenesis to sperm-oocyte fusion. Mammalian testis metabolism aimed at ensuring proper spermatogenesis and spermiogenesis defense against the (lipo)peroxidative stresses has been investigated for many years (41,42), examining both the enzymatic and nonenzymatic scavenging systems. Enzymatic activities have been monitored (catalase, superoxide dismutase, peroxidases), as well as molecular (tocopherol, ascorbate, carotenoids, quinones, GSH) and single element cofactors, such as selenium. Se deficiency has long been recognized as one of the major factors responsible for alterations of male germ cell maturation (41,43–46). Se-containing proteins and/or enzymes have therefore been actively considered and characterized in the mammalian reproductive tract (47,48).

The transit of mammalian spermatozoa from caput to cauda epididymis involves a sequence of complex maturation processes, mainly mediated by the epididymal environment. The final result is the transformation of a nonmotile, nonfertile cell into a potentially fertile one. These transformations chiefly involve chemical and physical modifications of the lipid assemblage of the plasma and outer acrosomal membrane (1,49–52). A specific protection against peroxidative damage of PUFA-rich membranes and their functions is therefore compulsory for maturing spermatozoa. Human spermatozoa exhibit both spontaneous lipoperoxidation (53) and a well-balanced antiperoxidative capacity, just sufficient to accomplish fertilization (54). μM H_2O_2 produced *in vitro* on human spermatozoa appears to be the most toxic ROS owing to its capacity to cross membranes, inhibit glucose 6P dehydrogenase, GPx, SOD, and decrease PUFA concentration (55). Epididymal sperm cells are well equipped with enzymatic activities, which can reduce H_2O_2 and other potentially harmful ROS. Superoxide dismutase (SOD, E.C. 1.15.1.1), GSH peroxidase (GPx or GPx-1 or c-GPx, E.C.1.11.1.9, tetrameric), and GSH reductase (GR, E.C. 1.6.4.2) are certainly present in epididymal spermatozoa (see 56 for a survey). The activity of the catalase (CAT, E.C. 1.11.1.6) is however still under debate (57–60). Phospholipid hydroperoxide glutathione peroxidase (PHGPx or GPX-4, E.C. 1.11.1.19, the 20 kDa monomeric form of the Se-enzymes GPxs) (61) was recently discovered by the authors to be active in epididymal sperm cells (62,63).

As reported in Table 14.1 (56), there is a significant statistical difference of the specific activities between caput and cauda epididymal isolated sperm cells for PHGPx, GPx, and SOD, with activities about 2–3-fold higher in the caput sperms.

A more detailed picture of PHGPx specific activity, separately monitored in the sperm heads and tails, is given in Figure 14.2. The hystograms clearly indicate that the catalytic ability of the protein, as would be expected on the basis of the data in Table 14.1, is lowest in the cauda fractions, but acrosomal/chromatin-associated (*heads*) PHGPx is more active than mitochondrial-associated (*tails*) PHGPx. This again suggests that the ability to reduce phospholipid hydroperoxides diminishes during epididymal transit. This may seem irrational, however other functions later discussed will shed light on the process. The concurrent probe of PHGPx protein distribution is

TABLE 14.1
Specific Activities in Rat Epididymal Sperm Cells[a]

	PHGPx*	GPx*	GR*	CAT[+]	SOD°
Whole epididymis	1.58 (0.39)	4.40 (0.88)	1.40 (0.18)	7.54 (1.18)	0.59 (0.11)
Caput	3.32 (0.53)	8.09 (1.02)	1.49 (0.24)	8.72 (1.60)	0.76 (0.26)
Cauda	0.95 (0.27)[a]	3.41 (0.38)[b]	1.33 (0.23)[d]	5.30 (2.80)[d]	0.44 (0.09)[c]

aPHGPx, phospholipid hydroperoxyde glutathione peroxidase; GPx, glutathione peroxidase; GR, glutathione reductase; CAT, catalase; SOD, superoxide dismutase. Values are presented as mean (SD) of 5–10 separate measurements. Units: * nmol NADPH/min.10^6 cells; + nmol O_2/min.10^6 cells; °U/10^6 cells. Significance: [a] $P < 0.0005$, [b] $P < 0.005$, [c] $P < 0.05$, [d] not significant in comparison to the caput epididymis spermatozoa corresponding value.

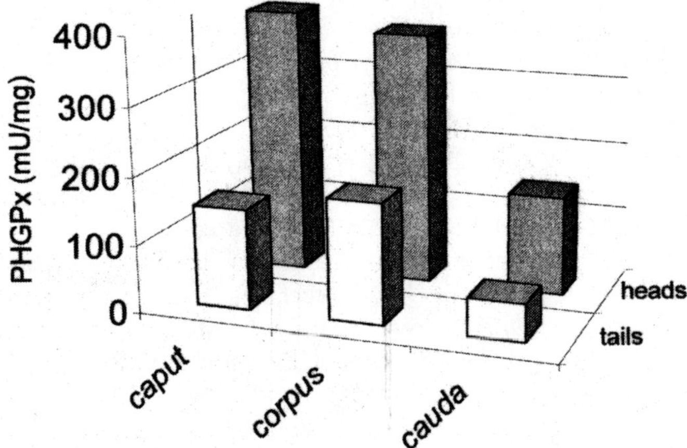

Fig. 14.2. PHGPx specific activity in rat caput-, corpus-, and cauda-epididymal sperm fractions.

reported in Figure 14.3. The immunogold spots shown in panel A depict the typical distribution in the acrosome membrane, into the chromatin, and at the level of the midpiece mitochondrial membranes. No signal at all was detected in the principal pieces (panel B) (63).

The presence and distribution of PHGPx in testis cells and spermatozoa, compared with other enzymes, is remarkable for a number of different reasons. First, the testis exhibits the highest specific activity of PHGPx so far monitored in any tissue: up

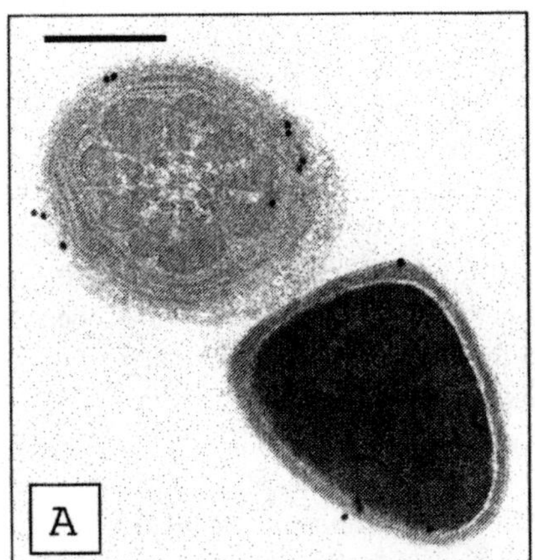

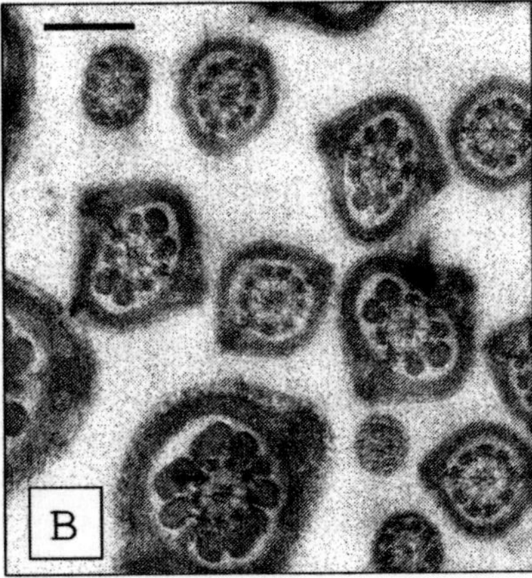

Fig. 14.3 Immunogold localization of PHGPx in 6-month-old rat epididymal spermatozoa. A: head midpiece (tranversally cut); B: principal pieces (tranversally cut). Bar: 300 nm.

to two orders of magnitude higher than that for brain or liver, for example (64,65). The enzyme activity in testis is, moreover, gonadotropin-dependent and expressed in the testis only after puberty (64,66,67). Roles for PHGPx in addition to its already established antioxidant function have been recently suggested. In different somatic cells PHGPx is, in fact, involved in the inactivation of 5-lipoxygenase. It works by lowering the level of the fatty acid hydroperoxides required for the full functioning of the lipoxygenase, thus resulting in a modulation of leukotrienes (68,69). A similar effect has been demonstrated for purified 15-lipoxygenase (70).

The intriguing novelty in the functional ambit concerns PHGPx's ability to oxidize thiol groups other than those of GSH or other small molecules. We demonstrated, in fact, that the enzyme specifically oxidizes the reduced –SH groups of isolated epididymal caput sperm protamine (62). This is an exciting result if the role of these unique sperm-proteins, which progressively substitute histones during spermiogenesis, is considered. In mammals these proteins are rich in cysteine residues, whose oxidation is crucial for the correct assembly and condensation of the mature sperm cell chromatin (71). The protamine-dependent compactness and resilience of the DNA protect it until fusion with the oocyte DNA. The selective PHGPx activity toward caput protamine thiols must therefore be carefully taken into account; given the higher enzyme specific activity in epididymal caput spermatozoa (Table 14.1), a key function of PHGPx in the oxidation of the caput protamines thiol groups could be envisaged. On the other hand, disulfide bond formation and chromatin condensation are already concluded in the cauda epididymis, and this could correlate well with the parallel decrease in PHGPx activity there (Table 14.1).

On the whole, these new roles can be viewed as a wider capability of the enzyme to modulate a "peroxide tone" thanks to the regulation of the ratio of the endogenous oxidized/reduced forms of hydroperoxides and thiol-bearing molecules, as already envisaged by some authors (69,72), and also for the DNA compaction mechanism (73).

The very recent additional function suggested for PHGPx in the midpiece mitochondria of the mature rat spermatozoa is as a structural molecule, as an enzymatically inactive, oxidatively cross-linked, insoluble protein (74). This new role may explain the Se-deficiency dependent alterations of spermatozoa. These data agree well with the results reported in Fig. 14.2, indicating that only the mature sperm tail PHGPx (*cauda*) is less endowed with catalytic activity. In fact, it was recently reported that a group of infertile men with oligoasthenozoospermia showed a dramatically decreased level of mitochondrial PHGPx expression in their cells, as well as morphologically and functionally abnormal midpiece mitochondria (75).

Another aspect of the GSH-linked enzymes (mainly PHGPx) concerns male aging. We recently examined 36 to 365 day old specimens of rat testis cells and epididymal spermatozoa, considering both specific activity and protein expression (63). Figure 14.4 reports the two distinct maxima reached by the specific activity in 3-month-old testis and 6-month-old sperm cells, respectively. Aging therefore causes a lowering of enzyme activity in testis cells. This occurs earlier and more markedly

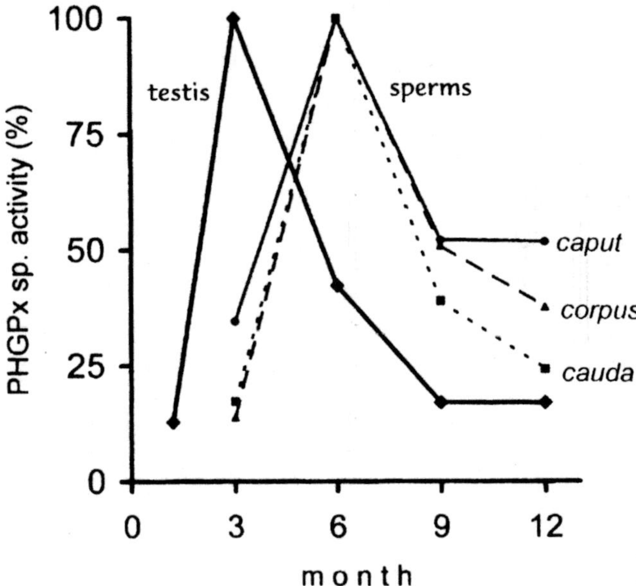

Fig 14.4. PHGPx specific activity (percent) in rat testis homogenate and caput-, corpus-, and cauda-epididymal sperm cells at vaious age.

than in spermatozoa. It has already been demonstrated that PHGPx protein expression in a given tissue shows a pattern often not superimposable with the catalytic activity (76). In testis cells, protein expression is at its maximum at 6 months (63), when the specific activity is already decreasing (Fig. 14.4). More intriguing is protein behavior in the epididymal sperm cell subfractions, reported in Figure 14.5. Only activity in the mitochondrial location (tail extract) increases continuously from 3 to 12 months, whereas chromatin-linked PHGPx (head + DNAse extract) and, chiefly, acrosomal PHGPx decrease consistently after 6 months. If one considers that the role of PHGPx in midpiece mitochondria has been defined as more structural (74) in comparison to its more catalytic role in the acrosome (56), one could suggest that aging is more detrimental to the proper acrosomal functioning than to other pHGPx-dependent mechanisms.

Nonenzymatic systems should be examined in strict connection with enzymatic activities. The couple GSH/GSSG is, for example, one of the most important nonenzymatic molecules, at least if one considers its links with the above-mentioned GSH-dependent enzymes (see Fig. 14.1). The reducing equivalents necessary for regeneration of GSH by GR are provided by NADPH and glucose-6P-dehydrogenase activity, which has been indicated as the limiting step in the reductive pathway (77).

GSH production in spermatogenic cells is dependent upon Sertoli cells and based on the interaction between different cell types (78,79). However, there are contradictory reports of the amount present in sperm cells (80,81). In principle, its presence in

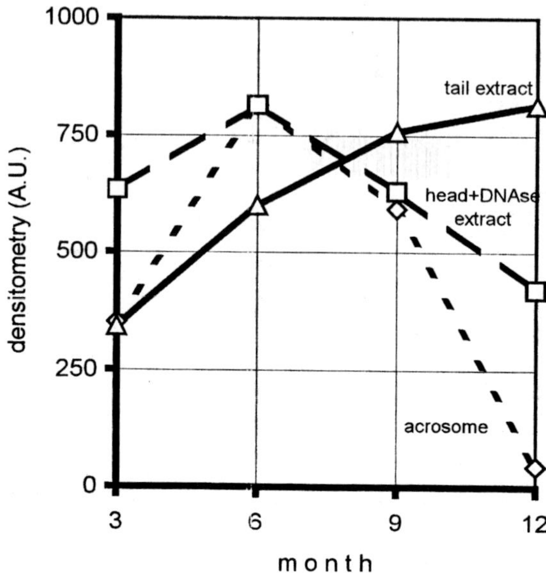

Fig. 14.5. Western blot analysis of PHGPx in rat epididymal sperm cells subfractions.

sperm cells should be expected, although for PHGPx other thiol-containing substrates may exist. The limited and easily auto-oxidable quantity of GSH, the sensitivity and accuracy of the assay, and the purity of sperm cell preparations are the main reasons for the discrepancies in its detection. Our data (56) indicate in rats a value of about 35 pmol GSH/10^6 sperm cells, without appreciable differences between caput and cauda epididymis spermatozoa. This value is similar to those reported for goat, rabbit, ram, dog, boar, and human specimens (81). Recently Ochsendorf *et al.* (82) reported for human sperm cells a value of about 30 pmol GSH/10^6 cells. In any case there is scant and scattered information if we consider that GSH can play a demonstrated therapeutical role in selected cases of male infertility, as described in detail later on. The monitoring of GSH-dependent enzymes would therefore be useful to define a link, on a metabolic and molecular basis, between this therapeutic agent and catalytic acitvities and distribution in normal and pathologic human specimens. Our recent, very preliminary, data indicate that GPx, PHGPx, and GR do not change their specific activity in asthenozoospermic human ejaculates compared to control samples.

Alpha-tocopherol and ascorbate are two other fundamental scavenger molecules capable of interrupting radical propagation. The lipophylic nature of tocopherol and the water solubility of ascorbate therefore provide protection in any cellular domain. The two vitamins can also interact; ascorbate can in fact regenerate the ROS-oxidated tocopheryl radical. Studies on the possible therapeutic use of vitamin E in mammalian infertility have been privileged up to now (83,84), rather than studies concerning its physiological distribution and role in germ cells and spermatozoa.

Table 14.2 reports the content and distribution of alpha-tocopherol in isolated rat epididymal spermatozoa (85). It is present in the plasma and acrosomal membrane and the mid-piece mitochondria (tails). This indicates the continuity of its presence from germ cell (85) to maturing spermatozoa. More interesting, from the point of view of epididymal maturative processes, is the finding that cauda spermatozoa contain only about 25% of the vitamin E level found in caput sperm cells.

The course of the specific activities of PHGPx, GPx, and SOD in epididymal sperm cells (Table 14.1) seems identical to that of vitamin E. This does not seem to be a coincidence and deserves further consideration. Our results clearly indicate the presence of a stronger endogenous protective equipment (enzymes and tocopherol) in epididymal caput spermatozoa, which are still immature, that weakens at the cauda level, where the sperm cells are mature. This may seem unexpected but suggests a functional difference in the protective processes in the two spermatozoa populations. In this framework other data indicate, moreover, that caput and cauda sperm cells react differently to peroxidative damage (56); the resulting decrease in vitamin E is, in fact, always more marked in cauda epididymal spermatozoa, where PHGPx, GPx, and SOD activities and alpha-tocopherol content are lower than in caput.

All these results can be well correlated with the already mentioned (1) changes of sperm cell plasma and acrosomal membranes during the passage from caput to cauda epididymis (higher PUFA and cholesterol content, higher asymmetry). All these conditions render the membranes more susceptible to alterations, and the cauda epididymal spermatozoa are therefore potentially capable of undergoing acrosomal reaction (1,86). The lower protective equipment present in the cauda epididymal sperm cells can be viewed in relation to this. Moreover, as spermatozoa enter into the seminal plasma, other scavenger molecules already present can assume protective role (87–90) up to the final event of the fusion with the oocyte.

On the basis of these findings, it is clear that the key domains of maturing epididymal spermatozoa (acrosome, chromatin, mitochondria) display effective scavenger systems, whose concentration, distribution, and binding are finely tuned by the sperm cell itself and/or by the epididymal fluid (90,91).

TABLE 14.2

Vitamin E In Rat Epididymal Spermatozoa[a]

Epididymal spermatozoa	3.42 (1.22)[a]
Caput spermatozoa	8.26 (1.79)[a]
Cauda spermatozoa	2.17 (0.37)[a,c]
Heads	0.92 (0.007)[a]
Sperm plasma and acrosomal membranes	351.11 (8.35)[b]
Tails	1.32 (0.035)[a]

[a]Values are mean (SD) of 3–12 separate measurements (HPLC and fluorometric detection). Units: [a] pmoles/10^6 cells (or 10^6 heads, or 10^6 tails) and [b] pmoles/mg protein. Significance: [c] $P < 0.0005$, in comparison to *caput* spermatozoa.

Seminal Fluid and ROS Damage

In contrast with the situation in other cells, the high concentration of unsaturated lipids in mature spermatozoa is related to a scarcity of various oxyradical scavenger mechanisms, also due to an almost complete absence of cytoplasm in mature sperm cells. However, the powerful antioxidant system found in seminal plasma compensates for this lack. It has been shown that, unlike other biological fluids, important SOD, catalase, and GSH peroxidase activities occur in seminal plasma. Additionally, it contains significant concentrations of antioxidants such as ascorbic acid, tocopherol, and GSH (87).

The antioxidant system is highly integrated. SOD, a metallo-enzyme, transforms the superoxide anion radical into hydrogen peroxide. Ceruloplasmin can have a similar scavenger effect. The hydrogen peroxide produced during this reaction must be removed by catalase and/or GSH peroxidase (GPx). If it is not completely eliminated, the Fenton reaction takes place in the presence of transition metals, and toxic hydroxyl radicals are produced. The chain-breaking antioxidant in membranes is Vitamin E, and its oxidation gives the tocopheryl radical, which is reduced by ubiquinone or ascorbic acid. Ascorbyl radicals, produced by the oxidation of Vitamin C, can be reduced by GSH, producing thiyl radicals and oxidized glutathione, which are then regenerated by GSH reductase. As a consequence, the entire system needs to work in harmony. A change to just one component can lead to a potentially damaging ROS accumulation (92).

Antioxidant systems in seminal plasma contain a relatively high GSH concentration. Utilizing its thiolic group, it reacts directly with hydrogen peroxide, superoxide anions, and hydroxyl radicals and reacts with alkoxyl radicals and hydroperoxides to produce alcohols (14).

In other biological systems, the GSH redox cycle helps protect cells against oxidative damage (93–95). It is usually present in millimolar concentrations in cytosol and the nucleus but is more dilute in blood serum and other biological fluids (14,87). Its presence in significant concentrations has been linked to both the liquefaction process of seminal plasma and the Vitamin C redox cycle. Oxidation of ascorbic acid to dehydroascorbic acid generates both ascorbyl radicals and hydrogen peroxide. As there is a low catalase concentration in spermatozoa and seminal plasma, removal of generated hydrogen peroxide is mainly dependent on GSH and GSH peroxidase (93).

The damage to sperm function caused by radicals and toxic compounds is well documented. The negative effects of ROS on sperm function are particularly well known (96–99). In mammalian cells, alteration of the membrane's fatty acid pattern has various effects, such as changes in the activity of different lipid-dependent enzymes and in resistance of spermatozoa to physical or chemical stress (100).

The risk that spermatozoa may undergo lipid peroxidation can be assessed with a spectrophotometric assay to test malonildialdeyde generation promoted with ferrous and ascorbate ions in the presence of thiobarbituric acid (TBA) (97). This measures ferrous ion-catalyzed breakdown of preexisting lipid hydroperoxides in the sperm plasma membrane and subsequent propagation of a lipid peroxidation chain reaction through generation of peroxyl and alkoxyl radicals (101). Many andrological pathologies, such as varicocele, infections, and germ-free genital tract inflammation, have been linked with a heightened risk of lipid peroxidation (29). These pathologies are the cause of many biological and clinical effects, such as modifications in microcirculation, venous stasis, and subsequent hypoxia, leucocyte activation, and cell necrosis. These all increase ROS in the semen. In fact, levels of radical oxygen species have been found to be higher in the male partner of infertile couples suffering from selected andrological conditions (97,99,102).

The harmful effects of ROS on *in vitro* spermatozoa, and its implications for IVF programs, have been the subject of many studies. However, ROS have also been found to initiate *in vitro* physiological sperm functions, such as capacitation and hyperactivated motility (103–105). These positive effects are dependent on the equilibrium between ROS and the scavenger systems. In fact, if semen characteristics are discounted and sperm preparation methods are not chosen on a case-by-case basis, there are large differences in the results of sperm selection techniques for assisted reproduction (106). The culture media and additives used for sample preparation must be chosen accordingly. For example, pentoxifylline stimulates *in vitro* iron-induced lipid peroxidation, which generally aids membrane fluidity and physiological destabilization. However, it can also induce a destructive peroxidation chain reaction with fragile spermatozoa or after too long an incubation period (107). It has recently been reported that the high ROS concentration seen in oligozoospermic patients may be of intracellular origin (108). This may explain both the fragility of these patients' sperm during *in vitro* treatment and the lack of efficacy of antioxidants added to the *in vitro* culture media in inhibiting ROS induced damage (109).

Scavenger Therapies

It is normally impossible to identify the true etiology of dyspermia. Many nonhormonal therapies have therefore been used for direct action on spermatozoa with the hope of improving their quality. As diagnosis in this field is so difficult, the use of these therapies is understandable. Various treatments have been employed, but carnitine, phosphatidilcholine, callicreine, penthossiphylline, and vitamins A, E, and C (15,82,83,110) are the most common. It is too often the case that infertile, dyspermic patients are referred to an andrologist years after sperm damage has been caused by the underlying pathology. Under these conditions, the simplest and most practical therapy is to prescribe a drug aimed at seminal parameter improvement, theoretically acting directly on gamete production or epididymal maturation. The often uncontrolled studies performed in support of such therapies frequently produce controversial data.

As previously discussed, several scavenging systems act to minimize the harmful effects of ROS and other toxic compounds to spermatozoa and seminal plasma. Those known are basically enzymes, proteins (albumin), GSH, vitamins E and C, taurine and hypotaurine, and mercapturic acids (111). Among the latter, GSH seems to be one of the most indicated drugs due to its known antitoxic and antioxidant actions in other degenerative pathologies (cirrhosis, neoplasia, and consequences of antiblastic therapies). Under experimental conditions sulfydryl compounds (cysteine, GSH, ergothioneine) in semen were found to have an important role in maintenance of sperm motility and metabolism (15) and, in isolated rat spermatids, GSH has prevented damage from exposure to peroxidizing agents (112). The pharmacology of exogenous GSH administration has not yet been fully studied, although it is unlikely that the polar molecule can cross the cell membranes. However, it has been shown in laboratory animals that GSH administration reduces stress-induced gastric injury with no change in antioxidant tissue concentration (93).

GSH as a Therapy

One of the most important reasons for selecting GSH as a therapeutic agent is its physiologically significant presence in seminal plasma. Although it is unable to cross cell membranes, after systemic administration its concentration increases in biological fluids, especially in seminal plasma (113).

The use of GSH in sperm pathology and its mechanism of action was the subject of a small, two-month pilot study on GSH (114). 600 mg/day i.m. was administered to a group of eleven patients with dyspermia associated with chronic epididymitis (2 patients), prostate-bladder germ-free chronic inflammation (6 patients), varicocele (2 patients), and antisperm antibodies (1 patient). Standard semen analysis (115) and computer analysis of sperm motility was performed before treatment and after 30 and 60 days of treatment. The therapy had a statistically significant effect on sperm motility patterns and sperm morphology. In particular, between baseline and 60-day analyses there was a significant difference in percentage of forward motility and the parameters of the sperm motility computer analysis (velocity, linearity, ALH, and BCF). A significant reduction in the percentage of atypical forms was also seen. Sperm motility improved, especially in patients with chronic epididymitis or varicocele. Four of the six patients with prostate-vesicular chronic inflammation also showed improvement. No changes were seen in semen parameters or in antibody titer in the patient with antisperm immune pathology (114). Given these encouraging results, treatment was extended in a controlled trial to a larger patient group with selected andrological pathologies.

We (113) conducted a placebo controlled double blind cross-over trial on a selected group of twenty infertile patients, ten with unilateral varicocele and ten with germ-free genital tract inflammation. The same seminological studies were performed as in the pilot study (microscopic semen analysis and computer sperm motion analysis conducted monthly). All patients were followed up for a two-month wash-out period. They then received either GSH or placebo for two months before crossing over to the alternative therapy for a further two months. Patients were randomly and blindly assigned to treatment with one i.m. injection every other day of either GSH 600 mg or an equal volume of a placebo. Criteria for clinical selection were two years infertility (with a gynecologically normal partner), age range 20–40 years, no systemic or hormonal pathologies, no history of cryptorchidism, no testicular hypotrophy, no detectable genital infections, and no antisperm antibodies. Of paramount importance were the criteria for seminological inclusion: the group showed homogeneous sperm concentration, motility, and morphology at the beginning of the study. No variations were seen in semen volume and leukocyte concentration.

The effect of GSH on sperm variables (Table 14.3) was already significant after one month of treatment. This improvement continued (although with a slow decrease) during the placebo period. All patients showed a significant increase in sperm concentration and a highly significant improvement in sperm motility, kinetic parameters, and morphology. This improvement was not only statistically but also biologically and clinically significant.

No significant differences were seen between germ free genital tract inflammation and varicocele patients. ROS production in these pathologies has a pathogenetic role in both the sperm cell membrane and the metabolic spermatozoa alterations resulting in hypomotility and teratozoospermia. This may explain the therapy's effect on sperm motility and kinetic patterns. Additionally, a more complex action is suggested by the significant reduction in percentage of atypical forms observed. It is possible that GSH affects sperm membrane maturation and the cell's biochemical constitution. This would have to be a post-spermatocyte effect as the treatment period was specifically chosen to be shorter than a complete spermatogenetic cycle, and positive results were in any case first seen after the first month of treatment. The improvements in sperm motility and morphology continued after treatment had stopped. This implies that GSH also could act indirectly, improving GSH peroxidases metabolic condition of the testicular-epididymal environment. Finally, the slight increase in sperm concentration may be due to reduced post-testicular sperm phagocytosis in consequence of the improved sperm structure. No side effects or significant modifications to hormonal patterns were observed in the group.

GSH (and SOD) use has also been suggested for treatment of oligozoospermia, with the purpose of avoiding possible sperm damage induced by contact of healthy sperm with pathological semen components during *in vitro* manipulation for assisted reproduction (104).

To study its *in vitro* action, GSH was tested directly on human sperm. Semen samples were selected from cryobank donors and infertile patients with and without leucospermia. The latter were selected with the aim of evaluating sperm damage predicted to be caused by leucocyte-produced ROS (116,106). Samples were examined by microscopic semen and computerized sperm motion analysis and tested on basal semen and post-rise spermatozoa from layer and pellet-swim up in Tyrode's solution (TIR) alone or with 1mg/mL added GSH. In leucospermic cases, *in vitro* GSH was evaluated on basal semen, diluted semen (1:1 semen − TIR + GSH), and post rise spermatozoa after layer and pellet-swim up.

No significant differences were seen in the sperm parameters between basal and TIR/GSH-diluted semen or between layer swim up with and without GSH in the media. A significant difference was seen only in sperm forward motility in leucosper-

TABLE 14.3

Sperm Parameter Variations during the Placebo Cross-Over Trial of Glutathione Therapy in Male Infertility (See Reference 113)

		Sperm Concentration 10^6/ml	Total motility%	Forward motility %	Morphology % atypical	Velocity μ/sec	Linearity Index 1–10	ALH μ	BCF Hz
GROUP 1	Base	26.35 (12.64)	28.00 (10.37)	12.00 (5.20)	57.20 (8.72)	28.03 (3.55)	2.70 (0.35)	2.48 (0.20)	11.09 (0.47)
	Glu I	30.20 (10.73)	38.50 (10.55)	26.50 (8.51)	48.10 (7.52)	42.80 (5.31)	4.30 (0.69)	3.55 (0.25)	12.93 (0.40)
	Glu II	29.80 (10.64)	38.00 (11.60)	27.50 (8.58)	48.20 (7.84)	43.70 (5.40)	4.35 (0.67)	3.52 (0.30)	12.84 (0.44)
	Pla I	30.00 (19.71)	32.50 (12.96)	20.00 (8.82)	50.8 (5.22)	38.8 (4.85)	3.79 (0.85)	3.35 (0.30)	12.64 (0.47)
	Pla II	28.20 (11.63)	28.50 (12.70)	18.5 (8.83)	53.4 (7.57)	36.1 (5.69)	3.50 (0.89)	2.98 (0.23)	12.25 (0.48)
GROUP 2	Base	27.56 (15.69)	24.83 (9.70)	10.50 (4.30)	63.20 (6.62)	28.80 (1.91)	2.69 (0.44)	2.55 (0.17)	11.12 (0.59)
	Pla I	27.40 (14.10)	26.00 (9.07)	10.50 (2.84)	62.50 (6.19)	28.60 (3.90)	2.61 (0.32)	2.44 (0.22)	11.05 (0.58)
	Pla II	28.10 (13.10)	26.50 (10.29)	10.00 (4.71)	62.50 (6.38)	28.70 (2.63)	2.64 (0.47)	2.53 (0.17)	11.10 (0.56)
	Glu I	31.40 (13.64)	35.50 (4.38)	28.50 (4.12)	52.10 (5.61)	47.20 (4.94)	4.78 (0.59)	3.67 (0.31)	12.98 (0.45)
	Glu II	31.10 (13.40)	37.00 (4.83)	29.50 (4.97)	52.40 (6.47)	47.10 (0.74)	4.78 (0.60)	3.67 (0.35)	12.96 (0.47)

[a]Values are presented as mean with standard deviation in parentheses. Base: values are mean (SD) of the three seminal analyses of the wash out period; Glu I: values are mean (SD) after 1 month of glutathione therapy. Glu II: values are mean (SD) after 2 months of glutathione therapy; Pla I: values are mean (SD) after 1 month of placebo; Pla II: values are mean (SD) after 2 months of placebo

mic samples treated with pellet swim up. In these samples, the presence of GSH in the migration media led to an increase in sperm forward motility (117). The results suggest that GSH protects sperm motility during pelleting, thus preventing possible damage from seminal ROS produced by leucocytes or damaged spermatozoa.

PUFA as Markers of Sperm Pathology: A Rationale for GHS Therapy

To further investigate these findings we explored the mechanisms through which GSH may act on sperm function. Oxidative stress can be defined as a situation in which pro-oxidants outnumber anti-oxidants, leading to free radical production and resulting in lipoperoxidation. Phospholipid PUFAs, of paramount importance in membrane constitution and function, are one of the main targets of this process. To study how GSH acts, the alterations it produces in (i) semen variables and lipoperoxidation sperm membrane risk (evaluated by TBA assay) and (ii) the pattern of phospholipid fatty acids from blood serum and red blood cell membranes were studied in infertile patients with unilateral varicocele and germ free genital tract inflammation. Red blood cells are in fact considered as representative of the constitution of general cell membranes and these were used due to the extreme difficulty of evaluating the fatty acid pattern of sperm membrane phospholipids in severely oligozoospermic patients.

Sperm concentration, motility, morphology, and kinetic variables were found to significantly improve even after 30 days' therapy. It can be seen that GSH therapy acts on the epididymis to enhance sperm maturation and discourage their reabsorption. These improvements were related to an increase in phospholipid PUFA levels in red blood cells and a decrease in lipoperoxide levels in sperm, as revealed by TBA assay. In fact, lipoperoxidative potentials in spermatozoa of patients studied before (T0) and at completion of (T60) glutathione therapy were 14.98 and 11.84 nmoles MDA/10^8 spermatozoa respectively, with a statistically significant difference (t = 9.358 P < 0.001).

It seems that GSH's therapeutic action is at least partly related to its protective effect on the cell membrane's lipid components. GSH probably acts as a free radical scavenger (both enzymatically and directly) in the epididymis, inhibiting lipoperoxidation generated by vascular or inflammatory pathologies. This theory is supported by the significant reduction in lipoperoxide levels in seminal plasma detected by the TBA test. In addition, the greater sperm cell concentration after one month of therapy (without variation in semen volume) suggests a reduction in sperm damage and consequent epididymal reabsorption rather than a variation in spermatogenesis (29). In fact, experimental data show that rat spermatids use GSH-dependent mechanisms to combat oxidative stress (112,65). These results may point to an impairment of the desaturase enzymes in the patients studied, possibly caused by genetic factors or unknown acquired pathologies, resulting in chronic systemic damage to all cell membranes. This constitutional cell membrane alteration may exacerbate the damage caused by ROS generated subsequent to vascular or inflammatory processes in the epididymis, facilitating dyspermia. Biochemical modifications to lipid membrane constitution may explain the seminal parameter values following GSH therapy.

However, subjects with systemic lipid membrane disturbances associated with andrological pathologies (*e.g.,* varicocele and inflammation) quite possibly express this membrane damage in their sperm and have a tendency to develop dyspermia. This could confirm experimental data from rats fed with a poor diet exploiting PUFA deficiency in serum and semen (35,118).

Two small patient groups with unilateral varicocele, associated or not with dyspermia ("Var-inf" and "Var-norm"), and a control group ("Control") of healthy fertile subjects were selected to test this theory (Table 14.4). A significant difference between red blood cell membrane PUFA of the Control group and the Var-norm patients was found. In contrast, a significant decrease of PUFA unsaturation in the red blood cells membranes of most Var-inf patients was seen (119). It is remarkable that normozoospermic varicocele patients show PUFA levels similar to normal, fertile men, whereas dyspermic varicocele patients demonstrate a significant PUFA deterioration.

There may be a pathogenetic relationship between damage to the male gamete and lower ROS resistance of the sperm plasma membrane and the vascular pathology of the testicular-epididymal region. If results are confirmed by a long-term follow up study, establishment of a predictive index on the risk of varicocele-induced dyspermia will be possible. Following prediction, predisposition surgery could then be recommended only to young patients with PUFA alterations in their red blood cell or other representative cells.

Conclusions

Sperm cells have an active lipid metabolism. The high PUFA content in their membranes and the significant quantities of free fatty acids and carnitine in seminal plasma clearly demonstrate that lipids are important energy sources and a structural necessity for sperm cells.

TABLE 14.4

Fatty Acids Concentration (Percentages) in Red Blood Cells of Controls Subjects (Controls) and Varicocele (Var) Patients Splitted in Norm and Inf[a]

Fatty acids	Controls mean (SD)	Var-norm mean (SD)	Var-inf mean (SD)	Contr vs. Var-norm T	sig	Var-norm vs. Var-inf t	sig
Palmitic	23.60 (0.26)	25.42 (2.41)	28.45 (4.80)	−5.367	0.001	−1.715	0.108
Stearic	14.71 (0.36)	20.7 (2.05)	22.9 (3.00)	−19.864	0.001	−1.728	0.106
Oleic	25.54 (0.95)	22.71 (2.51)	27.4 (3.80)	6.304	0.001	−2.961	0.010
Linoleic	9.78 (0.94)	12.95 (2.20)	13.04 (4.50)	−5.737	0.001	−0.055	0.957
Di-homo-γ-linolenic	1.37 (0.09)	1.99 (0.50)	0.86 (0.40)	−8.402	0.001	4.424	0.001
Arachidonic	15.13 (0.95)	15.49 (2.92)	6.70 (2.50)	−0.730	0.468	5.807	0.001
Docosahexaenoic	4.10 (0.16)	3.10 (0.70)	1.20 (0.40)	9.297	0.001	5.600	0.001

[a]Legend: mean (SD); T = student *t* test; sig = probability index.

The high PUFA levels and the need to protect the highly specialized membrane domains require efficient scavenger systems, for example, as sperm migrate through and mature in the epididymal tract. These antioxidant enzymatic and nonenzymatic systems are highly diversified but are generally based on the GSH/GSSG couple. Interesting new roles, going beyond a merely protective one, have recently been postulated for enzymes such as PHGPx, whose activity and expression change during sperm cell maturation and aging.

Peroxidation in maturing sperm cells is now demonstrated as having two roles, depending on the quantity of ROS present at a given time. It is already known that low ROS concentrations are involved in the physiological control of various sperm functions (39). Studies of enzymatic systems for ROS production/elimination should be viewed not only as protective but also as a regulatory activity. These systems may act to help provide the best conditions for sperm maturation. For example, specific epididymal sperm protamine oxidation may be a role in addition to the normal scavenger activity of PHGPx.

Seminal plasma is an excellent nutritive and protective medium for sperm cells because it possesses higher concentrations of antioxidants than do other biological fluids or blood serum. Only alteration of its anti-/pro-oxidant equilibrium or increased sperm membrane fragility following *in vitro* manipulation cause it to become aggressive. GSH and similar scavengers are therefore indicated for treatment of such cases, as they are able to restore the physiological constitution of PUFA in the cell membrane.

The composition and disequilibrium of sperm membrane seem sensitive markers of both sperm membrane function and increase in fragility. It would be extremely useful to demonstrate if the high n-3 PUFA (22:6n-3) percentage in the sperm membrane is necessary for fertilizing capacity and if there is a correlation between systemic lipid metabolism and sperm cell functions.

With respect to the metabolic pathway of essential fatty acids, our results on the differences between immature germ cells and various sperm populations suggest that long-chain PUFA are actively produced during maturation of sperm cells after testicular release. The high carnitine concentration in the human epididymis supports the theory of post-testicular fatty acid metabolism, as has already been demonstrated in other mammals (120). However, an alternative hypothesis of intra-testicular production of spermatozoa at different stages of maturation, deriving from spermatogenesis producing sperm with different degrees of PUFA unsaturation, is also possible. A final theory is that of post-testicular long-chain PUFA peroxidation occurring as a result of epididymal micro-environments capable of modifying relative PUFA percentages in different sperm populations.

Acknowledgments

This work was supported by grants from the University of Rome "La Sapienza," from the University of Trieste, and financial support provided by the Ministry of University (Rome).

REFERENCES

1. Nolan, J.P., and Hammerstedt, R.H. (1997) Regulation of Membrane Stability and the Acrosome Reaction in Mammalian Sperm, *Faseb. J. 11*, 670–682.

2. Miescher, F. (1878) Die Spermatozoen einiger Wirbeltiere; ein Beitrag zur Histochemie, *Verh Naturforsch. Ges. Basel. 6*, 138–143.

3. Miescher, F. (1897) Die Histochemischen und Physiologischen Arbeiten von Friedrich Miescher, *Vogel, Leipzig* pp. 243–262.

4. Koelliker, A. (1856) Physiologische Studien Uber die Samenflussigkeit Z, *Wiss. Zool. 7*, 201–207.

5. Matthews, A. (1897) Zur Chemie der Spermatozoen. Hoppe Seylers Z, *Physiol. Chem. 23*, 399–406.

6. Sano, M. (1922) Phosphatides in the Fish Sperm, *J. Biochem. 1*, 1–25.

7. Muller, C.P., and Krueger, G.R.F. (1986) Modulation of Membrane Proteins by Vertical Phase Separation and Membrane Lipid Fluidity. Basis for a New Approach to Tumor Immunotherapy, *Anticancer Res. 6*, 1181–1194.

8. Yeagle, P.L. (1989) Lipid Regulation of Cell Membrane Structure and Function, *Faseb. J. 3*, 1833–1842.

9. Langlais, J., Kan, F.W.K., Granger, L., Raymond, L., Bleau, G., and Roberts, K.D. (1988) Identification of Sterol Acceptors that Stimulate Cholesterol Efflux from Human Spermatozoa during *in Vitro* Capacitation, *Gamete Res. 12*, 183–224.

10. Myles, D.G., and Primakoff, P. (1984) Localized Surface Antigens of Guinea Pig Sperm Migrate to new Regions Prior to Fertilization, *J. Cell Biol. 99*, 1634–1641.

11. Primakoff, P., Hyatt, H., and Myles, D.G. (1985) A Role for the Migrating Sperm Surface Antigen PH20 in Guinea Pig Sperm Binding to the Egg Zona Pellucida, *J. Cell Biol. 101*, 2239–2244.

12. Lenzi, A., Gandini, L., Lombardo, F., Micara, G., Culasso, F., and Dondero, F. (1992) *In Vitro* Sperm Capacitation to Treat Antisperm Antibodies Bound to the Sperm Surface, *Am. J. Reprod. Immunol. 28*, 51–55.

13. Dondero, F., Lenzi, A., Gandini L., and Lombardo, F. (1995) Study of ASA-Reactive-Acrosome-Antigens from Epididymal Sperm Maturation to *in Vitro* Capacitation, *Regional Immunol. 6*, 290–297.

14. Mann, T. (1964) *The Biochemistry of Semen and of the Male Reproductive Tract*, Methuen Pubb, London.

15. Mann, T, and Lutwak-Mann, C. (1981) *Male Reproductive Function and Semen*, pp. 495, Springer-Verlag, Berlin.

16. Mattews, C.H., and Van Holde, K. (1990) Lipid Metabolism, in *Biochemistry 2/e*, pp. 613–655, Benjamin-Cummings Pub., Menlo Park, CA, USA.

17. Cornwell, D.G., and Moriski, N. (1984) Fatty Acid Paradoxes in the Control of Cell Proliferation: Prostaglandins, Lipid Peroxides and Cooxidation Reactions, in *Free Radicals in Biology VI*, Pryor, W.A. (Ed.), pp. 95–147, Academic Press, New York, USA.

18. Israelachvili, J.N., Marcelja, S., and Horn, R.G. (1980) Physical Principles of Membrane Organization, *Quart. Rev. Biophys. 13*, 121–200.

19. Fleming, A.D., and Yanagimachi, R. (1981) Effects of Various Lipids on the Acrosome Reaction and Fertilizing Capacity of Guinea Pig Spermatozoa with Special Reference to the Possible Involvement of Lysophospholipid in the Acrosome Reaction, *Gamete Res. 4*, 253–273.

20. Meizel, S., and Turner, K.O. (1983) Stimulation of an Exocytotic Event, the Hamster Sperm Acrosome Reaction by cis-Unsaturated Fatty Acids, *Febs. Lett. 161*, 315–318.

21. Muller, K., Pomarski, T., Muller, P., Zachowski, A., and Hermann, A. (1994) Protein-Dependent Translocation of Aminophospholipids and Asymmetric Transbilayer Distribution of Phospholipids in the Plasma Membrane of Ram Sperm Cells, *Biochemistry 33*, 9968–9974.

22. Infante, J.P. (1986) Vitamin E and Selenium Participation in Fatty Acid Desaturation. A Proposal for an Enzymatic Function of These Nutrients, *Mol. Cell Biochem. 69*, 93–108.

23. Scott, T.W., Voglmayr, J.K., and Setchell, B.P. (1967) Lipid Composition and Metabolism in Testicular and Ejaculated Ram Spermatozoa, *Biochem. J. 102*, 456–462.

24. Poulos, A., Brown-Woodman, P.D.C., White, I.G., and Cox, R.I. (1975) Changes in Phospholipids of Ram Spermatozoa during Migration through the Epididymis and Possible Origin of Prostaglandin F2 in Testicular and Epididymal Fluid, *Biochem. Biophys. Acta 12*, 388–403.

25. Wolf, D.E., Hagopian, S.S., Lewis, R.G., Voglmayr, J.K., and Fairbanks, G. (1986) Lateral Regionalization and Diffusion of a Maturation-Dependent Antigen in the Ram Sperm Plasma Membrane, *J. Cell Biol. 102*, 1826–1831.

26. Cowan, A.E., Primakoff, P., and Myles, D.G. (1986) Sperm Exocytosis Increases the Amount of Ph-20 Antigen on the Surface of Guinea-Pig Sperm, *J. Cell Biol. 103*, 1289–1297.

27. Gaunt, S.J., Brown, C.R., and Jones, R. (1983) Identification of Mobile and Fixed Antigens on the Plasma Membrane of Rat Spermatozoa Using Monoclonal Antibodies, *Exp. Cell Res. 144*, 275–284.

28. Hall, J.C., Hadley, J., and Doman, T. (1991) Correlation between Changes in Rat Sperm Membrane Lipids, Protein, and the Membrane Physical State during Epididymal Maturation, *J. Androl. 12*, 76–87.

29. Lenzi, A., Picardo, M., Gandini, L., Lombardo, F., Terminali, O., Passi, S., and Dondero, F. (1994) Glutathione Treatment of Dyspermia: Effect on the Lipoperoxidation Process, *Hum. Reprod. 9*, 2044–2050.

30. Jones, R., Mann, T., and Sherins, R. (1979) Peroxidative Breakdown of Phospholipids in Human Spermatozoa, Spermicidal Properties of Fatty Acid Peroxides, and Protective Action of Seminal Plasma, *Fertil. Steril. 31*, 531–537.

31. Poulos, A., and White, I.G. (1973) The Phospholipid Composition of Human Spermatozoa and Seminal Plasma, *J. Reprod. Fertil. 35*, 265–277.

32. Gandini, L., Lenzi, A., Lombardo, F., Pacifici, R., and Dondero, F. (1999) Immature Germ Cell Separation Using a Modified Discontinuous Percoll Gradient Technique in Human Semen, *Hum. Reprod. 14*, 1022–1027.

33. Lenzi, A., Gandini, L., Maresca, V., Dondero, F., and Picardo, M. (2000) Fatty Acids Composition of Spermatozoa and Immature Germ Cells, *Mol. Hum. Reprod. 6*, 226–231.

34. Picardo, M., Grammatico, P., De Luca, C., Passi, S., and Nazzaro-Porro, M. (1990) Differential Effect of Azelaic Acid in Melanoma Cell Cultures, *Pigment Cell Res. 20*, 142–149.

35. Leath, W.M.F., Northop, C.A., Harrison, F.A., and Cox, R.W. (1983) Effect of Linoleic Acid and Linolenic Acid on Testicular Developments in the Rat, *Q. J. Exp. Physiol. 68*, 221–231.

36. Aitken, R.J. (1991) Reactive Oxygen Species and Human Sperm Function, in *Comparative Spermatology 20 Years After*, Bacetti, B., Raven Press—Serono series, vol. 75, pp. 787–792.

37. Pryor, W. (1984) The Role of Free Radical Reactions in Biological Systems, in *Free Radicals in Biology*, Pryor, W., pp. 1–15.

38. Ochsendorf, F.R. (1999) Infections in the Male Genital Tract and Reactive Oxygen Species, *Hum. Reprod. Update 5*, 399–442.

39. Griveau, J.F., and Le Lannou, D. (1997) Reactive Oxygen Species and Human Spermatozoa: Physiology and Pathology, *Int. J. Androl. 20*, 61–69.

40. Bize, I., Santander, G., Cabello, P., Driscoll D., and Sharpe, C. (1991) Hydrogen Peroxide is Involved in Hamster Sperm Capacitation *in Vitro, Biol. Reprod. 44*, 398–403.

41. Wu, S.H., Oldfield, J.E., Whanger, P.D., and Weswig, P.H. (1973) Effect of Se, Vitamin E, and Antioxidants on Testicular Function in Rats, *Biol. Reprod. 8*, 625–629.

42. Robinson, B.S., Johnson, D.W., and Poulos, A. (1992) Novel Molecular Species of Sphingomyelin Containing 2-Hydroxylated Polyenoic Very-Long-Chain Fatty Acids in Mammalian Testes and Spermatozoa, *J. Biol. Chem. 267*, 1746–1751.

43. Behne, D., Hofer, T., von Berswordt Wallrabe, R., and Egler, W. (1982) Se in the Testis of the Rat: Studies on Its Regulation and Its Importance for the Organism, *J. Nutr. 112*, 1682–1687.

44. Wallace, E., Calvin, H.I., Ploetz, K., and Cooper, G.W. (1987) Functional and Developmental Studies on the Role of Se in Spermatogenesis, in *Selenium in Biology and Medicine*, Combs, G.F., Levander, O.A., Spallholz, J.E., and Oldfield, J.E., AVI Publ Co., Westport, Conn., part A, pp. 181–186.

45. Behne, D., Weiler, H., and Kyriakopoulos, A. (1996) Effects of Se in Deficiency on Testicular Morphology and Function in Rats, *J. Reprod. Fertil. 106*, 291–297.

46. Wu, A.S.H., Oldfield, J.E., Shull, L.R., and Cheeke, P.R. (1979) Specific Effect of Se Deficiency on Rat Sperm, *Biol Reprod 20*, 793–8.

47. McConnell, K.P., Burton, R.M., Kute, T., and Higgins, P.J. (1979) Selenoproteins in Rat Testis Cytosol, *Biochim. Biophys. Acta 588*, 113–119.

48. Smith, D.G., Senger, P.L., McCutchan, J.F., and Landa, C.A., (1979) Se and GPx Distribution in Bovine Semen and ^{75}Se Retention by the Tissues of the Reproductive Tract in the Bull, *Biol. Reprod. 20*, 377–383.

49. Seligman, J., Kosower, N.S., Weissenberg, R., and Shalgi, R. (1994) Thiol-Disulfide Status of Human Sperm Proteins, *J. Reprod. Fertil. 101*, 435–43.

50. Yanagimachi, R. (1988) Mammalian Fertilization, in *The Physiology of Reproduction*, Knobil, E., Neill, J., Ewing, L.L., Greenwald, G.S., Market, C., and Pfaff, W., Raven Press, New York, pp. 135–185.

51. Seligman, J., Shalgi, R., Oschry, Y., and Kosower, N.S. (1991) Sperm Analysis by Flow Cytometry Using the Fluorescent Thiol Labelling Agent Monobromobimane, *Mol. Reprod. Dev. 29*, 276–281.

52. Eddy, E.M. (1988) The Spermatozoon, in *The Physiology of Reproduction*, Knobil, E., Neill, J., Ewing, L.L., Greenwald, G.S., Market, C., Pfaff, W., Raven Press, New York, pp. 27–68.

53. Fisher, H.M., and Aitken, R.J. (1997) Comparative Analysis of the Ability of Precursor Germ Cells and Epididymal Spermatozoa to Generate Reactive Oxygen Metabolites, *J. Exp. Zool. 277*, 390–400.

54. Storey, B.T. (1997) Biochemistry of the Induction and Prevention of Lipoperoxidative Damage in Human Spermatozoa, *Mol. Hum. Reprod. 3*, 203–213.

55. Griveau, J.F., Dumont, E., Renard, P., Callegari, J.P., and Le Lannou, D. (1995) Reactive Oxygen Species, Lipid Peroxidation and Enzymatic Defense Systems in Human Spermatozoa, *J. Reprod. Fertil. 103*, 17–26.

56. Tramer, F., Rocco, F., Micali, F., Sandri, G., and Panfili, E. (1998) Antioxidant Systems in Rat Epididymal Spermatozoa, *Biol. Reprod. 59*, 735–758.

57. Zini, A., De Lamirande, E., and Gagnon, C. (1993) Reactive Oxygen Species in Semen of Infertile Patients: Levels of Superoxide Dismutase- and Catalaselike Activities in Seminal Plasma and Spermatozoa, *Int J Androl. 16*, 183–188.

58. Gu, W., and Hecht, N.B. (1996) Developmental Expression of Glutathione Peroxidase, Catalase and Manganese Superoxide Dismutase mRNAs during Spermatogenesis in the Mouse, *J. Androl. 17*, 256–262.

59. Jeulin, C., Soufir, J.C., Weber, P., Laval-Martin, D., and Calvayrac, R. (1989) Catalase Activity in Human Spermatozoa and Seminal Plasma, *Gamete Res. 24*, 185–196.

60. Oberley, T.D., Oberley, L.W., Slattery, A.F., Lauchner, L.J., and Elwell, J.H. (1990) Immunohystochemical Localization of Antioxidant Enzymes in Adult Syrian Hamster Tissues and during Kidney Development, *Am. J. Physiol. 137*,199–214.

61. Maiorino, M., Gregolin, C., and Ursini, F. (1990) Phospholipid Hydroperoxide Glutathione Peroxidase, *Methods Enzymol. 186*, 448–457.

62. Godeas, C., Tramer, F., Micali, F., Soranzo, M.R., Sandri, G., and Panfili, E. (1997) Distribution and Possible Novel Role of PGHPx in Rat Epididymal Spermatozoa, *Biol. Reprod. 57*, 1502–1508.

63. Tramer, F., Micali, F., Sandri, G., Bertoni, A., Lenzi, A., Gandini, L., and Panfili, E. (2002) Enzymatic and Immunochemical Evaluation of PHGPx in Testes and Epididymal Spermatozoa of Rats of Different Ages, *Int. J. Androl. 25*, 72–83.

64. Roveri, A., Casasco, A., Maiorino, M., Dalan, P., Calligaro, A., and Ursini, F. (1992) PHGPx of Rat Testis: Gonadotropin Dependence and Immunochemical Identification, *J. Biol. Chem. 267*, 6142–6146.

65. Godeas, C., Sandri, G., and Panfili, E. (1994) Distribution of PHGPx in Rat Testis Mitochondria, *Biochim. Biophys. Acta 1191*, 147–150.

66. Giannattasio, A., Girotti, M., Williams, K., Hall, L., Bellastella, A. (1997) Puberty Influences Expression of PHGPx in Rat Testis: Probable Hypophysis Regulation of the Enzyme in Male Reproductive Tract, *J. Endocr. Invest 20*, 439–444.

67. Maiorino, M., Wissing, J.B., Brigelius-Flohè, R., Calabrese, F., Roveri, A., Steinert, P., Ursini, F., and Flohè, L. (1998) Testosterone Mediates Expression of Selenoprotein PHGPx by Induction of Spermatogenesis and Not by Direct Transcriptional Gene Activation, *Faseb. J. 12*, 1359–1370.

68. Imai, H., Narashima, K., Arai, M., Sakamoto, H., Chiba, N., and Nakagawa, Y. (1998) Suppression of Leukotriene Formation in RBL-2H3 Cells that Overexpressed PHGPx, *J. Biol. Chem. 273*, 1990–1997.

69. Weitzel, F., and Wendel, A. (1993) Selenoenzymes Regulate the Activity of Leukocyte 5-Lipoxygenase Via the Peroxide Tone, *J. Biol. Chem. 268*, 6288–6292.

70. Schnurr, K., Belkner, J., Ursini, F., Schewe, T., and Kuehn, H. (1996) The Selenoenzyme PHGPx Controls the Activity of the 15-Lipoxygenase with Complex Substrates and Preserves the Specificity in the Oxygenation Products, *J. Biol. Chem. 271*, 4653–4658.

71. Balhorn, R., Corzett, M., Mazrimas, J., and Watkins, B. (1991) Identification of Bull Protamines Disulfide, *Biochemistry 30*, 175–181.

72. Brigelius-Flohè, R., Auman, K.D., Bloeckert, H., Gross, G., Kiess, M., Kloeppel, K.D., Maiorino, M., Roveri, A., Schuckelt, R., Ursini, F., Wingender, E., and Flohè, L. (1994) PHGPx. Genomic DNA, cDNA, and Deduced Aminoacid Sequence, *J. Biol. Chem. 269*, 7342–7348.

73. Aitken, R.J., Gordon, E., Harkiss, D., Twigg, J.P., Milne, P., Jennings, Z., and Irvine, D.S. (1998) Relative Impact of Oxidative Stress on the Functional Competence and Genomic Integrity of Human Spermatozoa, *Biol. Reprod. 59*, 1037–1046.

74. Ursini, F., Heim, S., Kiess, M., Maiorino, M., Roveri, A., Wissing, J., and Flohè, J. (1999) Dual Function of the Selenoprotein PHGPx during Sperm Maturation, *Science 285*, 1393–1396.

75. Imai, H., Suzuki, K., Ishizaka, K., Ichinose, S., Oshima, H., Okayasu, I., Emoto, K., Umeda, M., and Nakagawa, Y. (2001) Failure of the Expression of PHGPx in the Spermatozoa of Human Infertile Males, *Biol. Reprod. 64*, 674–683.

76. Roveri, A., Maiorino, M., and Ursini, F. (1994) Enzymatic and Immunological Measurements of Soluble and Membrane-Bound PHGPx, *Methods Enzymol. 233*, 202–212.

77. Storey, B.T., Alvarez, J.G., and Thompson, K.A. (1998) Human Sperm Glutathione Reductase Activity *in Situ* Reveals Limitation in the Glutathione Antioxidant Defense System Due to Supply of NADPH, *Mol. Reprod. Dev. 49*, 400–407.

78. Li, L., Seddon, A.P., Meister, A., and Risley, M.S. (1989) Spermatogenic Cell-Somatic Cell Interactions Are Required for Maintenance of Spermatogenic Cell Glutathione, *Biol. Reprod. 40*, 317–331.

79. Den Boer, P.J., Mackenbach, P., and Grootegoed, J.A. (1989) Glutathione Metabolism in Cultured Sertoli Cells and Spermatogenic Cells from Hamster, *J. Reprod. Fertil. 87*, 391–400.

80. Bauchè, F., Fouchard, M.H., and Jègou, B.(1994) Antioxidant Systems in Rat Testicular Cells, *Febs. Lett. 349*, 392–396.

81. Li, T.K. (1975) The Glutathione and Thiol Content of Mammalian Spermatozoa and Seminal Plasma, *Biol. Reprod. 12*, 641–646.

82. Ochsendorf, F.R., Buhl, R., Bästlein, A., and Beschman, H. (1998) Glutathione in Spermatozoa and Seminal Plasma of Infertile Men, *Hum. Reprod. 13*, 353–359.

83. Kessopoulou, E., Powers, J.H., Sharma, K.K., Pearson, M.J., Russell, J.M., Cooke, I.D., and Barrat, C.L. (1995) A Double-Blind Randomized Placebo Cross-Over Controlled Trial Using the Antioxidant Vitamin E to Treat Reactive Oxygen Species Associated with Male Infertility, *Fertil. Steril. 64*, 825–831.

84. Suleiman, S.A., Ali, M.E., Zaki, Z.M., el-Malik, E.M., and Nasr, M.A. (1996) Lipid Peroxidation and Human Sperm Motility: Protective Role of Vitamin E, *J. Androl. 17*, 530–537.

85. Godeas, C., Tramer, F., Sandri, G., and Panfili, E. (1966) Rat Testis Mitochondrial PHGPx Does Not Protect Endogenous Vitamin E Against Fe^{2+}-Induced (Lipo)Peroxidation, *Biochem. Mol. Med. 58*, 221–226.

86. Williams, R.M., Graham, J.K., and Hammerstedt, R.H. (1991) Determination of the Capacity of Ram Epididymal and Ejaculated Sperm to Undergo the Acrosomal Reaction and Penetrate Ova, *Biol. Reprod. 44*, 1080–1091.

87. Daunter, B., Hill, R., Hennessey, J., and Mackay, E.V. (1981) Preliminary Report: A Possible Mechanism for the Liquefaction of Human Seminal Plasma and Its Relationship to Spermatozoa Motility, *Andrologia 13*, 131–141.

88. Gagnon, C., Iwasaki, A., De Lamirande, E., and Kowalski, N. (1991) Reactive Oxygen Species and Human Spermatozoa, *Ann. NY Acad. Sci. 637*, 436–444.

89. Gagnon, C., and Iwasaki, A., (1992) Formation of Reactive Oxygen Species in Spermatozoa of Infertile Patients, *Fertil. Steril. 57*, 409–416.

90. Hinton, B.T., Palladino, M.A., Rudolph, D., and Labus, J.C. (1995) The Epididymis as Protector of Maturing Spermatozoa, *Reprod. Fertil. Dev. 7*, 731–745.

91. Zini, A., and Schlegel, P.N. (1997) Identification and Characterization of Antioxidant Enzyme mRNAs in the Rat Epididymis, *J. Androl. 20*, 86–91.

92. Poli, G., Albano, E., and Dianzani, M.U. (1993) Free Radicals: From Basic Science to Medicine. *Molecular and Cell Biology Updates Series*, Birkauser Verlag, Basel, Switzerland.

93. Inoue, M., Hirota, M., Sugi, K., Kawamoto, S., Ando, Y., Watanabe, N., and Morino, Y. (1989) Dynamic Aspects of Glutathione Metabolism and Transport during Oxidative Stress, in *Glutathione Centennial. Molecular Perspectives and Clinical Implications*, Taniguchi, N., Higashi, T., Sakamoto, Y., and Meister, A., Academic Press, New York, pp. 381.

94. Giblin, F.J., McCready, J.P., Reddan, J.R., Dziedzic, D.C., and Reddy, V.N. (1985) Detoxification of H_2O_2 by Cultured Rabbit Lens Epithelial Cells: Participation of the Glutathione Redox Cycle, *Exp. Eye Res. 40*, 827–840.

95. Meister, A. (1989) On the Biochemistry of Glutathione, in *Glutathione Centennial. Molecular Perspectives and Clinical Implications*, Taniguchi, N., Higashi, T., Sakamoto, Y., Meister, A., Academic Press, New York, pp. 1–31.

96. Aitken, R.J., and Clarkson, J.S. (1987) Cellular Basis of Defective Sperm Function and Its Association with the Genesis of Reactive Oxygen Species by Human Spermatozoa, *J. Reprod. Fertil. 81*, 459–469.

97. Aitken, R.J., Clarkson, J.S., and Fishel, S. (1989) Generation of Reactive Oxygen Species, Lipid Peroxidation, and Human Sperm Function, *Biol. Reprod. 40*, 183–187.

98. Alvarez, J.G., Touchtone, J.C., Blasco, L., and Storey, B.T. (1987) Spontaneous Lipid Peroxidation and Production of Superoxide and Hydrogen Peroxide in Human Spermatozoa: Superoxide Dismutase as Major Protectant Against Oxygen Toxicity, *J. Androl. 8*, 338–348.

99. D'Agata, R., Vicari, E., Moncada, M.L., Sidotti, G., Calogero, A.E., Fornito, M.C., Minacapilli, G., Mongioi, A., and Polosa, P. (1990) Generation of Reactive Oxygen Species in Subgroups of Infertile Men, *Int. J. Androl. 13*, 344–351.

100. Merril, A.H. (1989) Lipid Modulator of Cell Function, *Nutr. Rev. 47*, 161–169.

101. Aitken, R.J., Harkiss, D., and Buckingham, D. (1993) Analysis of Lipid Peroxidation Mechanisms in Human Spermatozoa, *Mol. Reprod. Develop 35*, 302–315.

102. Mazzilli, F., Rossi, T., Marchesini, M., Ronconi, C., and Dondero, F. (1994) Superoxide Anion in Human Semen Related to Seminal Parameters and Clinical Aspects, *Fertil. Steril. 62*, 862–8.

103. De Lamirande, E., and Gagnon, C. (1993) Human Sperm Hyperactivation in Whole Semen and Its Association with Low Superoxide Scavenging Capacity in Seminal Plasma, *Fertil. Steril. 59*, 1291–1295.

104. Griveau, J.F., and Le Lannou, D. (1994) Effects of Antioxidants on Human Sperm Preparation Tecniques, *Int. J. Androl. 17*, 225–231.

105. Griveau, J.F., Renard, P., and Le Lannou, D. (1994) An *in Vitro* Promoting Role for Hydrogen Peroxide in Human Sperm Capacitation, *Int. J. Androl. 17*, 300–307.

106. Mortimer, D. (1991) Sperm Preparation Techniques and Iatrogenic Failures of *in Vitro* Fertilization, *Hum. Reprod. 2*, 173–176.

107. Gavella, M., and Lipovac, V. (1994) Effect of Pentoxifylline on Experimentally Induced Lipid Peroxidation in Human Spermatozoa, *Int. J. Androl. 17*, 308–313.

108. Gomez, E., Buckingham, D.W., Brindle, J., Lanzafame, F., Irvine, D.S., and Aitken, R.J. (1996) Development of an Image Analysis System to Monitor the Retention of Residual Cytoplasm by Human Spermatozoa: Correlation with Biochemical Markers of the Cytoplasmic Space, Oxidative Stress, and Sperm Function, *J. Androl. 17*, 276–287.

109. Twigg, J., Fulton, N., Gomez, E., Irvine, D.S., and Aitken, R.J. (1998) Analysis of the Impact of Intracellular Reactive Oxygen Species Generation on the Structural and Functional Integrity of Human Spermatozoa: Lipid Peroxidation, DNA Fragmentation and Effectiveness of Antioxidants, *Hum. Reprod. 13*, 1429–1436.
110. Lanzafame, F., Chapman, M.G., Guglielmino, A., Gearon, C.M., and Forman, R.G. (1984) Pharmacological Stimulation of Sperm Motility, *Hum. Reprod. 9*, 192–199.
111. Halliwell, B., and Gutteridge, J.M.C. (1989) *Free Radicals in Biology and Medicine*, 2nd edn., pp. 152–157, pp. 253–259, Clarendon Press, Oxford.
112. Den Boer, P.J., Poot, M., Verkerk, A., Jansen, R., Mackenbach, P., and Grootegoed, J.A. (1990) Glutathione-Dependent Defense Mechanisms in Isolated Round Spermatids from the Rat, *Int. J. Androl. 13*, 26–38.
113. Lenzi, A., Culasso, F., Gandini, L., Lombardo, F., and Dondero, F. (1993) Placebo Controlled, Double Blind, Cross-Over Trial of Glutathione Therapy in Male Infertility, *Hum. Reprod. 8*, 1657–1662.
114. Lenzi, A., Lombardo, F., Gandini, L., Culasso, F., and Dondero, F. (1992) Glutathione Therapy for Male Infertility, *Arch. Androl. 29*, 65–68.
115. WHO Laboratory Manual for the Examination of Human Semen and Semen-Cervical Mucus Interaction (1999), 4th edn., Cambridge University Press, Cambridge.
116. Aitken, R.J., and West, K.M. (1990) Analysis of the Relationship between Reactive Oxygen Species Production and Leukocyte Infiltration in Fractions of Human Semen Separated on Percoll Gradients, *Int. J. Androl. 13*, 433–451.
117. Gandini, L., Lenzi, A., Lombardo, F., and Dondero, F. (1993) Glutathione: *In Vitro* Effects on Human Spermatozoa, in *Neuroendocrine and Intragonadal Regulation of Testicular Function*, Marrama, P., pp. 165–169.
118. Brenner, R.R. (1984) Effect of Unsaturated Fatty Acids on Membrane Structure and Enzyme Kinetics, *Prog. Lip. Res. 23*, 69–96.
119. Lenzi, A., Picardo, M., Gandini, L., and Dondero, F. (1996) Lipids of the Sperm Plasma Membrane: From Polynsaturated Fatty Acids Considered as Markers of Sperm Function to Possible Scavenger Therapy, *Hum. Reprod. Update 2*, 246–256.
120. Coniglio, J.C. (1994) Testicular Lipids, *Progr. Lipid Res. 33*, 387–401.

Chapter 15

Comparative Aspects of Lipid Peroxidation and Antioxidant Protection in Avian Semen

Peter F. Surai, Brian K. Speake, and Nick H.C. Sparks

Antioxidant and Lipid Research Group, Avian Science Research Centre, SAC, Auchincruive, Ayr, KA6 5HW, United Kingdom

Abstract

Avian spermatozoa are characterized by high proportions of polyunsaturated fatty acids (PUFA) in the phospholipid fraction of their membranes. This feature is associated with increased susceptibility of spermatozoa to free radical attack and lipid peroxidation. Therefore antioxidant protection is a vital element in maintaining sperm membrane integrity, motility, and fertilizing ability. It has been suggested that natural antioxidants (vitamin E, ascorbic acid, and glutathione) together with antioxidant enzymes (superoxide dismutase and glutathione peroxidase) build an integrated antioxidant system in avian semen capable of protecting it against free radicals and toxic products of their metabolism. There are species-specific, age-related differences in the expression of antioxidant systems in avian semen. The antioxidant/prooxidant balance in avian semen is an important determinant of membrane integrity and functions, including sperm viability and fertilizing capacity. Vitamin E is considered to be an effective membrane-stabilizing antioxidant of avian semen and dietary supplementation of this vitamin is found to be effective in preventing lipid peroxidation in the spermatozoa. Enhancement of the antioxidant capacity of semen could present a major opportunity for improving male fertility. A regulating role of reactive oxygen species (ROS) in sperm capacitation and the acrosome reaction in mammalian species has been demonstrated; but their role for avian species reproduction remains to be elucidated.

Introduction

Avian spermatozoa are unique in structure and chemical composition and are characterized by high proportions of polyunsaturated fatty acids (PUFA) in the phospholipid fraction of their membranes (1). This feature of these highly specialized cells is a reflection of the specific needs of their membranes for high levels of fluidity and flexibility, which are necessary for sperm motility and fusion with the egg. This functional advantage conferred by PUFA is, however, associated with disadvantages in terms of the susceptibility of sperm to free radical attack and lipid peroxidation. Therefore, antioxidant protection is a vital element in maintaining sperm membrane integrity, motility, and fertilizing ability. It has been suggested (1) that natural antioxidants (vitamin E, ascorbic acid, and glutathione) together with antioxidant enzymes (superoxide dismutase and glutathione peroxidase) build an integrated antioxidant system in avian semen capable of protecting it against free radicals and toxic products of their metabolism. The delicate balance between free radical production and antioxidant defense is considered to be an important determinant of semen quality and in particular its fertilizing ability. The relationship between fatty acid profile and antioxidant protection in avian semen as well as the possibility of modulating these parameters by nutritional means are important points for consideration (2).

Mechanisms and Consequences of Lipid Peroxidation in Avian Semen

The most important effect of free radicals on cellular metabolism is due to their participation in lipid peroxidation reactions. The first step of this process is called the initiation phase, during which carbon-centered free radicals are produced from a precursor molecule. For example, a polyunsaturated fatty acid (LH) is converted to a radical by abstraction of a hydrogen atom:

$$LH \xrightarrow{\text{Initiator}} L* \qquad [1]$$

In the presence of oxygen these radicals (L*) react quickly with the oxygen to produce peroxyl radicals, thereby starting the next stage of lipid peroxidation, the propagation phase:

$$L* + O_2 \longrightarrow LOO* \qquad [2]$$

At this stage a relatively unreactive carbon-centered radical (L*) is converted to a highly reactive peroxyl radical. A resultant peroxyl radical can attack any available peroxidazable material producing hydroperoxide (LOOH) and a new carbon-centered radical (L*):

$$LOO* + LH \longrightarrow LOOH + L* \qquad [3]$$

Therefore lipid peroxidation is a chain reaction and a potentially large number of cycles of peroxidation could cause substantial damage to cells. In membranes, the peroxidazable material is represented by PUFA. It is generally accepted that the susceptibility of PUFA to peroxidation is proportional to the number of double bounds in the molecule. Therefore docosahexaenoic fatty acid (DHA, 22:6n-3), docosatetraenoic fatty acid (DTA, 22:4n-6), and arachidonic acid (AA, 20:4n-6) are among major substrates for peroxidation in the sperm membrane. It is necessary to underline that the same PUFA are responsible for maintenance of physiologically important membrane properties, including fluidity and permeability. Therefore, as a result of lipid peroxidation within the biological membranes, their structure and functions are compromised. Since reaction 3 is the rate-limiting step of this chain reaction, any substance that can reduce the concentration of peroxyl radicals will limit lipid peroxidation (3). The main biological chain-breaking antioxidants, vitamin E, vitamin C, and glutathione, act at this step.

It is interesting that toxicity of oxygen free radicals to human spermatozoa was reported more than 55 years ago (4), and the toxic effect of H_2O_2 on chicken semen was shown by Wales *et al.* (5). However, major attention to this subject came in 1970 after publication of several milestone papers by Jones and Mann based on the results of experiments conducted in the Agricultural Research Council's Unit of Reproductive Physiology and Biochemistry, University of Cambridge (6–11). These publications clearly showed that lipid peroxidation

- Takes place in mammalian spermatozoa
- Causes decline in motility of spermatozoa
- Irreversibly abolishes the fructolytic and respiratory activity of spermatozoa
- Increases release of intracellular enzymes from spermatozoa into medium
- Is the major biochemical cause of sperm senescence under storage conditions *in vitro*
- Causes predominant oxidation of 22:6n-3 and 20:4n-6 fatty acids

Furthermore, those authors also showed that the susceptibility of spermatozoa to peroxidation was increased in cells damaged prior to incubation and that peroxidized PUFA added to a washed sperm suspension immobilized the spermatozoa rapidly and permanently. Those publications presented results obtained with ram and human semen. However, results on lipid peroxidation in other mammalian species have also been published, including boar (12–15), bull (16–20), buffalo (21), rabbit (22), and horse (23,24). Furthermore, lipid peroxidation in human semen has been studied further in detail and several comprehensive reviews have discussed their findings (25–29). The conclusion is that lipid peroxidation in mammalian semen is considered to be one of the most important factors causing infertility in man as well as causing decreased sperm quality during the storage of semen from farm animals.

Research on lipid peroxidation in avian semen started much later in comparison to mammalian species. This is probably because such research has largely been driven by a practical need to understand molecular mechanisms of semen deterioration during storage for further artificial insemination. In poultry production, however, artificial insemination was introduced several decades later than for mammalian species, and its practical usage is related mainly to turkey production. Therefore, a publication by Fujihara and Howarth showing that, during incubation at 41°C, chicken spermatozoa produced a thiobarbituric acid-reactive product and that susceptibility to peroxidation was enhanced by the addition of ascorbate was a starting point in research related to lipid peroxidation in avian semen (30). The authors concluded that chicken spermatozoa, following ejaculation and exposure to air, could undergo peroxidation with a consecutive decrease in their viability. The conclusion was very important for future improvement of techniques for avian semen storage *in vitro*. Further evidence for lipid peroxidation in avian semen was presented by Wishart (31), who found that the formation of high concentrations of malondialdehyde (MDA) during a 5-hour aerobic incubation of chicken semen was associated with a partial or complete loss of fertilizing ability. Most importantly, the fertilizing ability of samples that produced low or negligible concentrations of MDA remained unimpaired (31). Semen samples incubated under anaerobic conditions produced only a negligible amount of MDA. There was a considerable (70-fold) variability between individual males in relation to MDA production (31). This could be explained as a result of compositional and functional differences in sperm membranes among individual male chickens (32).

Independently of the work conducted in the United Kingdom by Wishart (31), investigation of lipid peroxidation in turkey semen was started approximately at the same time in Ukraine (33,34). In particular, an induced (by Fe^{2+}) lipid peroxidation in turkey semen was used to assess semen susceptibility to lipid peroxidation since the initial level of peroxides in fresh or even stored semen was shown to be comparatively low. At that time an idea of the possible protective effects of natural antioxidants in the male diet on the lipid peroxidation in the semen was developed (34). In particular, it was shown that dietary supplementation of male turkeys with vitamin E was associated with a significant decrease in semen susceptibility to lipid peroxidation. This work was further developed by Cecil and Bakst (35), who showed that during aerobic storage of turkey spermatozoa, lipid peroxidation was time- and temperature-dependent. The authors also suggested that turkey spermatozoa are more sensitive to lipid peroxidation than semen from other species. It seems likely that lipid peroxidation in semen is also age dependent. For example, Donoghue and Donoghue (36) reported that MDA concentrations were 10-fold higher in semen from older turkey males (56 wk of age) than from younger ones (30 wk of age). This is in agreement with the data of Kelso *et al.* (37), which indicates a fall in the antioxidant defense (activity of glutathione peroxidase, GSH-Px) of chicken spermatozoa between 25 and 60 weeks of age. Accumulation of thiobarbituric acid reactive substances (TBARS) in duck semen as a result of lipid peroxidation has also recently been described (38). It seems likely that MDA accumulation is associated with mid-piece abnormality in human spermatozoa (39) and with a decrease in the fertilizing capacity of chicken (31) and turkey (35) spermatozoa.

The molecular mechanisms of lipid peroxidation in avian semen have received little attention. Recently, it has been shown that during sperm storage, lipid peroxidation is associated with a significant decrease in PUFA concentration in spermatozoa. In particular, the main PUFA in chicken semen (22:4n-6) was most susceptible to peroxidation. Its proportion in the phospholipid fraction was significantly decreased as a result of incubation of chicken sperm for 12 h at 20°C (Fig. 15.1; 40). The inclusion of a promotor of lipid peroxidation (Fe^{2+}) in the incubation medium further increased the rate of lipid peroxidation, significantly decreasing the proportions of not only 22:4n-6

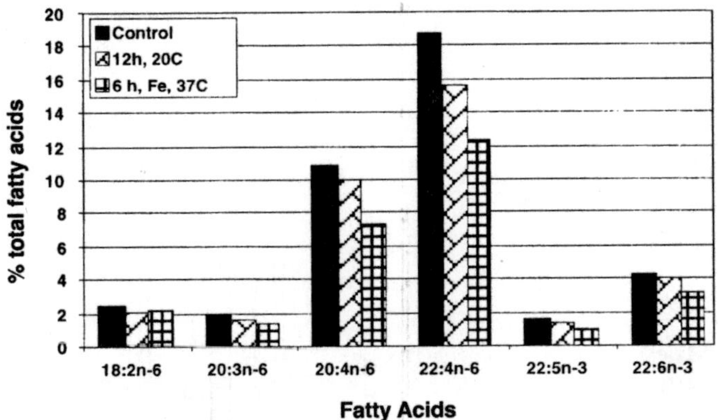

Fig. 15.1. Effect of lipid peroxidation on main PUFA in chicken spermatozoa. Chicken semen was incubated 12 h at 20°C or 6 h at 37°C in the presence of iron. Adapted from Surai *et al.*, 1998.

but also 20:4n-6, 22:5n-3, and 22:6n-3 in the phospholipid fraction of the spermatozoa. The confirmation of the suggestion that the loss of PUFA was due to peroxidation came from the data showing simultaneous accumulation of TBARS in the semen (40). Recently, it has been shown that the total lipid content, the proportion of total phospholipids, and the levels of phosphatidylcholine (PC), phosphatidylethanolamine (PE), and sphingomyelin (Sph) were significantly decreased in chicken semen during *in vitro* storage, and this was associated with a reduction in the proportion of motile, viable, and morphologically normal cells (41). Similarly, in turkey spermatozoa incubated at 37°C in the presence of exogenous Fe^{2+}, a significant decrease in PS (by 47%) and PE (by 35%), the two most unsaturated fractions of avian spermatozoa, was observed (42,43). Storage of diluted turkey semen for 48 h at 4°C was also associated with a decrease in total phospholipid content, PC, and, to a lesser extent, Sph, phosphatidylserine (PS), and phosphatidylinositol (PI) (44). The significance of the decreased concentration of these phospholipids needs further investigation. However, PS appears to be an important phospholipid fraction in avian spermatozoa, having the highest degree of unsaturation (38,45), decreasing during aging (46), and showing a significant positive correlation with the fertilizing ability of chicken semen during the reproductive cycle (47).

As a result of lipid peroxidation in turkey spermatozoa due to a 1-h incubation at 37°C in the presence of Fe^{2+}, there was a significant decrease in the levels of the main PUFA, 22:4n-6, 20:4n-6, 22:6n-3, and 22:3n-9 (Fig. 15.2), and in proportions of PE and PS fractions (Fig. 15.3). Inclusion of vitamin E into the incubation medium decreased PUFA peroxidation and prevented decline in PE and PS fractions in turkey spermatozoa (Fig. 15.2 and 15.3). Similarly, studies using liposomes have shown that 22:6n-3, 22:5n-3, 22:4n-6, and 20:4n-6 were very susceptible to peroxidation in an *in vitro* system (48). Therefore, the mechanisms by which reactive oxygen species

                          P.F. Surai et al.

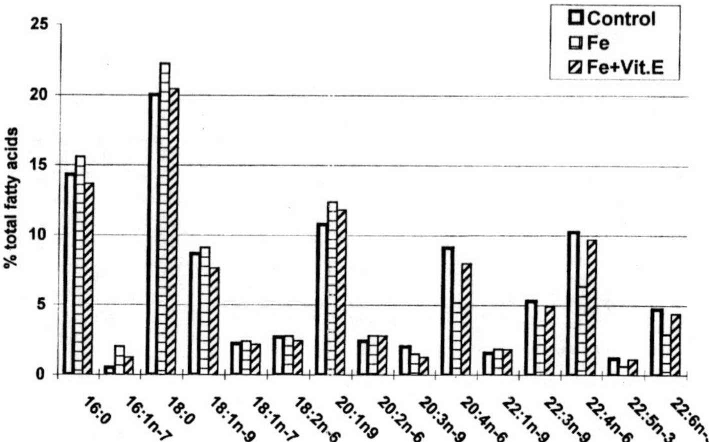

Fig. 15.2. Effect of lipid peroxidation and vitamin E on fatty acid profile of turkey spermatozoa. Turkey semen was incubated in presence of Fe^{2+} or Fe^{2+} + vitamin E at 37°C. Adapted from Maldjian *et al.*, 1998.

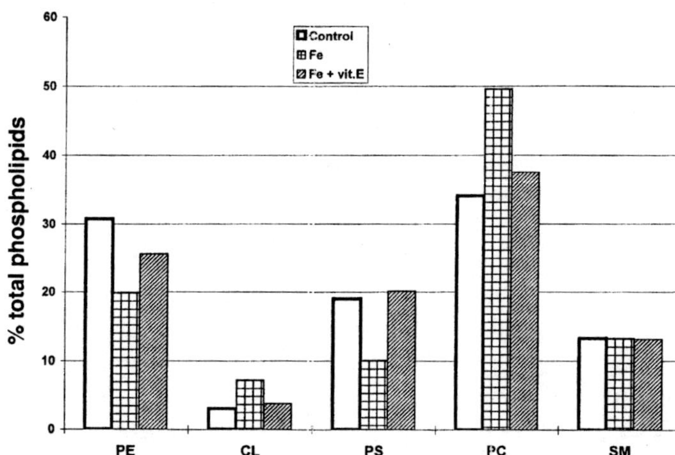

Fig. 15.3. Effect of lipid peroxidation and vitamin E on phospholipid composition of turkey spermatozoa. Turkey semen was incubated in presence of Fe^{2+} or Fe^{2+} + vitamin E at 37°C. Adapted from Maldjian *et al.*, 1998.

(ROS) disrupt sperm function probably involve the peroxidation of PUFA in the sperm plasma membrane. For example, it has been shown that in human spermatozoa, lipid peroxidation damages the cell plasma membrane, leading to loss of cytoplasmic components and hence to cell death—a process that is considered to play an important role in the pathophysiology of male infertility (39). A negative correlation between MDA production and sperm motility was observed in human semen (49). However, sperm storage at refrigeration temperature is not always associated with lipid peroxidation. For example, in contrast to the above-mentioned observations, storing turkey semen for 48 h at 4°C did not significantly affect the fatty acid profile nor the level of free cholesterol, but the motility, viability, and morphological integrity of spermatozoa significantly decreased (44).

However, lipid peroxidation is not restricted to damage to membranes, and other detrimental consequences for cell metabolism have been described as well (1):

- chromatin destabilization
- marked alterations in the DNA-protein complex
- changes in the activities of various enzymes, including cytochrome oxidase, lactate dehydrogenase, and glucose-6-phosphate dehydrogenase
- disruption of mitochondria functions
- inhibition of the synthesis of DNA, RNA, and proteins
- increase of DNA fragmentation
- modification of the cytoskeleton
- alteration in the sperm axoneme
- inhibition of sperm-oocyte fusion

It is necessary to stress that most of the studies on mechanisms and consequences of lipid peroxidation have been associated with mammalian (mainly human) spermatozoa with much less emphasis on avian semen. Nevertheless, lipid peroxidation in avian semen without doubt would have similar consequences. For example, H_2O_2 and organic hydroperoxides had toxic effects on avian sperm motility (Fig. 15.4). On a molar basis, H_2O_2 was about 3 times more powerful in terms of decreasing spermatozoa motility than cumene hydroperoxide. The difference in the toxicity is probably due to higher permeability of plasma membranes for H_2O_2 than for organic hydroperoxides. At the same time, the susceptibility of chicken spermatozoa to H_2O_2 toxicity was much higher than that in mammalian spermatozoa (5).

To understand species-specific differences in lipid peroxidation in spermatozoa, it is necessary to consider an antioxidant/pro-oxidant balance in semen. For example, duck spermatozoa are characterized by increased unsaturation of lipids and decreased vitamin E concentration (Fig. 15.5) in comparison to chicken spermatozoa (38). However, the susceptibility of duck spermatozoa to peroxidation was not different from that of chicken spermatozoa (Fig. 15.6).

Antioxidant Protection in Avian Semen

The antioxidant protection in avian semen is poorly characterized. Recently, it has been suggested that the antioxidant system of the spermatozoa includes three major levels of antioxidant defense (1,50) responsible for maintenance of spermatozoan functions in various stress conditions, including sperm dilution, storage, and deep freezing. Superoxide dismutase (SOD) together with GSH-Px and metal-binding pro-

 P.F. Surai et al.

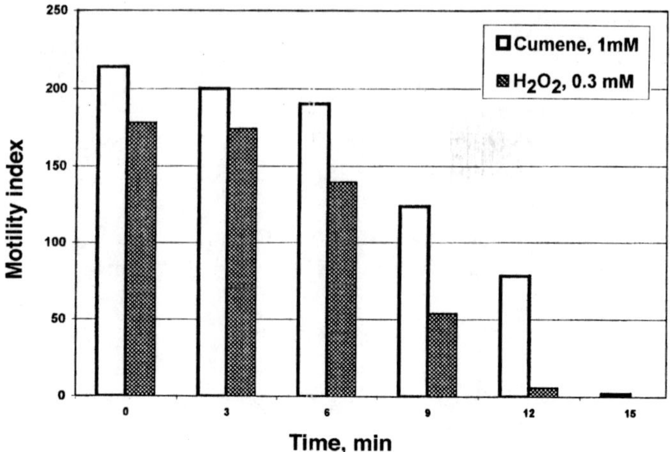

Fig. 15.4. Effect of cumene hydroperoxide or hydrogen peroxide on chicken semen motility.

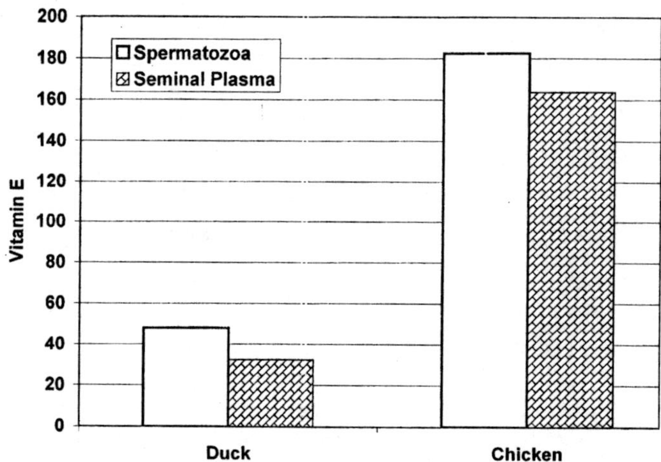

Fig. 15.5. Vitamin E concentration in chicken and duck spermatozoa (ng/10^9) and seminal plasma (ng/ml). Adapted from Surai *et al.,* 2000.

teins comprise the first level of antioxidant defense responsible for prevention and restriction of free radical formation (1). However, the first level of antioxidant defense is not sufficient to prevent the initiation of lipid peroxidation.

Natural antioxidants (vitamin E, ascorbic acid, glutathione), together with additional actions of GSH-Px, build the second level of antioxidant defense dealing with prevention and restriction of chain formation and propagation. Lipid peroxidation can

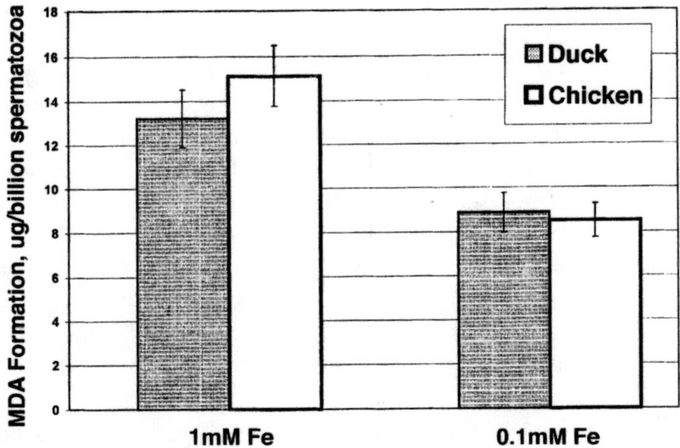

Fig. 15.6. Malondialdehyde formation in duck and chicken semen as a result of Fe-stimulated lipid peroxidation. Adapted from Surai *et al.*, 2000.

be kept under control until these antioxidants are used up and the chain reaction becomes uncontrolled, resulting in damage to cellular constituents and structures.

The third level of defense is based on the enzymatic system responsible for repair or/and removal of damaged molecules from the cell. It seems likely (51) that this level of antioxidant defense in the spermatozoa is either not present or is very inefficient.

First Level of Antioxidant Defense in Avian Semen: Superoxide Dismutase (SOD)

Since the superoxide radical is the main free radical produced under physiological conditions in the cell (52), superoxide dismutase (SOD; EC 1.15.1.1) is considered to be the main element of the first level of intracellular antioxidant defense (50). This enzyme dismutates the superoxide radical in the following reaction:

$$O_2^- + O_2^- + 2H^+ \xrightarrow{\text{SOD}} H_2O_2 + O_2$$

There are three different forms of this enzyme in mammalian and avian species (53). The main form is Mn-SOD, which is located in mitochondria (54), a prime site of superoxide radical production (55). Therefore, the expression of Mn-SOD is considered to be essential for the survival of aerobic life and the development of cellular resistance to oxygen radical-mediated toxicity (56).

The second form of the enzyme, Cu,Zn-SOD, is located in the cytosol. The third SOD, so-called extra-cellular SOD is a secretory, Cu,Zn-enzyme found in the interstitial spaces of tissues and in extra-cellular fluids (54). A fourth form of the enzyme, Fe-SOD, is present in various bacteria, blue-green algae, and protozoa but is not found in animal tissues (53). Cu,Zn-SOD was purified from chicken liver and shown to have two subunits with a molecular weight of 16,000 for each (57).

In spite of the importance of SOD in protecting cells against lipid peroxidation, its activity in avian semen has received only limited attention. For example, when a comparative study of SOD activity was conducted in spermatozoa from boar, rabbit, stallion, donkey, ram, bull, man, and chicken, it was shown that donkey sperm had the highest and chicken spermatozoa the lowest activity (58). Subsequently, turkey spermatozoa were shown to contain even lower SOD activity than chicken spermatozoa and it was suggested that, due to inadequate SOD activity, lipid peroxidation may be a significant factor in poor semen quality and lowered fertility in the turkey (59). The total SOD activity of human seminal plasma was 20 times higher than in blood plasma; human spermatozoa also contained exceptionally large amounts of Cu,Zn-SOD but little Mn-SOD (60).

Our recent data indicate that in seminal plasma of five avian species, only Cu,Zn-SOD was detected (Fig. 15.7 and 15.8; 40,61). There are species-specific differences in SOD activity in the seminal plasma, with the highest SOD activity recorded in turkey and guinea fowl and the lowest activity in duck (Fig. 15.8). Total antioxidant activity of the seminal plasma was also the highest in turkey (Fig. 15.8). In the spermatozoa both forms of SOD are expressed with significant species-specific differences (Fig. 15.7). For example, in goose spermatozoa, the activity of Cu,Zn-SOD was more than twice that of Mn-SOD. An opposite distribution between different forms of SOD was found in guinea fowl, where Mn-SOD was more than twofold higher compared to Cu,Zn-SOD (Fig. 15.9). In the chicken, about 67% of total semen SOD activity was detected in the spermatozoa and only 33% in the seminal plasma (40). The biological meaning and physiological consequences of such species-specific differences in SOD activity and distribution need further clarification.

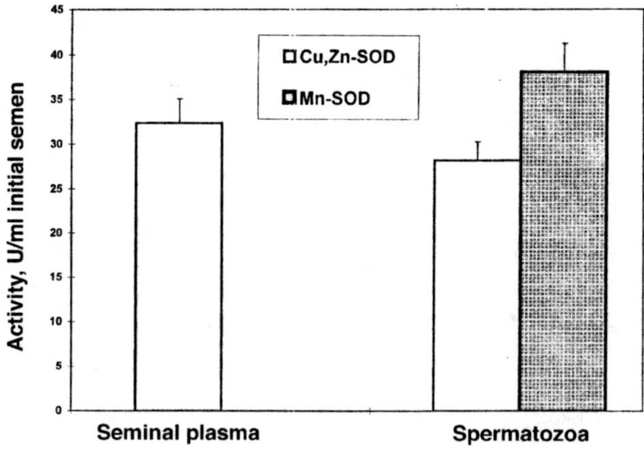

Fig. 15.7. Distribution of SOD in chicken spermatozoa and seminal plasma. Adapted from Surai *et al.*, 1998a.

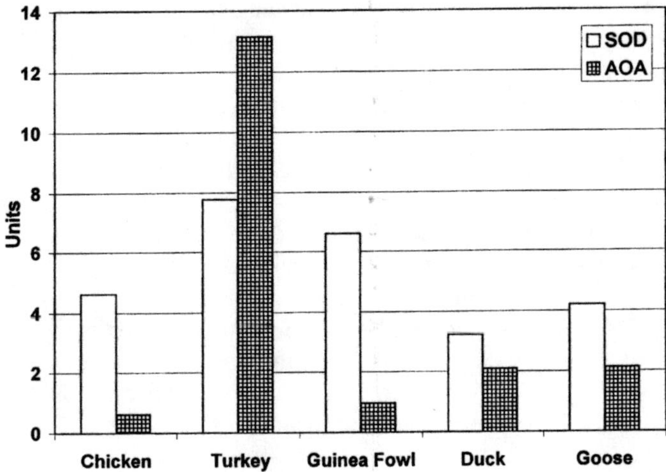

Fig. 15.8. Superoxide dismutase and total antioxidant activity in avian seminal plasma. Adapted from Surai *et al.,* 1998a.

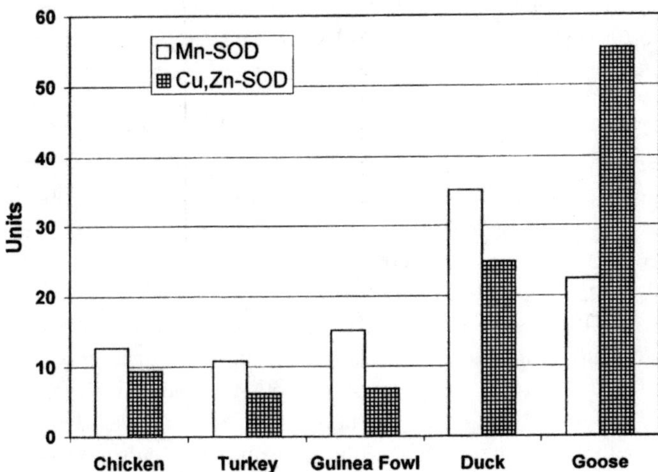

Fig. 15.9. Superoxide dismutase activity in avian spermatozoa. Adapted from Surai *et al.,* 1998a.

Se and GSH-Px

The essentiality of selenium for male fertility was shown in the early 1980s (62–65). This conclusion was based on the results of a range of different experiments with mammals showing the following:

- In mild deficiency, Se is preferentially retained in rat testes (62).
- Mammalian semen is considered to contain the highest selenium concentration of all other body tissues (66).
- In the human, a significant positive correlation in the selenium concentration was demonstrated between the different reproductive organs, with the testis having the highest concentrations of this element (67).
- Progressive selenium deficiency was associated with morphological alterations of spermatids and spermatozoa (63) with subsequent complete disappearance of mature germinal cells (68).
- In selenium-deficient mice, the proportion of abnormal sperm ranged from 6.8 to 49.6%, whereas in the control group it was only 4.0–15.0%. The most frequently occurring abnormalities in sperm shape were found in the sperm head. However there was also a tendency of increasing abnormalities in other spermatozoa regions, including neck, mid-piece, and tail (69).
- In human semen, selenium was found mainly (more than 85%) in the seminal plasma and sperm motility was maximal when semen Se levels were between 50 and 69 ng/mL (70).

There are species-specific differences in the Se level in semen. For example, the seminal plasma level of Se was lowest in the human and the stallion, higher in ram and boar, and highest in the bull (71). Selenocysteine is shown to be the main form of Se in rat sperm and selenocysteine and selenomethionine were found in ovine sperm (72).

It is generally accepted that Se participates in various physiological functions as an integral part of a range of selenoproteins. The selenoprotein family includes at least 20 eukaryotic proteins (73). Expression of individual eukaryotic selenoproteins is characterized by high tissue specificity, depends on Se availability, can be regulated by hormones, and if compromised contributes to various pathological conditions (73). Most of the selenoproteins contain a single selenocysteine residue per polypeptide chain (74). GSH-Px and thioredoxin reductase (TR) are the most abundant antioxidant Se-containing proteins in mammals (75). The best characterized among selenoproteins is the GSH-Px family. In mammals it includes five members. The first member of this family, the so-called classical GSH-Px, was described in 1973 (76,77). The second selenoperoxidase, the phospholipid hydroperoxide glutathione peroxidase (PHGSH-Px), was discovered 9 years later (78) and characterized in 1985 (79). Next, plasma glutathione peroxidase (pGSH-Px) was described in 1987 (80,81). The fourth selenoperoxidase, gastrointestinal glutathione peroxidase (GI-GSH-Px), was characterized in 1993 (82; for review see 83). Recently, a fifth member of Se-dependent glutathione peroxidases, a specific sperm nuclei GSH-Px (sn-GSH-Px), was characterized (84,85). In particular, this selenoenzyme has been identified in rat testes (84) to be a 34-kDa selenoprotein. It was localized in the spermatid nuclei and found to comprise about 80% of total Se present. It was identified as specific to the sperm nuclei GSH-Px with similar properties to PH-GSH-Px (85). The authors showed that it differs from PH-GSH-Px in its N-terminal sequence. In rats, sn-GSH-Px is highly expressed in the nuclei of the late spermatids, where it is the only selenoprotein present (85). In Se-depleted rats the concentration of sn-GSH-Px decreased to a third of the normal level and chromatin condensation was severely disturbed (85).

The various GSH-Px are characterized by different tissue specificity and are expressed from different genes (86,87). The major function of these peroxidases is considered to be the removal and detoxification of hydrogen peroxide and lipid hydroperoxides (54,86). Since hydrogen peroxide is considered an intracellular messenger (88) and redox regulation can play a basic role in the activation of key transcription factors (89,90), it has been suggested that regulation of the delicate regional redox balance is one of the main functions of glutathione peroxidases (87). In contrast, the main function of sn-GSH-Px is protamine thiol cross-linking during sperm maturation (85).

Glutathione peroxidases are found in all mammalian tissues in which oxidative processes occur (73). The major role of these enzymes includes the reduction of hydrogen peroxide and organic peroxides to water and the corresponding alcohol, respectively. This is an important step in preventing production of reactive oxygen radicals. In general, the cytoplasmic GSH-Px is considered an "emergency enzyme" (73) responsible for prevention of detrimental effects of oxidative stress.

Maintenance of cellular redox state is another important function of the GSH-Px enzymes and GSH-Px forms are involved in such physiological events as differentiation, signal transduction, and regulation of pro-inflammatory cytokine production (91). Peroxynitrite scavenging by GSH-Px (92) could also play a prominent role in cell signal transduction events. Participation of GSH-Px enzymes in regulating biosynthesis of leukotrienes, thromboxanes, and prostaglandins is responsible for the modulation of inflammatory reactions, whereas PH-GSH-Px can bring about cytokine-induced transcriptional gene activation (for review see 73).

In general, different forms of GSH-Px perform their protective functions in concert, with each providing antioxidant protection at different sites of the body. For example, GI-GSH-Px could be considered to be a barrier against hydroperoxide resorption (87). Furthermore, in the gastrointestinal tract there are at least three more selenoproteins including plasma GSH-Px, selenoprotein P, and thioredoxin reductase (93). Plasma GSH-Px is an important antioxidant in plasma, which together with selenoprotein P and other antioxidant compounds maintain antioxidant protection. On the other hand, PH-GSH-Px is an important antioxidant inside biological membranes, where lipid peroxidation occurs and lipid hydroperoxides are produced.

GSH-Px activity ultimately depends on Se provision in the diet. However, some forms of GSH-Px Se are only synthesized when the Se supply is optimal. There are substantial differences among different forms of GSH-Px with regard to response to Se deficiency (87). The selenoproteins retained in tissues for longer periods during progressive Se deficiency are considered to have higher physiological significance in comparison to those whose activities rapidly decline. In this respect, the main GSH-Px forms rank as follows (87):

GI-GSH-Px > PH-GSH-Px > Plasma GSH-Px = Cytosolic GSH-Px.

There is also a range of other selenoproteins identified, but their functions are less obvious (94,95). In relation to the antioxidant defense in avian sperm provided by GSH-Px, two other selenoproteins are of great importance: thioredoxin reductase (TR) and sperm capsular selenoprotein. Recently it has been appreciated that the redox status of the cell is a major determinant of many different pathways, including gene regulation (96). A thiol redox system consisting of the glutathione system (glutathione/glutathione reductase/glutaredoxin/glutathione peroxidase (97,98) and a thioredoxin system (thioredoxin/thioredoxin peroxidase/thioredoxin reductase) are believed to be the major players in this regulation (99,100). Together they supply electrons for deoxyribonucleotide formation, antioxidant defense, and redox regulation of signal transduction, transcription, cell growth, and apoptosis (101,102). Interestingly, TR can reduce not only thioredoxin but also oxidized glutathione (103). Therefore, these two systems are linked much more closely than previously considered. Experiments with yeast mutants lacking both the mitochondrial thioredoxin system and the mitochondrial peroxyredoxin system suggest an important role for thioredoxin, TR, and peroxyredoxin in the protection against oxidative stress (104).

It is interesting that sperm-specific thioredoxin (Sptrx) was recently identified and characterized in humans (105). The authors showed Sptrx mRNA to be expressed only in round and elongating spermatids, whereas the Sptrx protein is located in the cytoplasmic droplets of ejaculated sperm, suggesting that it might be an important factor in regulating critical steps of human spermatogenesis. Furthermore, a second member of this family, called Sptrx-2 and specifically expressed in human sperm cells, has been identified and characterized (106) and is considered to be a novel component of the human sperm axonemal organization. It seems likely that it is just the beginning of a deeper understanding of roles of new proteins in sperm function. For example, mouse Sptrx-1 has been cloned and characterized (107) as being similar to that described for the human and showing protein disulphide reducing activity in an enzymatic assay coupled to NADPH and TR. Therefore, it is just a matter of time before TR in the sperm is characterized and its essential role in sperm antioxidant protection is shown.

Sperm capsule selenoprotein (SCS) is localized in the mid-piece of the spermatozoa, where it stabilizes the integrity of the sperm flagella (108) and recently has been identified as PH-GSH-Px (109). However, recently it has been shown that the pertinent genes of rats and mice did not contain any TGA codons within the translated regions and, as a result, the essentiality of SCS for sperm function was questioned (73).

Unfortunately there are no data available concerning Se content in avian semen. However, GSH-Px was found to be expressed in chicken seminal plasma and spermatozoa (Fig. 15.10). There are species-specific differences in activity and distribution of GSH-Px in avian semen. For example, on the one hand, in seminal plasma total GSH-Px activity was the highest in turkey and lowest in duck and goose (Fig. 15.11). In spermatozoa, on the other hand, the highest GSH-Px activities were found for goose and duck, and much lower GSH-Px activity was recorded for guinea fowl, turkey, or chicken (Fig. 15.12). Recently, it was shown that despite a high proportion of PUFA

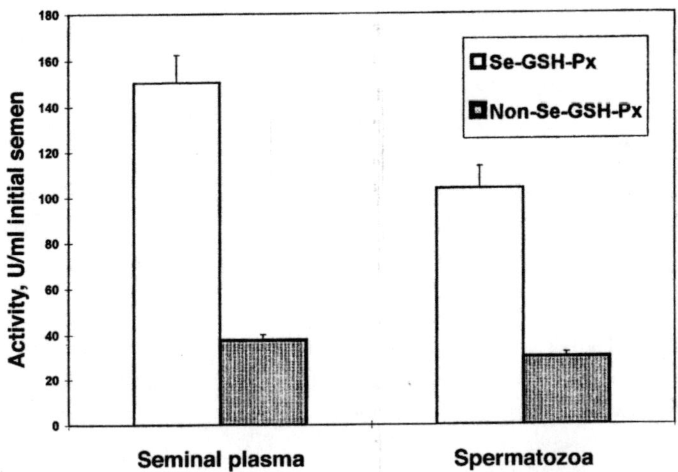

Fig. 15.10. Distribution of GSH-Px in chicken spermatozoa. Adapted from Surai *et al.,* 1998.

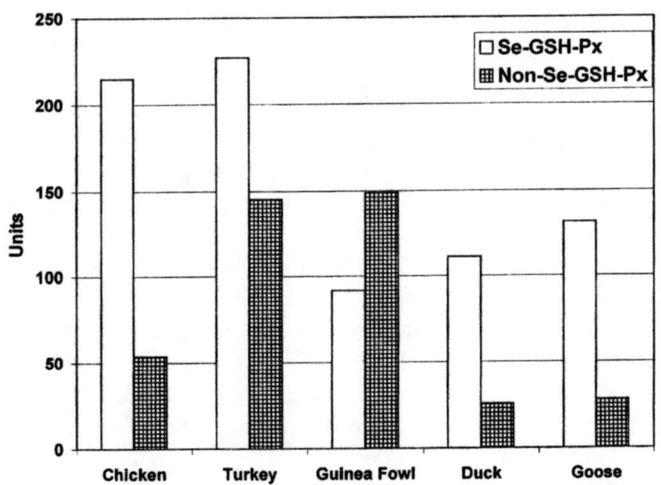

Fig. 15.11. GSH-Px activity in avian seminal plasma. Adapted from Surai *et al.,* 1998a.

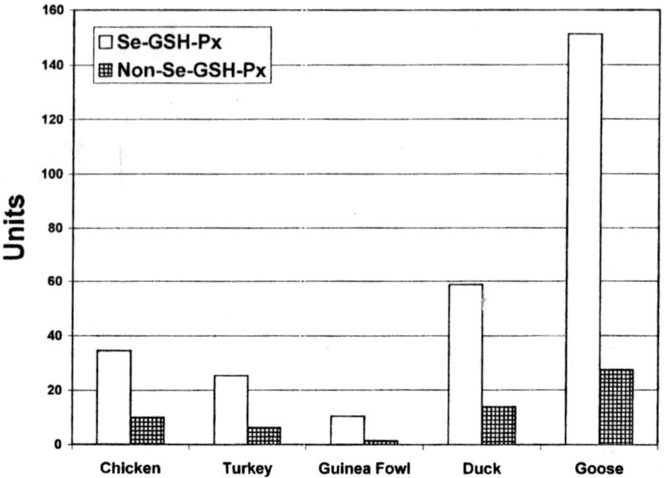

Fig. 15.12. GSH-Px activity in avian spermatozoa. Adapted from Surai *et al.,* 1998a.

and a low level of vitamin E, duck spermatozoa have the same susceptibility to lipid peroxidation as chicken spermatozoa (38). It has been suggested that an increased activity of Se-GSH-Px in duck semen compensates for the relatively low concentrations of other antioxidants.

It seems likely that GSH-Px is a universal antioxidant for spermatozoa because lipid hydroperoxides are extremely toxic for this kind of cell. For example, GSH-Px activity was found to be expressed in the semen of several mammalian species, including ram, dog, human, goat, and bull (110–112). However, there are species-specific differences in expression of this enzyme in semen. In bulls, for example, GSH-Px is exclusively associated with the seminal plasma and not found in spermatozoa (113,114). In contrast, GSH-Px activity in seminal plasma was low in man and ram and absent in boar and stallion (71). It has been shown that approximately two thirds of GSH-Px activity in bull semen was non-Se-GSH-Px (115). In the same experiment it was found that the MDA level was negatively correlated with Se-GSH-Px activity, and it has been suggested that Se-GSH-Px plays a role in protecting the acrosome membranes against disruption.

If selenium is limited in the diet (which is the case in many countries in the world), then dietary supplementation of this trace element should have a beneficial effect on the antioxidant defense in various tissues, including sperm. This was confirmed in our studies. Inclusion of Se in the diet of male chickens significantly increased Se-GSH-Px activity in the liver, testes, spermatozoa, and seminal plasma (Fig. 15.13 and 15.14; 116). As a result, a significant decrease in the sperm and tissue susceptibility to lipid peroxidation was observed. This protective effect was more expressed in stored semen as compared to fresh. In this respect, it is extremely important that an inducible form of the enzyme (Se-GSH-Px) represents more than 75% of

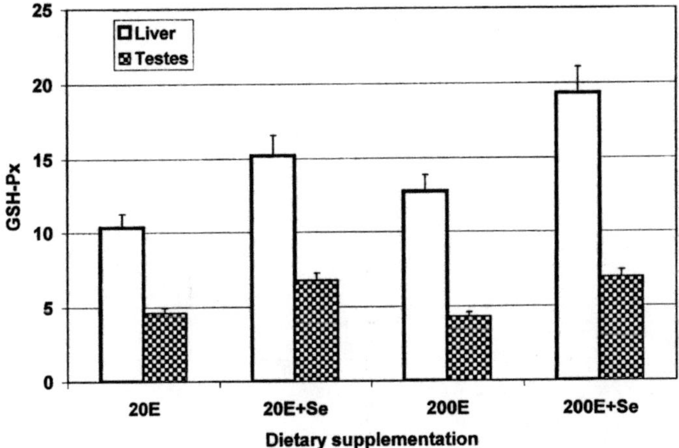

Fig. 15.13. Effect of vitamin E and vitamin E+ selenium on GSH-Px activity in chicken liver and testes. Adapted from Surai *et al.,* 1998b.

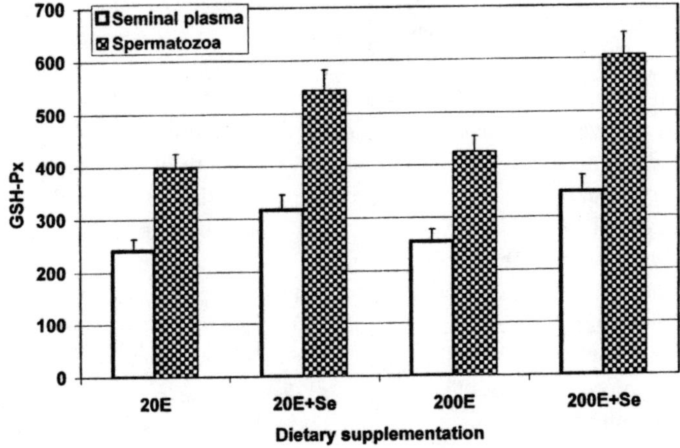

Fig. 15.14. Effect of vitamin E and vitamin E+ selenium on GSH-Px activity in chicken semen. Adapted from Surai *et al.,* 1998b.

the total enzymatic activity in chicken spermatozoa and more than 60% in the testes and liver of cockerels. A similar stimulating effect of Se-supplementation on GSH-Px activity in sows has been found at a level of 0.5 mg Se/kg in the diet (117).

Unfortunately, data on the effect of Se supplementation of avian males on functional characteristics of spermatozoa and their fertilizing ability are very limited. Recently, Edens (118) showed that, when cockerels were fed on a basal diet contain-

TABLE 15.1

Spermatozoal Abnormalities (%) in Semen from Cockerels Fed on a Basal Diet or Diets Supplemented with Either Sodium Selenite or Selenomethionine[a]

Sperm morphology	Basal diet	Selenite	Selenomethionine
Normal sperm	57.9	89.4	98.7
Bent midpiece	18.7	6.2	0.7
Swollen midpiece	1.6	0.4	0.1
Ruptured midpiece	0.9	0.1	0.0
Swollen head	1.3	0.2	0.2
Corkscrew head	15.4	1.8	0.2
Coiled	3.2	0.8	0.0
Fragment/other	1.0	1.1	0.1

[a]Adapted from Edens (118).

ing 0.28 ppm Se without additional dietary supplementation of this trace element, the percentage of normal spermatozoa was only 57.9% (Table 15.1), and two major abnormalities seen were bent mid-piece (18.7%) and corkscrew head (15.4%). When this diet was supplemented with an additional 0.2 ppm Se in the form of selenite, the percentage of normal spermatozoa increased to 89.4% and abnormalities in the form of bent mid-piece and corkscrew head were decreased to 6.2 and 1.8%, respectively. However, when organic selenium was included in the cockerel's diet in the same amount, semen quality was further improved and those abnormalities decreased to 0.7 and 0.2%, and the percentage of normal spermatozoa increased to 98.7%. These results clearly showed that the form of dietary Se supplementation is a crucial factor of its efficiency, with organic selenium being much more effective than selenite. We suggested an explanation for this difference (119) based on an evolutionary approach because in nature birds will have only one form of selenium in their diet, organic selenium, mainly as selenomethionine, which is an integral part of any food item. Therefore, it seems that the digestive system of birds became adapted to this form of selenium, and as a result, there is a principal difference between organic and inorganic selenium in terms of their assimilation from the diet and use in the body with organic selenium being more effective (1).

Additional data from Edens (118) indicated that selenomethionine (0.3 ppm from 21 weeks of age) in the diet of Hubbard roosters improved semen quality to a greater extent than achieved by selenite at the same dose (Table 15.2). The sperm quality index significantly increased as well as the percentage of normal spermatozoa. At the same time, the proportions of various abnormalities in semen decreased. There was also a positive effect on fertility, which improved 0.56–1.03% by selenomethionine dietary supplementation. These experimental results confirmed the importance of selenium in maintaining chicken semen quality and specifically showed the advantages of organic selenium.

Similar positive responses of dietary Se supplementation have been seen with mammals, including cattle and humans (120–124), where Se supplementation enhances the *in vitro* motility and oxygen uptake of sperm.

TABLE 15.2
Effects of Sodium Selenite or Selenomethionine of Productive Parameters of Hubbard Breeder Hens[a]

	Farm 1		Farm 2	
Variable	Selenite	SeMet	Selenite	SeMet
Egg production, %	82.87	85.46	84.22	84.74
Fertility, %	96.12	96.68	96.23	97.26
Daily settable eggs	8799	9111	8379	8647
Hatchability, %	83.10	84.40	82.40	82.64

[a]Adapted from Edens (118).

Second Level of Antioxidant Defense—Vitamin E

Vitamin E is considered as the main antioxidant of biological membranes (125). It reacts with free radicals as follows:

$$\text{Vitamin E} + \text{R–OO}^* \longrightarrow \text{Vitamin E}^* + \text{ROOH}$$

Vitamin E concentration in membranes is relatively low, comprising less that 1 mol per 1000 mol of phospholipid (126). Nevertheless, due to its location inside the membrane on the water/lipid interface, vitamin E is able to effectively scavenge free radicals. Recently, the idea of vitamin E recycling from its oxidized form has received substantial attention. Vitamin E is considered to be recycled from its oxidized radical form by means of ascorbate, glutathione, cysteine, ubiquinols, lipoic acid, estrogens, carotenoids, and some other reductants. Therefore, the antioxidant protection in the cell depends not only on the vitamin E concentration and location but also relies on effective recycling. Indeed, if the recycling is effective then even low vitamin E concentrations are able to maintain high antioxidant protection in physiological conditions. One such example could be chicken embryonic brain (127). In this tissue, products of lipid peroxidation are almost undetectable in physiological conditions despite the very low vitamin E concentration. However, whether tocopherol recycling takes place in semen is not clear and this topic awaits investigation.

Vitamin E was first detected in turkey semen in 1981, and it has been shown that most α-tocopherol is located in the cells and only a very low concentration of this vitamin was detected in the seminal plasma (128). A similar distribution of vitamin E was shown for chicken semen with about 88% of the semen's vitamin E located in the spermatozoa (40). In general, depending on dietary supplementation, vitamin E concentration in chicken semen varied from 0.46 μg/mL (without vitamin E supplementation) up to 1.04–1.20 μg/mL (vitamin E dietary supplementation at level of 200 mg/kg) (45,116). It seems likely that vitamin E concentration in semen as well as in other tissues depends on the fatty acid profile of the diet. For example, when maize oil (5%) was included in the cockerel diet supplemented with 40 mg/kg vitamin E, the concentration of α-tocopherol in the semen was 1.1 μg/mL (129). However, tuna oil dietary supplementation decreased vitamin E concentration in the semen by more than

30% (129). α-Tocopherol is considered to be the main vitamin E form in spermatozoa, since the proportion of γ-tocopherol found in the spermatozoa was only 5–7% of total vitamin E (45). It is interesting that there are species-specific differences in vitamin E concentration in avian semen. For example, in duck spermatozoa vitamin E concentration was almost 3 times lower compared to chickens (38). In duck semen, most vitamin E was also located in spermatozoa. It is not clear at present if the vitamin E concentration in semen is associated with the fatty acid profile of the spermatozoa. When vitamin E is incorporated into sperm membranes, a high number of double bonds in the lipid fraction would increase the membrane's capacity to accommodate vitamin E.

The associations between sperm vitamin E content and spermatozoan physiological and biochemical characteristics have so far received only limited attention. An increased vitamin E concentration in turkey spermatozoa was associated with improved motility, viability, and fertilizing ability after artificial insemination (33,130). An increased vitamin E concentration in chicken semen was associated with improved spermatozoa progressive motility (131). In contrast, increased vitamin E supplementation of the pheasant diet was associated with decreased fertility, although the fertilizing persistence was longer with vitamin E supplementation (132).

Vitamin E concentration in spermatozoa is a reflection of its dietary supplementation. For example, inclusion of increased vitamin E doses in the turkey diet was shown to increase α-tocopherol concentration in spermatozoa (33,133). It has been suggested that vitamin E could be considered as a natural stabilizer of spermatozoa membranes. To test this hypothesis two main approaches were used. First, the release of glutamic-oxalacetic transaminase (GOT) from spermatozoa was used as a marker of sperm membrane integrity. We showed that during sperm storage *in vitro* the GOT activity increased in the medium and decreased in the spermatozoa (134). Similar changes in GOT activity were also observed in chicken spermatozoa during a freeze-thaw procedure (135), and a highly significant ($r = 0.99$) correlation was found between GOT activity in seminal plasma and the percentage of dead spermatozoa (136). The second approach was based on the inclusion of low concentrations of detergent (Triton X-100) in the sperm storage medium to induce sperm membrane damage. This treatment significantly increased the release of GOT from spermatozoa (137).

Therefore, the results of our experiments have shown the following:

- Turkey spermatozoa enriched with vitamin E released less GOT into the medium during sperm storage compared to the control group (138).
- During sperm cryopreservation a protective effect of increased vitamin E concentration in the spermatozoa was observed (139).
- An increased level of vitamin E in the turkey spermatozoa was associated with a reduction in susceptibility to Fe^{2+}-induced lipid peroxidation (34). This effect of vitamin E was confirmed with chicken semen (45).
- For inhibition of lipid peroxidation in the turkey spermatozoa, the efficiency of vitamin E, incorporated into the sperm membranes as a result

of its increased level in the diet, was almost 500 times higher than α-tocopherol inclusion in the diluent (128). Similar results were seen with chicken semen (129).

- Prevention of lipid peroxidation could be an important mechanism of the stabilizing effect of vitamin E on sperm membranes.

Thus it has been proved that vitamin E plays a role as a biological stabilizer of the sperm plasma membrane (1,33,50,140,141). Increasing the α-tocopherol content of the membrane was shown to make spermatozoa more resistant to the "unnatural" stresses incurred during artificial insemination, short-term storage, and cryopreservation (133,142). Increased dietary vitamin E supplementation of the goose (from 5 to 40 mg/kg diet) was associated with increased fertilizing ability of spermatozoa when used for artificial insemination (143).

It has been shown that inclusion of vitamin E in the chicken diet at the level of 200 mg/kg was associated with an almost twofold increase of α-tocopherol concentrations in whole semen, spermatozoa, and seminal plasma compared with that at 20 mg/kg supplementation (Fig. 15.15). However, vitamin E incorporation into spermatozoa membranes has a limit, since further increase in dietary vitamin E, from 200 to 1000 mg/kg, did not change α-tocopherol concentration in the semen (Fig. 15.16). As mentioned above, this could be a reflection of the limiting ability of the sperm membranes to incorporate vitamin E.

The dietary-induced increase in the α-tocopherol content of semen did result in a significant reduction in the susceptibility of the semen to lipid peroxidation. In fact, the susceptibility of semen to peroxidation displayed a very high negative correlation ($r = -0.998$) with the α-tocopherol content of the semen. The susceptibility of testes homogenates to *in vitro* peroxidation was also reduced by the dietary supplementation

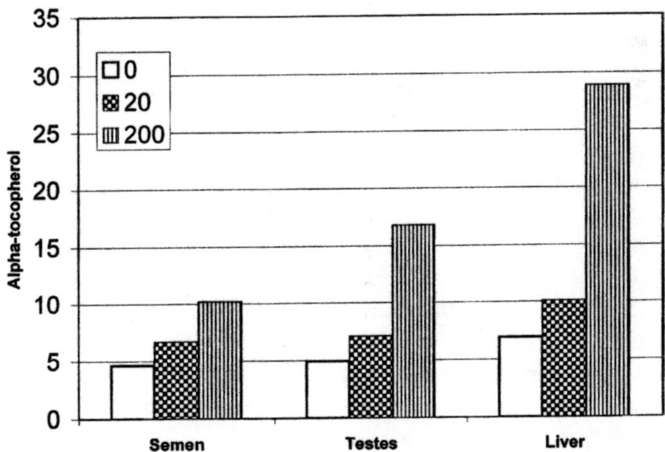

Fig. 15.15. Effect of dietary vitamin E on alpha-tocopherol concentration in semen (μg/mL), testes and liver (μg/g) of cockerels. Adapted from Surai *et al.*, 1997.

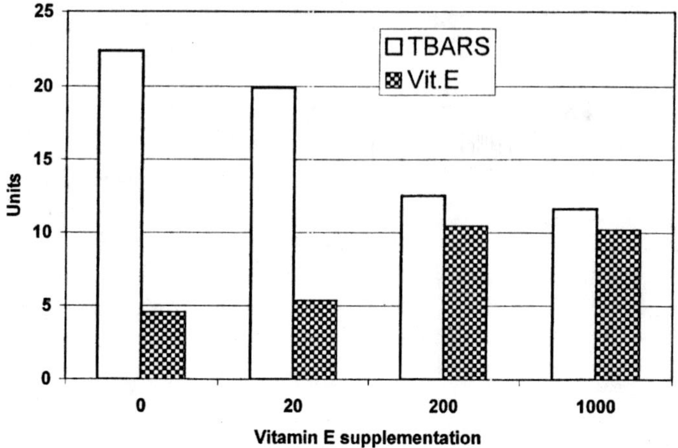

Fig. 15.16. Effect of dietary vitamin E on lipid peroxidation in chicken semen. Adapted from Surai *et al.,* 1997.

with α-tocopherol (116). During storage, the susceptibility of spermatozoa to lipid peroxidation significantly increased, probably due to initiation of spontaneous lipid peroxidation (35). In such conditions, the protective effect of vitamin E enrichment of the spermatozoa has been clearly demonstrated (116). Thus even the relatively limited enhancement of semen α-tocopherol content that was achieved by dietary means was found to produce significant benefits by reducing the susceptibility of the semen to lipid peroxidation.

Positive effects of increased vitamin E supplementation were recorded in mammalian species as well, including rams (144,145), boars (14), rats (146,147), bulls (148), and men (149–151).

Ascorbic Acid

Vitamin C (ascorbic acid, AA) acts as a potent water-soluble antioxidant in biological fluids by scavenging biologically relevant ROS and reactive nitrogen species (RNS; 152). In fact, AA is considered to be the most effective aqueous-phase antioxidant in human blood plasma (153). In cytosol, AA also acts as a primary antioxidant scavenging ROS and RNS (154). An indirect antioxidant role of AA is associated with the recycling of other antioxidants. In addition to vitamin E recycling, AA can regenerate such antioxidants as GSH, urate, and β-carotene from their respective radical species (152). A particularly important function of AA and GSH is their ability to neutralize hydroxyl radicals, since there are no enzymatic systems to scavenge it (155).

AA concentration in chicken semen was shown to be 210.2 ± 16.4 μM (40). On a molar basis, this concentration was more than 2.5 times higher than glutathione and more than 100-fold higher than α-tocopherol. AA was almost equally distributed

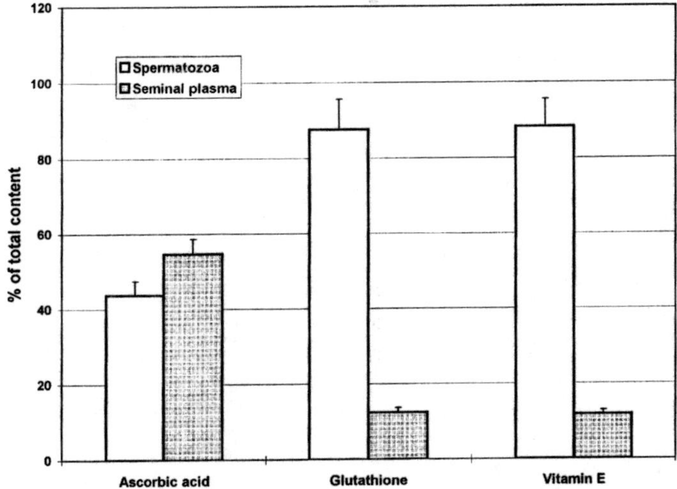

Fig. 15.17. Antioxidant distribution in chicken semen. Adapted from Surai *et al.,* 1998.

between the spermatozoa and seminal plasma (Fig. 15.17). These data suggest that AA plays an important role as a water-soluble antioxidant in avian seminal plasma.

Effects of AA on the animal reproductive system have recently been reviewed by Luck *et al.* (156) and main points of that review are as follows:

- There are direct effects of ascorbate deficiency on male fertility in laboratory and farm species, including bulls, guinea pigs, and rabbits.
- Ascorbate affected both the integrity of the tubular structure and the functionality of sperm.
- Ascorbate deficiency is associated with low sperm count, increased numbers of abnormal spermatozoa, reduced motility, and agglutination.

In human seminal plasma, ascorbate contributes to antioxidant protection almost twice as much as urate, and thiol levels are about one third of ascorbate (157). It is interesting that AA is accumulated in human and rat seminal plasma 5–10-fold compared with the serum level (158,159). In the seminal plasma of infertile men the AA concentration was found to vary widely, in a range of 93–954 µmol/L (160). Ascorbate levels in seminal plasma of asthenozoospermic individuals exhibiting ROS activity are significantly reduced (157). AA concentration in human seminal plasma was shown to be 612 µM, was negatively correlated with ROS production, and was positively correlated with the percentage of spermatozoa with normal morphology (161). AA also protects against endogenous oxidative DNA damage in human sperm (162). In bulls, the sperm motility correlated with the ascorbate concentration (163).

In cockerels housed under hot and humid tropical conditions, semen volume, motile sperm per ejaculate, and sperm number per ejaculate were significantly increased by AA supplementation at a level of 500 mg/kg (164).

Glutathione

Glutathione (GSH) is the most abundant nonprotein thiol in avian and mammalian cells and is considered to be an active antioxidant in biological systems, providing cells with their reducing milieu (165). Cellular GSH plays a key role in many biological processes (166):

- the synthesis of DNA and proteins
- cell growth and proliferation
- regulation of programmed cell death
- immune regulation
- the transport of amino acids
- xenobiotic metabolism
- redox-sensitive signal transduction

Furthermore, GSH thiolic group can react directly with (28, 167) the following:

- H_2O_2
- superoxide anion
- hydroxyl radicals
- alkoxyl radicals
- hydroperoxides

Therefore, a crucial role for GSH is as free radical scavenger, particularly effective against the hydroxyl radical (168). Usually, a low GSH concentration in tissues is associated with increased lipid peroxidation (169). Furthermore, in stress conditions, GSH prevents the loss of protein thiols and vitamin E (170) and plays an important role as a key modulator of cell signaling (171). Birds are able to synthesize glutathione.

GSH concentration in chicken semen has been shown to be 83.7 ± 9.12 μM (40), equivalent to about 2.34 nmol/10^8 spermatozoa. Similarly, in the rat, GSH concentration was reported to be 3.5 nmol/10^8 spermatozoa (172). These data are consistent with those for spermatozoa of goat, rabbit, ram, dog, boar, and human (110). Recently, in human spermatozoa, GSH concentrations were reported to be 3.49 nmol/10^8 spermatozoa (173). GSH concentration in bull spermatozoa was also similar: 3.1 nmol/108 spermatozoa (115). GSH was shown to play an important role in maintaining sperm motility and metabolism in experimental conditions (174). Adding GSH to the incubation medium had a preserving effect on equine sperm motility at the end of a 30-min incubation in the presence of a free radical-generating system (23). In an *in vitro* experiment, inclusion of GSH into the incubation medium caused a 57% decrease in lipid peroxidation in boar spermatozoa (14). GSH can also protect isolated rat spermatids from damage due to exposure to peroxidizing agents (175) and have a protective effect on rates of acrosome reaction and loss of motility over 24 h in human spermatozoa prepared by centrifugation (176). GSH was also effective in preventing the impairment of sperm motility observed in the presence of activated polymorphonuclea leukocytes (177). In contrast, addition of GSH to human sperm preparation medium had no significant effect on sperm progressive motility or baseline DNA integrity (178).

Metabolic Aspects of Antioxidant Defense

It is widely accepted that superoxide radical formation is usually the result of electron leakage from the mitochondrial electron transport chain due to uncoupled oxidative phosphorylation (55). There are also observations that leukocyte contamination of the semen is responsible for increased generation of free radicals. However, if semen contamination is minimal, metabolic differences between the species studied, especially in terms of mitochondrial oxidative phosphorylation activity (55), would determine differences in the rate of formation of superoxide radicals. Probably stress factors, responsible for uncoupling of oxidation and phosphorylation in mitochondria, could stimulate electron leakage and superoxide radical formation.

There is a relationship between species differences in free radical production in spermatozoa and their rate of oxidative metabolism. The rate of oxidative metabolism in chicken spermatozoa is very similar to that in turkey spermatozoa, although turkey spermatozoa are very dependent on oxidative metabolism to maintain optimal ATP levels (179). In this respect, the lower unsaturation of turkey sperm lipid could be an advantage in terms of prevention of lipid peroxidation. However, activities of antioxidant enzymes in turkey spermatozoa are also lower compared to chickens (61). Unfortunately, there are no data available on metabolic comparisons between other avian species.

Whereas the ratio of polyunsaturated fatty acids to antioxidants in the spermatozoa is a very important determinant of their survival *in vitro*, this could also be a factor in survival of spermatozoa in the oviduct. A unique feature of avian reproduction is spermatozoa storage within oviducal sperm storage tubules (SST; 180) for several weeks. Therefore, maintenance of membrane stability and prevention of lipid peroxidation during this high temperature (41°C) sperm storage could be an important strategy for avian species. In this respect the level of lipid unsaturation and fatty acid profile of the avian spermatozoa are different from those of mammals. Furthermore, turkey spermatozoa characterized by the lowest degree of lipid unsaturation have the longest fertile period in the SST. Therefore, an antioxidant role for the SST has been proposed (61).

There are also other unanswered questions in relation to species-specific features of fatty acid profile and antioxidant protection of avian spermatozoa. For example, duck spermatozoa containing the highest proportions of PUFA and characterized by the highest peroxidability index of their lipids, had a much lower vitamin E concentration compared to chickens (38). However the duck spermatozoa's susceptibility to peroxidation was similar to that of chicken spermatozoa (38), emphasizing an important role for the high activities of antioxidant enzymes in duck spermatozoa (61).

Therefore, species-specific features in carbohydrate metabolism and rate of mitochondrial oxidative phosphorylation are additional factors affecting free radical production in the semen. For example, our previous work (130) showed that chicken spermatozoa rely more on oxidative phosphorylation for energy production than waterfowl species. In fact, the lactate dehydrogenase (LDH) profile in spermatozoa of the chicken is opposite to that in duck or goose semen (Fig. 15.18 and 15.19). The

                                   P.F. Surai et al.

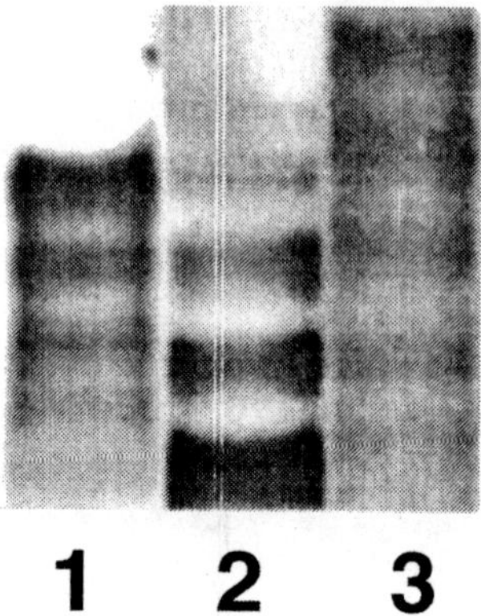

Fig. 15.18. Lactate dehydrogenase (LDH) profile in duck (1), chicken (2), and goose (3) spermatozoa. Adapted from Surai, 1991.

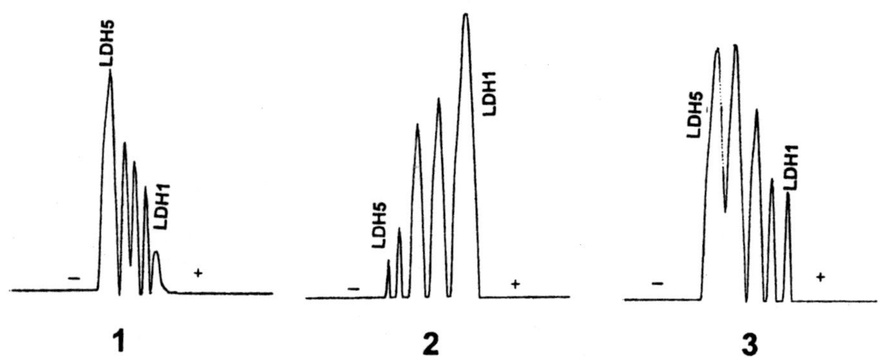

Fig. 15.19. Distribution of lactate dehydrogenase (LDH) isoenzymes in duck (1), chicken (2), and goose (3) spermatozoa. Adapted from Surai, 1991.

most active LDH isozymes in the chicken semen are LDH-1 and LDH-2, and the H-subunit of LDH comprises 81% of the total (Table 15.3), showing a clear preference for the Krebs Cycle and oxidative phosphorylation as a main route of energy production. It has been shown (181) that when cockerels with low cytochrome oxidase activity were removed from the flock, fertility was increased from 87.3 to 89.9%, confirming the importance of oxidative metabolism in maintenance of chicken semen quality.

In contrast, in duck and goose semen the main forms of LDH are LDH-5 and LDH-4, showing a preference for glycolytic energy production. This means that energy production in duck and goose semen is less dependent on oxidative phosphorylation, and so less free radicals may be generated in the mitochondria. It is interesting to

TABLE 15.3
Lactate Dehydrogenase (LDH) Isoenzyme Distribution on Avian Semen[a]

Species	LDH1, %	LDH2, %	LDH3, %	LDH4, %	LDH5, %	H-subunits, %
Chicken	53.14	23.52	17.77	4.53	1.05	80.8
Goose	3.92	7.34	19.74	30.67	38.34	26.95
Duck	4.89	8.82	13.46	18.65	54.13	22.93

[a]Adapted from (130) and (181)

note that the LDH profile in testes of cockerels and duck and goose (Fig. 15.20) is very similar to that observed in spermatozoa, with LDH1 and LDH2 being the major isoenzymes in cockerel's testes. However, LDH profile in breast muscle (mainly LDH5) or heart (mainly LDH1) of goose and chicken are very similar. Therefore the specific differences in LDH profile in testes and spermatozoa between chicken and waterfowl males need further investigation.

Since copulation in waterfowl could be conducted on the water surface, it could well be that protective mechanisms exist to prevent any water appearance in the reproductive tract and, therefore, the oxygen supply there could be lower in comparison to chicken. Furthermore, in the chicken and turkey, natural mating consists of semen deposition in the lower (abovarian) vagina due to the presence of a vestigial penis, which, in these species, prevents any vaginal penetration of the female at copulation

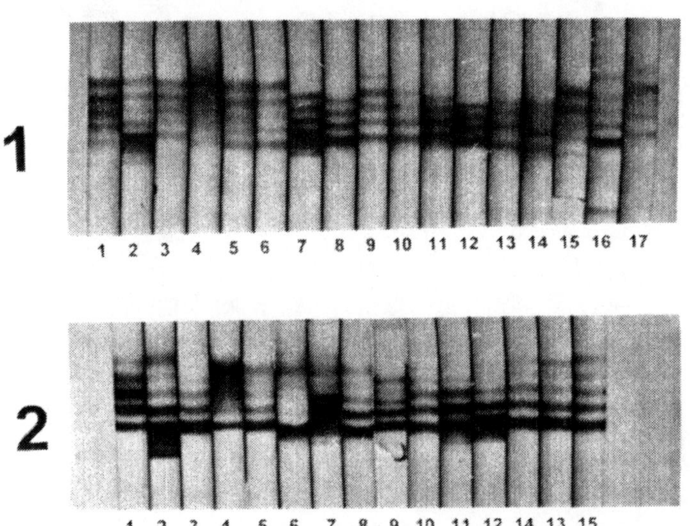

Fig. 15.20. Lactate dehydrogenase (LDH) profile (gel-electrophoresis) in various tissues of goose (1) and chicken (2) males. 1, liver; 2, heart; 3, testes; 4, breast muscle; 5, thigh muscle; 6, gizzard; 7, kidney; 8, lung; 9, spleen; 10, skin; 11, brain; 12, pancreas; 13, thyroid; 14, adrenals; 15, thymus; 16, blood hemolysate; 17, blood plasma.

(182). Spermatozoa in these species must therefore migrate through most of the luminal portion of the vagina before reaching the storage sites, a migration performed in the somewhat oxygenated environment of the vaginal mucosa. By contrast, in ducks the existence in the female of a nontubular vagina (presence of a double "S-like" portion) located approximately at mid-vagina, and in the male of a well-developed penis, suggest that ejaculated semen is deposited in the upper vagina (182), which, due to its anatomical specificities, is likely to be isolated from a direct contact with ambient air. Therefore, it has been suggested (38) that the antioxidant defense of duck spermatozoa is not, in the natural situation, as crucial as it is in the chicken and the turkey. However, increased activity of antioxidant enzymes in duck spermatozoa (38) could be another important factor on the antioxidant/pro-oxidant balances in semen.

In general there are three major features of avian semen that put it under pressure of oxidative stress:

- Limitations in antioxidant recycling. Because of very low activity or even absence of the hexose monophosphate shunt in avian spermatozoa (183), the production of NADPH, the coenzyme for glutathione reductase, is limited. This means that recycling in the chain vitamin E-vitamin C-GSH in the spermatozoa is limited as well. In such a situation, the primary defense preventing conversion of superoxide radical to more powerful radicals (for example, OH*) would be of great importance for spermatozoa survival.
- Sperm storage within oviductal sperm storage tubules (SST) at a body temperature of 41°C can be considered a risk factor for lipid peroxidation, and an antioxidant role of the SST has been proposed
- It is suggested that spermatozoa cannot carry out extensive biosynthetic repair of damage (51). Therefore, any damaging alteration to the membrane irreversibly alters sperm functions and the antioxidant protection is thus absolutely vital for maintaining the fertilizing ability of spermatozoa.

Conclusions

- Avian spermatozoa are rich in PUFA, which makes them vulnerable to lipid peroxidation, especially during *in vitro* manipulation. In particular, docosatetraenoic (22:4n-6) and arachidonic (20:4n-6) fatty acids are the most vulnerable to lipid peroxidation.
- Lipid peroxidation in semen is considered an important mechanism of impaired sperm quality and reduced fertilizing ability.
- Excessive free radical generation by spermatozoa could be induced by various factors, including the redox cycling of xenobiotics, excessive NADPH oxidase activity, the increased availability of transition metals, and impaired antioxidant protection due to dietary deficiencies, age, or genetic factors (27).

- Antioxidant systems of semen play an important role protecting spermatozoa membranes against the damaging effects of free radicals and toxic products of their metabolism.
- There are species-specific, age-related differences in the expression of antioxidant systems in avian semen.
- Sperm enrichment by DHA is shown to decrease antioxidant protection of the spermatozoa and cause lipid peroxidation. Dietary supplementation of increased vitamin E levels is found to be effective to prevent lipid peroxidation in such cases.
- Vitamin E is considered to be an effective membrane-stabilizing antioxidant of avian semen.
- An antioxidant function of SST has been suggested, and species-specific differences in strategy of antioxidant defense have been described.
- Enhancement of the antioxidant capacity of semen could present a major opportunity for improving male fertility.
- The antioxidant/pro-oxidant balance in avian semen is an important element in maintaining membrane integrity and functions, including sperm viability and fertilizing capacity. The antioxidant system can be suggested to be a crucial element of such a regulation.
- A regulating role of ROS in sperm capacitation and the acrosome reaction in mammalian species has been demonstrated; but their role for avian species reproduction remains to be elucidated. Clearly there is a need for further research to understand molecular mechanisms of lipid peroxidation and antioxidant protection in avian semen.

Acknowledgments

We are grateful to the Scottish Executive Environment and Rural Affairs Department for financial support and to the WPSA for the Research Award to Peter F. Surai.

References

1. Surai, P.F. (2002) *Natural Antioxidants in Avian Nutrition and Reproduction*, Nottingham University Press, Nottingham.
2. Surai, P.F., Fujihara, N., Speake, B.K., Brillard, J-P., Wishart, G.J., and Sparks, N.H.C. (2001) Polyunsaturated Fatty Acids, Lipid Peroxidation and Antioxidant Protection in Avian Semen—Review, *Asian-Australian J. Anim. Sci. 17*, 1024–1050.
3. Hogg, N. (1998) Free Radicals in Disease, *Seminars Reprod. Endocrin. 16*, 241–248.
4. McLeod, J. (1943) The Role of Oxygen in the Metabolism and Motility of Human Spermatozoa, *Am. J. Physiol. 138*, 512–518.
5. Wales, R.G., White, I.G., and Lammond, D.R. (1959) The Spermicidal Activity of Hydrogen Peroxide *in Vitro* and *in Vivo*, *J. Endocrin. 18*, 236–244.
6. Jones, R., and Mann, T. (1973) Lipid Peroxidation in Spermatozoa, *Proc. Roy. Soc., Lond. B. 184*, 103–107.
7. Jones, R., and Mann. T. (1976) Lipid Peroxides in Spermatozoa; Formation, Role of Plasmalogen, and Physiological Significance, *Proc. Roy. Soc, Lond. 193*, 317–333.

8. Jones, R., and Mann, T. (1977) Damage to Ram Spermatozoa by Peroxidation of Endogenous Phospholipids, *J. Reprod. Fert. 50*, 261–268.

9. Jones, R., and Mann, T. (1977a) Toxicity of Exogenous Fatty Acid Peroxides Towards Spermatozoa, *J. Reprod. Fert. 50*, 255–260.

10. Jones, R., Mann, T., and Sherins, R.J. (1978) Adverse Effects of Peroxidized Lipid on Human Spermatozoa, *Proc. Roy. Soc., Lond. 201*, 413–417.

11. Jones, R., Mann, T., and Sherins, R. (1979) Peroxidative Breakdown of Phospholipids in Human Spermatozoa, Spermicidal Properties of Fatty Acid Peroxides, and Protective Action of Seminal Plasma, *Fertil. Steril. 31*, 531–537.

12. Mrotek, J.J., Hoekstra, W.G., and First, N.L. (1966). Effect of Boar Semen Senility on Peroxidation of Semen Lipids, *J. Anim. Sci. 25*, 688–692.

13. Smutna, M., and Synek, O. (1979) Lipid Peroxidation in Semen of the Boar, *Acta Veterinar. Brno. 48*, 35–43.

14. Brzezinska-Slebodzinska, E., Slebodinski, A.B., Pietras, B., and Wieczorek, G. (1995) Antioxidant Effect of Vitamin E and Glutathione on Lipid Peroxidation in Boar Semen Plasma, *Biol. Trace Elem. Res. 47*, 69–74.

15. Cerolini, S., Maldjian, A., Surai, P.F., and Noble, R.C. (2000) Viability, Susceptibility to Peroxidation and Fatty Acid Composition of Boar Semen During Liquid Storage, *Anim. Reprod. Sci. 58*, 99–111.

16. Dawra, R.K., Sharma, O.P., and Makkar, H.P. (1983) Lipid Peroxidation in Bovine Semen, *Int. J. Fert. 28*, 231–234.

17. Beconi, M.T., Affranchino, M.A., Schang, L.M., and Beorlegui, N.B. (1991) Influence of Antioxidants on SOD Activity in Bovine Sperm, *Biochem. Int. 23*, 545–553.

18. Slaweta, R., T. Laskowska, T., and E. Szymanska, E (1988) Lipid Peroxides, Spermatozoa Quality and Activity of Glutathione Peroxidase in Bull Semen, *Acta Physiol. Pol. 39*, 207–214.

19. Oflaherty, C., Beconi, M., and Beorlegui, N. (1997) Effect of Natural Antioxidants, Superoxide Dismutase and Hydrogen Peroxide on Capacitation of Frozen-Thawed Bull Spermatozoa, *Androl. 29*, 269–275.

20. Beorlegui, N., Cetica, P., Trinchero, G., Cordoba, M., and Beconi, M. (1997) Comparative Study of Functional and Biochemical Parameters in Frozen Bovine Sperm, *Androl. 29*, 37–42.

21. Singh, P., Chand, D., and Georgie, G.C. (1989) Lipid Peroxidation in Buffalo (Bubalus bubalis L.) Spermatozoa: Effect of Added Vitamin C and Glucose, *Indian J. Exp. Biol. 27*, 1001–1002.

22. Castellini, C., Lattaioli, P., Bernardini, M., and Dal Bosco, A. (2000) Effect of Dietary Alpha-tocopheryl Acetate and Ascorbic Acid on Rabbit Semen Stored at 5 Degrees C, *Theriogenology 54*, 523–533.

23. Baumber, J., Ball, B.A., Gravance, C.G., Medina, V., and Davies-Morel, M.C.G. (2000) The Effect of Reactive Oxygen Species on Equine Sperm Motility, Viability, Acrosomal Integrity, Mitochondrial Membrane Potential, and Membrane Lipid Peroxidation, *J. Androl. 21*, 895–902.

24. Ball, B.A., and Vo, A. (2002) Detection of Lipid Peroxidation in Equine Spermatozoa Based Upon the Lipophilic Fluorescent Dye C11-BODIPY581/591, *J. Androl. 23*, 259–269.

25. Aitken, R.J. (1994) A Free Radical Theory of Male Infertility, *Reprod. Fert. Develop. 6*, 19–24.

26. Aitken, R.J. (1995) Free Radicals, Lipid Peroxidation, and Sperm Function, *Reprod. Fert. Develop. 7,* 659–668.

27. Aitken, R.J. (1999) The Human Spermatozoa—A Cell in Crisis? *J. Reprod. Fert. 115,* 1–7.

28. Lenzi, A., Gandini, L., Maresca, V., Rago, R., Sgro, P., Dondero, F., and Picardo, M. (2000) Fatty Acid Composition of Spermatozoa and Immature Germ Cells, *Molecul. Human Reprod. 6,* 226–231.

29. Lenzi, A., Gandini, L., Picardo, M., Tramer, F., Sandri, G., and Panfili, E. (2000) Lipoperoxidation Damage of Spermatozoa Polyunsaturated Fatty Acids (PUFA): Scavenger Mechanisms and Possible Scavenger Therapies, *Front. Bioscience 5,* 1–15.

30. Fujihara, N., and Howarth, B. (1978) Lipid Peroxidation in Fowl Spermatozoa, *Poult. Sci. 57:* 1766–1768.

31. Wishart, G.J. (1984) Effects of Lipid Peroxide Formation in Fowl Semen on Sperm Motility, ATP Content and Fertilising Ability, *J. Reprod. Fert. 71,* 113–118.

32. Fujihara, N., and Koga, O. (1992) Functional Differences in Sperm Membrane Among Individual Male Chickens, *Proc. 12th Intern. Congr. Anim. Reprod., The Netherlands,* Hague. Vol. 1, pp. 452–454.

33. Surai, P.F. (1983) Biochemical and Functional Changes in Turkey Tissues and Sperm as a Function of the Levels of Vitamins E and A in Feed, *Can. Sci. (PhD) Thesis.* Ukrainian Poultry Research Institute, Borky, Ukraine.

34. Surai, P.F. (1984) Lipid Peroxidation in Turkey Semen, *Ptitsevodstvo* (Kiev) *37,* 58–59.

35. Cecil, H.C., and Bakst, M.R. (1993) *In Vitro* Lipid Peroxidation of Turkey Spermatozoa, *Poult. Sci. 72,* 1370–1378.

36. Donoghue, A.M., and Donoghue, D.J. (1997) Effects of Water- and Lipid-Soluble Antioxidants on Turkey Sperm Viability, Membrane Integrity, and Motility During Liquid Storage, *Poult. Sci. 76,* 1440–1445.

37. Kelso, K.A., Cerolini, S., Noble, R.C., Sparks, N.H.C., and Speake, B.K. (1996) Lipid and Antioxidant Changes in Semen of Broiler Fowl From 25 to 60 Weeks of Age, *J. Reprod. Fert. 106,* 201–206.

38. Surai, P.F., Brillard, J-P., Speake, B.K., Blesbois, E., Seigneurin, F., and Sparks, N.H.C. (2000) Phospholipid Fatty Acid Composition, Vitamin E Content, and Susceptibility to Lipid Peroxidation of Duck Spermatozoa, *Theriogenology 53,* 1025–1039.

39. Aitken, R.J., Harkiss, D., and Buckingham, D. (1993) Relationship Between Iron-Catalyzed Lipid Peroxidation Potential and Human Sperm Function, *J. Reprod. Fert. 98,* 257–265.

40. Surai, P.F., Cerolini, S., Wishart, G.J., Speake, B.K., Noble, R.C., and Sparks, N.H.C. (1998b) Lipid and Antioxidant Composition of Chicken Semen and its Susceptibility to Peroxidation, *Poult. Avian Biol. Rev. 9,* 11–23.

41. Blesbois, E., Grasseau, I., and Hermier, D. (1999) Changes in Lipid Content of Fowl Spermatozoa after Liquid Storage at 2 to 5 Degrees C, *Theriogenology 52,* 325–334.

42. Surai, P.F., Cerolini, S., Maljian, A., Noble, R..C., and Speake, B.K. (1998) Effect of Lipid Peroxidation on the Phospholipid and Fatty Acid Composition of Turkey Spermatozoa: a Protective Effect of Vitamin E, *Proc. 50th Internat. Congress on Anim. Reprod.,* Milano, p. 603.

43. Maldjian, A., Cerolini, S., Surai, P.F., and Speake, B.K. (1998) The Effect of Vitamin E, Green Tea Extracts and Catechin on the *in Vitro* Storage of Turkey Spermatozoa at Room Temperature, *Poult. Avian Biol. Rev. 9,* 143–151.

44. Douard, V., Hermier, D., and Blesbois, E. (2000) Changes in Turkey Semen Lipids during Liquid *in Vitro* Storage, *Biol. Reprod. 63*, 1450–1456.

45. Surai, P.F., Kutz, E., Wishart, G.J., Noble, R.C., and. Speake, B.K. (1997) The Relationship between the Dietary Provision of α-Tocopherol and the Concentration of this Vitamin in the Semen of Chicken: Effects on Lipid Composition and Susceptibility to Peroxidation, *J. Reprod. Fert. 110*, 47–51.

46. Kelso, K.A., Cerolini, S., Speake, B.K., Cavalchini, L.G., and Noble, R.C. (1997) Effects of Dietary Supplementation with α-Linolenic Acid on the Phospholipid Fatty Acid Composition and Quality of Spermatozoa in Cockerel from 24 To 72 Weeks of Age, *J. Reprod. Fert. 110*, 53–59.

47. Cerolini, S., Kelso, K.A., Noble, R.C., Speake, B.K., Pizzi, F., and Cavalchini, L.G. (1997) Relationship between Spermatozoan Lipid Composition and Fertility during Aging of Chickens, *Biol. Reprod. 57*, 976–980.

48. Sevanian, A., and Hochstein, P. (1985) Mechanisms and Consequences of Lipid Peroxidation in Biological Systems, *Annual Rev. Nutr. 5*, 365–390.

49. Huang, Y.L., Tseng, W.C., Cheng, S.Y., and Lin, T.H. (2000) Trace Elements and Lipid Peroxidation in Human Seminal Plasma, *Biol. Trace Elem. Res. 76*, 207–215.

50. Surai, P.F. (1999) Vitamin E in Avian Reproduction, *Poult. Avian Biol. Rev. 10*, 1–60.

51. Hammerstedt, R.H. (1993) Maintenance of Bioenergetic Balance in Sperm and Prevention of Lipid Peroxidation: a Review of the Effect on Design of Storage Preservation Systems, *Reprod. Fert. Develop. 5*, 675–690.

52. Halliwell, B. (1994) Free Radicals and Antioxidants: A Personal View, *Nutr. Rev. 52*, 253–265.

53. Michalski, W. (1992) Resolution of Three Forms of Superoxide Dismutase by Immobilized Metal Affinity Chromatography, *J. Chromatogr., Biomed. Appl. 576*, 340–345.

54. Mates, J.M., and Sanchez-Jimenez, F. (1999) Antioxidant Enzymes and their Implications in Pathophysiologic Processes. *Front. Biosci. 4*, D339–D345 .

55. Halliwell, B., and Gutteridge, J.M.C. (1999) *Free Radicals in Biology and Medicine*, Third Edition, Oxford University Press, Oxford.

56. Fridovich, I. (1995) Superoxide Radical and Superoxide Dismutases, *Annual Rev. Biochem. 64*, 97–112.

57. Ozturk-Urek, R., and Tarhan, L. (2001) Purification and Characterization of Superoxide Dismutase from Chicken Liver, *Comp. Biochem. Physiol. 128B*, 205–212.

58. Mannella, M.R.T., and Jones, R. (1980) Properties of Spermatozoal Superoxide Dismutase and Lack of Involvement of Superoxides in Metal-Ion-Catalyzed Lipid Peroxidation Reactions in Semen, *Biochem. J. 191*, 289–297.

59. Froman, D.P., and Thurston, R.J. (1981) Chicken and Turkey Spermatozoal Superoxide Dismutase: A Comparative Study. *Biol. Reprod. 24*, 193–200.

60. Peeker, R., Abramsson, L., and Marklund, S.L. (1997) Superoxide Dismutase Isoenzymes in Human Seminal Plasma and Spermatozoa, *Mol. Human Reprod. 3*, 1061–10666.

61. Surai, P.F., Blesbois, E., Grasseau, I., Ghalah, T., Brillard, J-P.,Wishart, G., Cerolini, S., and Sparks, N.H.C. (1998) Fatty Acid Composition, Glutathione Peroxidase and Superoxide Dismutase Activity and Total Antioxidant Activity of Avian Semen, *Comp. Biochem. Physiol. 120B*, 527–533.

62. Behne, D., Hofer, T., von Berswordt-Wallrabe, R., and Elger, W. (1982) Selenium in the Testis of the Rat: Studies on its Regulation and its Importance for the Organism, *J. Nutr. 112*, 1682–1687.

63. Calvin, H.I., Grosshans, K., Musicant-Shikora, S.R., and Turner, S.I. (1987) A Developmental Study of Rat Sperm and Testis Selenoproteins, *J. Reprod. Fert. 81,* 1–11.

64. Wu, A.S., Oldfield, J.E., Shull, L.R., and Cheeke, P. (1979) Specific Effect of Selenium Deficiency on Rat Sperm, *Biol. Reprod. 20,* 793–798.

65. Hansen, J.C., and Deguchi, Y. (1996) Selenium and Fertility in Animals and Man—A Review, *Acta Vet. Scand. 37,* 19–30.

66. Behne, D., Duk, M., and Elger, W. (1986) Selenium Content and Glutathione Peroxidase Activity in the Testis of the Maturing Rat, *J. Nutr. 116,* 1442–1447.

67. Oldereid, N.B., Thomassen, Y., and Purvis, K. (1998) Selenium in Human Male Reproductive Organs, *Human Reprod. 13,* 2172–2176.

68. Behne, D., Weiler, H., and Kyriakopoulos, A. (1996) Effects of Selenium Deficiency on Testicular Morphology and Function in Rats, *J. Reprod. Fert. 106,* 291–297.

69. Watanabe, T., and Endo, A. (1991) Effects of Selenium Deficiency on Sperm Morphology and Spermatocyte Chromosomes in Mice, *Mutat. Res. 262,* 93–99.

70. Bleau, G., Lemarbre, J., Faucher, G., Roberts, K.D., and Chapdelaine, A. (1984). Semen Selenium and Human Fertility, *Fertil. Steril. 42,* 890–894 .

71. Saaranen, M., Suistomaa, U., and Vanha-Perttula, T. (1989) Semen Selenium Content and Sperm Mitochondrial Volume in Human and Some Animal Species, *Human Reprod. 4,* 304–308.

72. Alabi, N.S., Beilstein, M.A., and Whanger, P.D. (2000) Chemical Forms of Selenium Present in Rat and Ram Spermatozoa—*In Vivo* and *in Vitro* Studies, *Biol. Trace Elem. Res. 76,* 161–173.

73. Kohrle, J., Brigelius-Flohe, R., Bock, A., Gartner, R., Meyer, O., and Flohe, L. (2000) Selenium in Biology: Facts and Medical Perspectives, *Biol. Chem. 381,* 849–864.

74. Tujebajeva, R.M., Harney, J.W., and Berry, M.J. (2000) Selenoprotein P Expression, Purification, and Immunochemical Characterization, *J. Biol. Chem. 275,* 6288–6294.

75. Gladyshev, V.N., Jeang, K.T., Wootton, J.C., and Hatfield, D.L. (1998) A New Human Selenium-Containing Protein. Purification, Characterization, and cDNA Sequence, *J. Biol. Chem. 273,* 8910–8915.

76. Rotruck, J.T., Pope, A.L., Ganther, H.E., Swanson, A.B., Hafeman, D.G., and Hoekstra, W.G. (1973) Selenium: Biochemical Role as a Component of Glutathione Peroxidase, *Science 179,* 588–590.

77. Flohe, L., Gunzler, W.A., and Schock, H.H. (1973) Glutathione Peroxidase: A Selenoenzyme, *FEBS Lett. 32,* 132–134.

78. Ursini, F., Maiorino, M., Valente, M., Ferri, L., and Gregolin, C. (1982) Purification From Pig Liver of a Protein Which Protects Liposomes and Biomembranes from Peroxidative Degradation and Exhibits Glutathione Peroxidase Activity on Phosphatidylcholine Hydroperoxides, *Biochim. Biophys. Acta. 710,* 197–211.

79. Ursini, F., Maiorino, M., and Gregolin, C. (1985) The Selenoenzyme Phospholipid Hydroperoxide Glutathione Peroxidase, *Biochim. Biophys. Acta 839,* 62–70.

80. Maddipati, K.R., and Marnett, L.J. (1987) Characterization of the Major Hydroperoxide-Reducing Activity of Human Plasma. Purification and Properties of a Selenium-Dependent Glutathione Peroxidase, *J. Biol. Chem. 262,* 17398–403.

81. Takahashi, K., Avissar, N., Whitin, J., and Cohen, H. (1987) Purification and Characterization of Human Plasma Glutathione Peroxidase: A Selenoglyco-protein Distinct from the Known Cellular Enzyme, *Arch. Biochem. Biophys. 256,* 677–686.

82. Chu, F.F., Doroshow, J.H., and Esworthy, R.S. (1993) Expression, Characterization, and Tissue Distribution of a New Cellular Selenium-Dependent Glutathione Peroxidase, GSHPx-GI, *J. Biol. Chem. 268*, 2571–2576.

83. Wingler, K., and Brigelius-Flohe, R. (1999) Gastrointestinal Glutathione Peroxidase, Biofactors *10*, 245–249.

84. Behne, D., Rothlein, D., Pfeifer, H., and Kyriakopoulos, A. (2000) Identification and Characterization of New Mammalian Selenoproteins, *J. Trace Elem. Med. Biol. 14*, 117.

85. Pfeifer, H., Conrad, M., Roethlein, D., Kyriakopoulos, A., Brielmeier, M., Bornkamm, G.W., and Behne, D. (2001) Identification of a Specific Sperm Nuclei Selenoenzyme Necessary for Protamine Thiol Cross-Linking during Sperm Maturation, *FASEB J. 15*, 1236–1238.

86. Ursini, F., Maiorino, M., and Roveri, A. (1997) Phospholipid Hydroperoxide Glutathione Peroxidase (PHGPx): More Than an Antioxidant Enzyme? *Biomed. Environ. Sci. 10*, 327–332.

87. Brigelius-Flohe, R. (1999) Tissue-specific Functions of Individual Glutathione Peroxidases, *Free Rad. Biol. Med. 27*, 951–965.

88. Rhee, S.G. (1999) Redox Signaling: Hydrogen Peroxide as Intracellular Messenger, *Experim. Mol. Med. 31*, 53–59.

89. Jackson, M.J., McArdle, A., and McArdle, F. (1998) Antioxidant Micronutrients and Gene Expression, *Proc. Nutr. Soc. 57*, 301–305.

90. Dalton, T.P., Shertzer, H.G., and Puga, A. (1999) Regulation of Gene Expression by Reactive Oxygen, *Annu. Rev. Pharmacol.Toxicol. 39*, 67–101.

91. Ursini, F. (2000) The World of Glutathione Peroxidases, *J. Trace Elem. Med. Biol. 14*, 116.

92. Sies, H., Sharov, V.S., Klotz, L.O., and Briviba, K. (1997) Glutathione Peroxidase Protects Against Peroxynitrite-Mediated Oxidations. A New Function for Selenoproteins as Peroxynitrite Reductase, *J. Biol. Chem. 272*, 27812–27817.

93. Mork, H., Lex, B., Scheurlen, M., Dreher, I., Schutze, N., Kohrle, J., and Jakob, F. (1998) Expression Pattern of Gastrointestinal Selenoproteins—Targets for Selenium Supplementation, *Nutr. Cancer 32*, 64–70.

94. Holben, D.H., and Smith, A.M. (1999) The Diverse Role of Selenium within Selenoproteins: A Review, *J. Am. Diet. Assoc. 99*, 836–843.

95. Burk, R.F., and Hill, K.E. (1999) Orphan Selenoproteins, Bioessays *21*, 231–237.

96. Morel, Y. and Barouki, R. (1999) Repression of Gene Expression by Oxidative Stress, *Biochem. J. 342*, 481–496.

97. Holmgren, A. (1989) Thioredoxin and Glutaredoxin Systems, *J. Biol. Chem. 264*, 13963–13966.

98. Cotgreave, I.A., and Gerdes, R.G. (1998) Recent Trends in Glutathione Biochemistry-Glutathione-Protein Interactions: a Molecular Link between Oxidative Stress and Cell Proliferation? *Biochem. Biophys. Res. Commun. 242*, 1–9.

99. Holmgren, A. (2000) Redox Regulation by Thioredoxin and Thioredoxin Reductase, *Biofactors 11*, 63–64.

100. Holmgren, A. (2000) Antioxidant Function of Thioredoxin and Glutaredoxin Systems, *Antiox. Redox Signal. 2*, 811–820.

101. Mustacich, D., and Powis, G. (2000) Thioredoxin Reductase, *Biochem. J. 346*, 1–8.

102. Arner, E.S., and Holmgren, A. (2000) Physiological Functions of Thioredoxin and Thioredoxin Reductase, *Eur. J. Biochem. 267*, 6102–6109.

103. Sun, Q.A., Kirnarsky, L., Sherman, S., and Gladyshev, V.N. (2001) Selenoprotein Oxidoreductase with Specificity for Thioredoxin and Glutathione Systems, *Proc. Natl. Acad. Sci. USA 98*, 3673–3678.

104. Miranda-Vizuete, A., Damdimopoulos, A.E., and Spyrou, G. (2000) The Mitochondrial Thioredoxin System, *Antiox. Redox Signal. 2*, 801–810.

105. Miranda-Vizuete, A., Ljung, J., Damdimopoulos, A.E., Gustafsson, J.A., Oko, R., Pelto-Huikko, M., and Spyrou, G. (2001) Characterization of Sptrx, a Novel Member of the Thioredoxin Family Specifically Expressed in Human Spermatozoa, *Biol. Chem. 276*, 1567–31574.

106. Sadek, C.M., Damdimopoulos, A.E., Pelto-Huikko, M., Gustafsson, J.A., Spyrou, G., and Miranda-Vizuete, A. (2001) Sptrx-2, a Fusion Protein Composed of One Thioredoxin and Three Tandemly Repeated NDP-kinase Domains Is Expressed in Human Testis Germ Cells, *Genes to Cells: Devoted to Molecular and Cellular Mechanisms 6*, 1077–1090.

107. Jimenez, A., Oko, R., Gustafsson, J.A., Spyrou, G., Pelto-Huikko, M., and Miranda-Vizuete, A. (2002) Cloning, Expression and Characterization of Mouse Spermatid Specific Thioredoxin-1 Gene and Protein, *Mol. Hum. Reprod. 8*, 710–718.

108. Brown, K.M., and Arthur, J.R. (2001) Selenium, Selenoproteins and Human Health: A Review, *Public Health Nutr 4*, 593–599.

109. Ursini, F., Heim, S., Kiess, M., Maiorino, M., Roveri, A., Wissing, J., and Flohe, L. (1999) Dual Function of the Selenoprotein PHGPx During Sperm Maturation, *Science 285*, 1393–1396.

110. Li, K.T. (1975) The Glutathione and Thiol Content of Mammalian Spermatozoa and Seminal Plasma, *Biol. Reprod. 12*, 641–646.

111. Kantola, M., Saaranen, M., and Vanha-Perttula, T. (1988) Selenium and Glutathione Peroxidase in Seminal Plasma of Men and Bulls, *J. Reprod. Fert. 83*, 785–794.

112. Kelso, K.A., Redpath, A., Noble, R.C., and Speake, B.K. (1997b) Lipid and Antioxidant Changes in Spermatozoa and Seminal Plasma Throughout the Reproductive Period of Bulls, *J. Reprod. Fert. 109*, 1–6.

113. Brown, D.V., Senger, P.L., Stone, S.L., Froseth, J.A., and Becker, W.C. (1977) Glutathione Peroxidase in Bovine Semen, *J. Reprod. Fert. 50*, 117–118.

114. Smith, D.G., Senger, P.L., McCutchan, J.F., and Landa, C.A. (1979) Selenium and Glutathione Peroxidase Distribution in Bovine Semen and Selenium-75 Retention by the Tissues of the Reproductive Tract in the Bull, *Biol. Reprod. 20*, 377–383.

115. Slaweta, R., and Laskowska-Klita, T. (1985) Glutathione Content in the Semen of Bulls of the Lowland Black-White Breed, *Acta Physiol. Pol. 36*, 107–111.

116. Surai, P.F., Kostjuk, I.A., Wishart, G., MacPherson, A., Speake, B., Noble, R.C., Ionov, I.A., and Kutz, E. (1998c) Effect of Vitamin E and Selenium of Cockerel Diets on Glutathione Peroxidase Activity and Lipid Peroxidation Susceptibility in Sperm, Testes, and Liver, *Biol. Trace Elem. Res. 64*, 119–132.

117. Neumann, U.F., and Bronsch, K. (1988) Studies on the Optimum Supplementation of Non-Gravid and Gravid Sows, *J. Vet. Med., A 35*, 673–682.

118. Edens F.W. (2002) Practical Applications for Selenomethionine: Broiler Breeder Reproduction, in *Nutritional Biotechnology in the Feed and Food industries. Proceedings of 18th Alltech's Annual Symposium*, Lyons, T.P., and. Jacques, K.A., Nottingham University Press, Nottingham, pp. 29–42.

119. Surai P.F. (2000) Organic Selenium and the Egg: Lessons from Nature, *Feed Compound. 20*, 16–18.

120. Julien, W.E., and Murray, F.A. (1977) Effect of Selenium and Selenium with Vitamin E on *in Vitro* Motility of Bovine Spermatozoa, *Proc. American Soc. Anim. Sci., 69th Annual Meeting*, University of Wisconsin, Madison, p. 174.

121. Pratt, W. (1978) A Study of the Effect of *in Vitro* Supplementation of Sodium Selenite on the Metabolism of Bovine Sperm, M.S. Thesis, Ohio State University, Columbus, Ohio.

122. Vezina, D., Mauffette, F., Roberts, K.D., and Bleau, G. (1996) Selenium-Vitamin E Supplementation in Infertile Men—Effects on Semen Parameters and Micronutrient Levels and Distribution, *Biol. Trace Elem. Res. 53*, 65–83.

123. MacPherson, A., Scott, R., and Yates, R. (1993) The Effect of Selenium Supplementation in Subfertile Males, *Proc. 8th Internat. Symp. Trace Elements in Man and Animals*, Anke, M., Meissner, D., and Mills, C.F., Verlag Media Touristik, Germany, Jena, pp. 566–569.

124. Scott, R., MacPherson, A.,Yates, R.W.S., Hussain, B., and Dixon, J. (1998) The Effect of Oral Selenium Supplementation on Human Sperm Motility, *Brit. J. Urology 82*, 76–80.

125. Niki, E. (1996) α-Tocopherol, in *Handbook of Antioxidants*, Cadenas, E. and Packer, L., Marcel Dekker, New York, pp. 3–25.

126. Packer, L. (1992) Interactions among Antioxidants in Health and Disease: Vitamin E and Its Redox Cycle, *Proc. Soc. Exp. Biol. Med. 200*, 271–276.

127. Surai, P.F., Noble, R.C., and Speake, B.K. (1996) Tissue-Specific Differences in Antioxidant Distribution and Susceptibility to Lipid Peroxidation during Development of the Chick Embryo, *Biochim. Biophys. Acta* 1304, 1–10.

128. Surai, P.F. (1981) Fat-Soluble Vitamins in Turkey Sperm, *Proc. 2nd Conference of Young Scientists*, Zagorsk, USSR, pp. 55–56.

129. Surai, P.F., Noble, R.C., Sparks, N.H.C., and Speake, B.K. (2000a) Effect of Long-term Supplementation with Arachidonic and Docosahexaenoic Acids on Sperm Production in the Broiler Chicken, *J. Reprod. Fert. 120*, 257–264.

130. Surai, P.F. (1991) Nutritional and Biochemical Aspects of Vitamins in Poultry, Doctor Science (DSc) Thesis, Ukrainian Poultry Research Institute, Borky, Ukraine.

131. Franchini, A., Bergonzoni, M.L., Melotti, C., and Minelli, G. (2001) The Effect of Dietary Supplementation with High Doses of Vitamin E and C on the Quality Traits of Chicken Semen, *Arch. Geflugelkunde 65*, 76–81.

132. Romboli, I., Marzoni, M., Schiavone, A., and Carbas, S. (2000) Reproductive Performance of Pheasants Fed High Vitamin E Levels, *Proc. XXI World's Poultry Congr.*, Canada, Montreal, CD-ROM.

133. Surai, P., and Ionov, I. (1992) Vitamin E in Fowl Sperm, *Proc. 12th Intern. Congr. Anim. Reprod.*, The Hague, The Netherlands, vol. 1, pp. 535–537.

134. Surai, P.F., and Ionov, I.A. (1981) Changes in GOT Activity in Turkey Semen as a Result of Storage, *Nauchno-Tekhnicheskii Byulletin of the Ukrainian Research Poultry Institute 11*, 24–30.

135. Matsumoto, Y., Terada, T., and Tsutsumi, Y. (1985) Glutamic Oxalacetic Transaminase Releases from Chicken Spermatozoa during Freeze-Thaw Procedure, *Poult. Sci. 64*, 718–722.

136. Bilgili, S.F., Renden, J.A., and Sexton, K.J. (1985) Fluorometry of Poultry Semen: Its Application in the Determination of Viability, Enzyme Leakage and Fertility, *Poult. Sci. 64*, 1227–1230.

137. Surai, P.F. (1989) Detergent Treatment of Poultry Spermatozoa: Release of Some Enzymes, *Proc. 8th Internat. Symp. Current Problems of Avian Genetics*, Smolenice, Czechoslovakia, pp. 174–175.

138. Surai, P.F. (1982) The Effect of High Doses of Vitamin E in Turkey Male Diet on the GOT and LDH Activity in Stored Sperm, *Nauchno-Tekhnicheskii Byulletin of the Ukrainian Research Poultry Institute 12*, 24–29.

139. Surai, P.F. (1988) A Protective Effect of Fat-Soluble Vitamins during Turkey Sperm Cryopreservation, *Abstracts Internat. Conf. Achievements and Prospects of the Development of Cryobiology and Cryomedicine*, Ukraine, Kharkov, pp. 213–214.

140. Surai, P.F. (1983) Stabilizing Effect of Vitamins A and E on Turkey Sperm Membranes, *Ptitsevodstvo* (Kiev) *36*, 49–52.

141. Surai, P.F. (1989) Relations Between Vitamin E Concentration in Poultry Spermatozoa and Some Semen Biochemical and Physiological Characteristics, *Proc. 8th Internat. Sympos. Current Problems of Avian Genetics*, Smolenice, Czechoslovakia, pp. 171–173.

142. Surai, P.F. (1992) Vitamin E Feeding of Poultry Males, *Proc. XIX World's Poultry Congr.*, Amsterdam, The Netherlands, Vol. 1, pp. 575–577.

143. Surai, P. and Ionov, I. (1992) Vitamin E in Goose Reproduction, *Proc. 9th Internat. Sym. Waterfowl*, Pisa, Italy, pp. 83–85.

144. Gokcen, H., Camas, H., Erding, H., Asti, R., Cekgul, E., and Sener, E. (1990), Studies on the Effects of Vitamin E and Selenium Added to the Ration on Acrosome Morphology, Enzyme Activity, and Fertility of Frozen Ram Spermatozoa, *Doga Turk Veterinerlik ve Hayvancilik Dergisi 14*, 207–218.

145. Erdinc, H., Gokcen, H., Camas, H., and Cekgul, E. (1986) Sperm Production and Traits in Rams Fed Rations with Different Levels of Vitamin A and Vitamin E, *Veteriner Fakultesi Dergisi, Uludag Universitesi 5–7*, 97–101.

146. Hsu, P.C., Liu, M.Y., Hsu, C.C., Chen, L.Y., and Guo, Y.L. (1998) Effects of Vitamin E and/or C on Reactive Oxygen Species-Related Lead Toxicity in the Rat Sperm, *Toxicology 128*,169–179.

147. Lei, X.G., Ross, D.A., Parks, J.E., and Combs, G.F. Jr. (1997) Effects of Dietary Selenium and Vitamin E Concentrations on Phospholipid Hydroperoxide Glutathione Peroxidase Expression in Reproductive Tissues of Pubertal Maturing Male Rats, *Biol. Trace Element Res. 59*, 195–206.

148. Udala, J., Ramisz, A., Drewnowski, W., Lasota, B., and Radoch, W. (1995) Semen Quality of Bulls Treated with Selenium and Vitamin E, *Zeszyty Naukowe Akademii Rolniczej w Szczecinie, Zootechnika 32*, 57–63.

149. Geva, E., Bartoov, B., Zabludovsky, N., Lessing, J.B., Lerner-Geva, L., and Amit, A. (1996) The Effect of Antioxidant Treatment on Human Spermatozoa and Fertilization Rate in an *in Vitro* Fertilization Program, *Fertil. Steril. 66*, 430–434.

150. Kessopoulou, E., Powers, H.J., Sharma, K.K., Pearson, M.J., Russell, J.M., Cooke, I.D., and Barratt, C.L. (1995) A Double-blind Randomized Placebo Cross-Over Controlled Trial Using the Antioxidant Vitamin E to Treat Reactive Oxygen Species Associated Male Infertility, *Fertil. Steril. 64*, 825–831.

151. Suleiman, S.A., Ali, M.E., Zaki, Z.M., El-Malik, E.M., and Nasr, M.A. (1996) Lipid Peroxidation and Human Sperm Motility: Protective Role of Vitamin E, *J. Androl. 17*, 530–537.

152. Carr, A., and Frei, B. (1999) Does Vitamin C Act as a Pro-Oxidant under Physiological Conditions? *FASEB J. 13*, 1007–1024.

153. Frei, B., England, L., and Ames, B.N. (1989) Ascorbate Is an Outstanding Antioxidant in Human Blood Plasma, *Proc. Natl. Acad. Sci. USA 86*, 6377–6381 .

154. May, J.M. (1999) Is Ascorbic Acid an Antioxidant for the Plasma Membrane? *FASEB J. 13*, 995–1006.

155. Rice, M.E. (2000) Ascorbate Regulation and Its Neuroprotective Role in the Brain, *Trends Neurosci. 23*, 209–216.

156. Luck, M.R., Jeyaseelan, I., and Scholes, R.A. (1995) Ascorbic Acid and Fertility, *Biol. Reprod. 52*, 262–266.

157. Lewis, S.E.M., Boyle, P.M., Mckinney, K.A., Young, I.S., and Thompson, W. (1997) Comparison of Individual Antioxidants of Sperm and Seminal Plasma in Fertile and Infertile Men, *Fertil. Steril. 67*, 142–147.

158. Vaishwanar, P.S., and Deshkar, B.V. (1966) Ascorbic Acid Content and Quality of Human Semen, *Amer. J. Obstet. Gynecol. 95*, 1080–1082.

159. Pandi, J.K., Chowdhury, S.R., Dasgupta, P.R., Chowdhury, A.R., and Karr, A.B. (1966) Biochemical Composition of the Rat Testis Fluid, *Proc. Soc. Exp. Biol. Med. 121*, 899–902.

160. Gavella, M., Lipovac, V., Vucic, M., and Rocic, B. (1997) Evaluation of Ascorbate and Urate Antioxidant Capacity in Human Semen, *Androl. 29*, 29–35.

161. Thiele, J.J., Friesleben, H.J., Fuchs, J., and Ochsendorf, F.R. (1995) Ascorbic Acid and Urate in Human Seminal Plasma—Determination and Interrelationships with Chemiluminiscence in Washed Semen, *Human Reprod. 10*, 110–115.

162. Fraga, C.G., Motchnic, P.A., Shigenaga, M.K., Helbock, H.J., Jacob, R.A., and Ames, B.N. (1991) Ascorbic Acid Protects Against Endogenous Oxidative DNA Damage in Human Sperm, *Proc. Natl. Acad. Sci. USA 88*, 11003–11006.

163. Abdou, M.S.S., El-Guindi, M.M., El-Menouty, A.A., and Zaki, U. (1978) Some Biochemical and Metabolic Aspects of the Semen of Bovines Bubalus-bubalis and Bostaurus. Part 4. Ascorbic Acid Relationships, *Zeitschrift fur Tierzuchtung und Zuchtungsbiologie 94*, 192–197.

164. Monsi, A., and Onitchi, D.O. (1991) Effects of Ascorbic Acid (vitamin C) Supplementation on Ejaculated Semen Characteristics of Broiler Breeder Chickens under Hot and Humid Tropical Conditions, *Anim. Feed Sci. Technol. 34*, 141–146.

165. Meister, A. (1992) On the Antioxidant Effects of Ascorbic Acid and Glutathione, *Biochem. Pharmacol. 44*, 1905–1915.

166. Sen, C.K., and Packer, L. (2000) Thiol Homeostasis and Supplements in Physical Exercise, *Am. J. Clin. Nutr. 72* (suppl), 553S–669S.

167. Meister, A., and Anderson, M.E. (1983) Glutathione, *Annual Rev. Biochem. 52*, 711–760.

168. Bains, J.S., and Shaw, C.A. (1997) Neurodegenerative Disorders in Human: the Role of Glutathione in Oxidative Stress-Mediated Neuronal Death, *Brain Res. Rev. 25*, 335–358.

169. Thompson, K.H., Godin, D.V., and Lee, M. (1992) Tissue Antioxidant Status in Streptozotocin-Induced Diabetes in Rats. Effects of Dietary Manganese Deficiency, *Biol. Trace Elem. Res. 35*, 213–224.

170. Palamanda, J.R., and Kehrer, J.P. (1993) Involvement of Vitamin E and Protein Thiols in the Inhibition of Microsomal Lipid Peroxidation by Glutathione, *Lipids 278*, 427–431.

171. Elliott, S.J., and Koliwad, S.K. (1997) Redox Control of Ion Channel Activity in Vascular Endothelial Cells by Glutathione, *Microcirculation 4*, 341–437.

172. Tramer, F., Rocco, F., Micali, F., Sandri, G., and Panfili, E. (1998) Antioxidant Systems in Rat Epididymal Spermatozoa, *Biol. Reprod. 59*, 753–758.

173. Ochsendorf, F.R., Buhl, R. Bastlein, A., and Beschmann, H. (1998) Glutathione in Spermatozoa and Seminal Plasma of Infertile Men, *Human Reprod. 13*, 353–359.

174. Mann, T., ed. (1981) *Male Reproduction Function and Semen.* Springer-Verlag, Berlin.

175. Den Boer, P.J., Poot, M., Verkerk, A., Jansen, R., Mackenbach, P., and Grootegoed, J.A. (1990) Glutathione-Dependent Defense Mechanisms in Isolated Round Spermatids from the Rat, *Internat. J. Androl. 13*, 26–38.

176. Griveau, J.F., and Le Lannou, D. (1994) Effects of Antioxidants on Human Sperm Preparation Techniques, *Internat. J. Androl. 17*, 225–231.

177. Irvine, D.S. (1996) Glutathione as a Treatment for Male Infertility, *Rev. Reprod. 1*, 6–12.

178. Donnelly, E.T., McClure, N., and Lewis, S.E. (2000) Glutathione and Hypotaurine *in Vitro*: Effects on Human Sperm Motility, DNA Integrity and Production of Reactive Oxygen Species, *Mutagenesis 15*, 61–68.

179. Wishart, G.J. (1982) Maintenance of ATP Concentration in and Fertilizing Ability of Fowl and Turkey Spermatozoa *in Vitro*, *J. Reprod. Fertil. 66*, 457–462.

180. Bakst, M.R., Wishart, G.J., and Brillard, J-P. (1994) Oviducal Sperm Selection, Transport, and Storage in Poultry, *Poult. Sci. Rev. 5*, 117–143.

181. Surai, P.F. (1991). Comparison of Carbohydrate Metabolism in Semen of Cock, Turkey, Goose, and Drake, *Proc. 9th Internat. Sympos. Current Problems Avian Genetics*, Smolenice, Czechoslovakia, pp. 81–85.

182. Sauveur, B., and de Carville, H. (1990) Le Canard de Barbarie, INRA, Paris, pp. 114–115.

183. Sexton, T.J. (1974) Oxidative and Glycolytic Activity of Chicken and Turkey Spermatozoa, *Comp. Biochem. Physiol. 48B*, 59–65.

Chapter 16

The Effect of Antioxidants on Nicotine and Caffeine Induced Changes in Human Sperm—An *in Vitro* Study

Mehran Arabi[a], Sankar Nath Sanyal[b], Usha Kanwar[c], Ravinder Jit Kaur Anand[c]

[a]Department of Biology, Shahrekord University, Shahrekord, POB 115, Iran
[b]Department of Biophysics, Panjab University, Chandigarh - 160014, India
[c]Department of Zoology, Panjab University, Chandigarh - 160014, India

Abstract

We designed an experiment to study the effects of nicotine (0.5 and 1 mM), and caffeine (5, 7, and 9 mM) on membrane integrity, total phospholipid content, DNA integrity, and glutathione redox ratio and the effectiveness of antioxidants ascorbate, glutathione (GSH), and trolox, a water-soluble analog of vitamin E, in sperm cells of normospermic men. Lipoperoxidation (LPO) as an index of membrane integrity was found to be elevated in nicotine- and caffeine-treated samples against spontaneous LPO in the control spermatozoa samples. When ferrous ions were added to media, the rate of LPO was augmented. Ascorbate acted as a pro-oxidant in such samples. Total phospholipid content was depressed, and this depression was more prominent in nicotine than caffeine additions. The glutathione redox ratio (GSH/GSSG), with an inverse proportion to oxidative stress, was also markedly impaired in nicotine and caffeine additions. The single cell gel electrophoresis (SCGE), or Comet assay, checked the DNA integrity, and it revealed that nicotine and caffeine could induce strand breaks in the human sperm DNA ladder that were modulated or reversed by antioxidants. The percentage of cells with migrated DNA (sperm comets) was higher in the nicotine- than the caffeine-treated samples. Among the antioxidants used, trolox acted as a better antioxidant singly and with GSH. The elevated levels of TBARS and lowered redox ratio indicate that nicotine and caffeine imposed a severe and a mild oxidative stress, respectively, on human spermatozoa. Taken together, nicotine and caffeine can alter maturity and fertilizing ability of sperm cells and ultimately induce infertility.

Introduction

During the last several decades, the quality of human sperm and its fertility potential have decreased dramatically. This may suggest that the quality of semen has deteriorated partly due to the effects of increasing toxic factors in the environment (1,2).

Infertility in males may result from several primary biological impairments such as semen abnormalities or hormonal alterations (3). Male reproductive functions may also be altered by chronic exposure to bioactive compounds capable of crossing the blood-testis barrier following systemic absorption. Male infertility accounts for 40% of infertility problems (4). In addition to the endocrine aspects, a large number of toxicological substances and pharmacological and physical agents (*e.g.*, radiation damage) can cause reproductive intervention at the cellular and molecular level. Among these, the influence of reactive oxygen species (ROS) and related antioxidant treatments have become of increasing interest in recent times (5).

Oxygen (O_2) is a double-edged sword. Nobody can live without oxygen, but at the same time there is a darker side to the story as we are continuously exposed to oxygen toxicity. During evolution, the switch from energy generation by anaerobic metabolism to the use of O_2 as the electron sink was one of the most important events. The major ROS, superoxide anion ($^\bullet O_2^-$), hydrogen peroxide (H_2O_2), the hydroxyl radical ($^\bullet OH$), and peroxynitrite anion ($^\bullet ONOO^-$), are capable of adversely modifying cell functions, ultimately endangering the survival of the cell. The ROS are basically chemical species endowed with an unpaired electron that spread a sequence of radical reactions. There is considerable evidence that even 21% O_2 has slowly manifested the damaging effects on the survival of the organism. The effects observed vary considerably with the type of organism and its age, physiological state, and diet, such as the presence of varying amounts of vitamins E and C, transition metals, antioxidants, and polyunsaturated fatty acids (PUFA) in the diet (6).

In human semen, defective sperm cells and contaminating neutrophils are potential sources of ROS as oxidative agents (7,8). Human spermatozoa have been found to be extremely vulnerable to the attack of ROS because of their stage of differentiation (9) and the presence of PUFA in their membranes (10). PUFA are required for plasma membrane fluidity. The major PUFA in human sperm cells is docosahexaenoic acid (DHA, 22:6n-3) with six unsaturated double bonds per molecule. The best morphological pattern also corresponds to the highest content of DHA in the sperm populations (11). It has been confirmed that oxidation of membrane elements results in a dramatic loss of spermatozoal function, impairing the fertilizing capacity of the sperm cells. It may be noted that the production of ROS is a normal physiological process but an imbalance between ROS generation and scavenging activity is detrimental to the cells (10).

During the past decade evidence has accumulated to support a pivotal role of ROS in the pathogenesis of sperm dysfunction among men with infertility. In addition, certain lifestyle factors, such as tobacco smoking and environmental agents, may reduce the antioxidant capacity of seminal plasma and impair the secretion of the accessory sex glands (12–14).

Antioxidants are compounds that scavenge, dispose, and suppress the formation of oxygen free radicals in the medium, and they are used here to counter the possible oxidative stress in the drug-treated samples. The antioxidants have been used to combat infertility cases in the human population and may function as protectors to cell components against oxidative insult. A complex antioxidant system is present in spermatozoa and seminal plasma to scavenge oxygen radicals and prevent their damaging action under normal physiological conditions. Such a system embraces enzymatic activities, such as superoxide dismutase, catalase, and glutathione peroxidase, and also nonenzymatic antioxidants/scavengers, *e.g.,* water soluble (ascorbate, glutathione, and uric acid) and/or fat-soluble (vitamin E, caratenoids, and ubiquinones) natural compounds (15–19).

It has been shown that seminal plasma from infertile men has a significantly lower total antioxidant capacity than that from fertile men (20). Recently, there has been much debate regarding the potential advantage of antioxidant therapy in improving male fertility (21,22). The discovery that lipoperoxidation (LPO) is a causative mechanism in the etiology of defective sperm function is important because it has led to the use of antioxidants as a strategy to reverse the damage caused by oxidative stress (23).

Approximately one-third of the world's population ($\geq$15 years) smokes regularly (24). Cigarette smoking is known to be detrimental to health and fertility potential (25,26). Cigarette smoke contains several substances, including nicotine, carbon monoxide, benzo(a)pyrine, radioactive polonium, and other carcinogens and mutagens, that are harmful to germ cells (26,27). Numerous investigations have been conducted on the positive relationship between smoking and male infertility (28–32).

Nicotine is an alkaloid that is strongly alkaline in reaction and also very volatile. It is present together with a number of minor alkaloids in tobacco (27). In a series of experiments carried out by Wetscher *et al.* (33,34) it was shown that nicotine induced the oxidative stress in esophageal mucosa and pancreatic tissue of rat toward cellular damages. Cope (35) suggested that the effects of nicotine and/or cigarette smoke *in toto* on sperm motility are caused by ROS generated from leukocyte contamination of semen and that these effects can be inhibited by antioxidants.

Caffeine and its two major metabolites, theophylline(1,3-dimethylxanthine) and theobromine (3,7-dimethylxanthine), are three closely related alkaloids in the methylxanthine group that occur in plants widely distributed geographically. The caffeine is lipophilic in nature and readily crosses biological membranes. Its absorption into the bloodstream after oral ingestion is rapid and complete (36). Caffeine is reported to stimulate the motility and forward progression of ejaculated human spermatozoa (37,38). Caffeine has also been found to increase sperm velocity (39,40) and the percentage and viability of motile spermatozoa and metabolism when added to human semen, the effect being most dramatic with poor samples, *e.g.,* cryopreserved ones (37,41,42).

Materials and Methods

The semen samples were collected from healthy nonsmoking donors with normal characterizations according to WHO standards (24). The samples were washed with phosphate-buffered saline (PBS) (0.2 M, pH = 7. 2) and centrifuged (300g). The resulting pellet was used throughout the study. Nicotine and caffeine were obtained from Sigma Chemical Co. (St. Louis, MO).

The final concentrations of antioxidants were 1 mM ascorbate (Loba chemie, PB No. 2042, Mumbai, India), 5 mM glutathione (GSH) (Hi Media Laboratories Pvt. Ltd., Mumbai, India), and 0.02 mM trolox (Aldrich Chemical Co., Milwaukee, WI) were used. In all materials, the solvent used was PBS. The LPO was assessed by determination of thiobarbituric acid reactive substances (TBARS) in the media (43). The total phospholipid content was obtained by estimating Pi, and the GSH redox ratio was determined by calculating the amount of GSH/GSSG (reduced to oxidized glutathione) (44). The Comet assay technique was used to check the DNA integrity in sperm samples upon drug additions using acridine orange as a fluorescent dye to DNA breaks (45). Each cell with damaged DNA gives the appearance of a comet with a tail and head.

Discussion

LPO Rate

Irrespective of the clinical diagnosis and semen characteristics, the presence of seminal oxidative stress in infertile men suggests that ROS may play a major role in the pathophysiology of male infertility (46). ROS production is also energy dependent (47). A continuous decline in sperm viability in association with an increased ROS production was reported (48). LPO as a major manifestation of ROS-induced damage in cell populations is able to induce perturbation in the membrane (cellular and organellar) structure and function (49,50). Besides membrane effects, LPO can damage DNA and proteins, either through oxidation of DNA bases (primarily guanine via lipid peroxyl and alkoxyl radicals) or through covalent binding to malonyldialdehyde (MDA) resulting in strand breaks and cross-linking as well (10,50). There has been little attention to the possible impact of use of nicotine and caffeine on the membrane integrity and related processes in mammalian spermatozoa.

First, we examined the oxidant potential of nicotine (0.5 and 1 mM) and caffeine (5, 7, and 9 mM) on spermatozoa membranes. Nicotine, a major component of cigarette smoke that mimics many of the deleterious effects of tobacco, was found to augment the level of TBARS in media by about 51.5 and 78% ($P < 0.01$ and $P < 0.001$) (Table 16.1). Caffeine, an active compound in tea and coffee, also could propagate the LPO process in sperm samples by about 14, 20, and 30 % ($P > 0.05$, $P < 0.05$, and $P < 0.05$) (Table 16.2). Nicotine caused an increased chemiluminescence and formed LPO 3.3-fold in the rat esophageal mucosa in a dose- and time-dependent manner, which could be inhibited by addition of enzymatic antioxidants to the assay mixture (34). A recent study registered that caffeine at concentrations of 5–20 mM caused a sharp increase in the superoxide anion formation and DNA degradation in alveolar macrophages from rat lung. The study suggested that caffeine at moderate and high concentrations can induce apoptosis in rat alveolar macrophage culture (51).

TBARS content expressed as MDA makes a yellow-colored complex with TBA at 90°C. MDA is a stable peroxidation product of PUFA and usually shows covalent

TABLE 16.1

Effectiveness of antioxidant supplementations (alone/in combination) on nicotine-induced lipid peroxidation in human ejaculated spermatozoa[a]

Nicotine (mM)	Antioxidant Supplementation						
	None	AA	T	G	AA + T	AA + G	G + T
0	.332 ± .019	.117 ± .024	.113 ± .028	.144 ± .026	.107 ± .036	.108 ± .024	.091 ± .030
0.5	.503 ± .043	.314 ± .028	.265 ± .026	.377 ± .033	.281 ± .021	.320 ± .029	.340 ± .025
1	.591 ± .028	.385 ± .032	.270 ± .033	.502 ± .022	.349 ± .026	.401 ± .025	.396 ± .021
Correlation coefficient (r)	+0.983	+0.965	+0.880	+0.980	+0.969	+0.968	+0.939

[a]Each datum represents mean ± SD of three independent observations each made in triplicate. Mean values are n moles MDA · mg prot^{-1} · min^{-1}. The abbreviations indicate AA, 1mM ascorbic acid; T, 0.02 mM trolox; G, 5mM glutathione.

TABLE 16.2

Effectiveness of antioxidant supplementations (alone/in combination) on caffeine-induced lipid peroxidation in human ejaculated spermatozoa[a]

Caffeine (mM)	Antioxidant Supplementation						
	None	AA	T	G	AA + T	AA + G	G + T
0	.332 ± .019	.117 ± .024	.113 ± .028	.144 ± .026	.107 ± .036	.108 ± .024	.091 ± .030
5	.380 ± .334	.334 ± .028	.251 ± .026	.324 ± .021	.254 ± .039	.273 ± .033	.221 ± .028
7	.400 ± .028	.363 ± .033	.265 ± .025	.312 ± .032	.268 ± .022	.273 ± .027	.247 ± .034
9	.431 ± .026	.321 ± .031	.265 ± .039	.312 ± .025	.280 ± .036	.247 ± .028	.246 ± .024
Correlation coefficient (r)	+0.994	+0.875	+0.935	+0.880	+0.953	+0.838	+0.952

[a]Each datum represents mean ± SD of three independent observations each made in triplicate. Mean values are n moles MDA · mg prot^{-1} · min^{-1}. The abbreviations indicate AA, 1mM ascorbic acid; T, 0.02 mM trolox; G, 5mM glutathione.

binding and cross-linking to proteins and DNA as well (50). MDA formation varies considerably from one sample to another (52). A number of independent lines of evidence suggest a role of lipid peroxidation in the etiology of defective sperm functions (23,53,54). The seminal plasma and normal motile spermatozoa do not produce high levels of ROS under the normal conditions (10). It was speculated that nicotine and caffeine functioned as potent and mild oxidants, respectively, in promoting the rate of LPO by generating the ROS when added to the spermatozoa samples. In a report by Aitken and Clarkson it was proposed that the production of ROS by normal spermatozoa is partially dependent on normal or excessive function of a membrane-bound NADPH-oxidase (55). Peroxidation of membrane lipids, especially PUFA, leads to a disturbance in the membrane fluidity and hence its function, in other words LPO decreases the fluidity and increases the viscosity of the membrane (56).

The selective antioxidants ascorbate, GSH, and trolox were supplemented to the treated sperm samples. A depleted ascorbate level is observed in the presence of high levels of ROS and oxidative stress. It may, therefore, be safely labeled as an effective antioxidant against oxidative assault (57). The ubiquitous tripeptid reduced glutathione (GSH) is widely distributed in animal cells, plant cells, and microorganisms. In different biological systems, the GSH redox cycle plays an important role in protecting the cells against oxidative damage. Generally, GSH is present in millimolar concentrations in cytosol and the nucleus of sperm cells (58). Glutathione therapy has been proposed in various pathologic situations in which ROS could be involved in idiopathic infertility (10). Trolox as an aqueous analogue of α-tocopherol (lacking phytyl-chain) is able to move partially into the membrane lipid bilayer to quench the free radial and other peroxidized substances. Each molecule of trolox can trap two peroxyl radicals when oxidation is initiated in the lipid phase (59). It has been shown that trolox at a concentration of 40 μM protected the LDL oxidation significantly by reducing TBARS and conjugated diene production by about 43 and 80%, respectively (60).

Our results regarding the effectiveness of the antioxidants on the spontaneous or nicotine- and caffeine-induced lipoperoxidation in spermatozoa samples show that trolox was more effective than ascorbate and glutathione in lowering the level of TBARS in the assay mixture (Tables 16.1 and 16.2). Recently, it has been reported that trolox could bind to some proteins, such as human serum albumin, inhibit structural damage of these proteins, and act as a very potent protector following oxidative damage (60). In *in vitro* models, trolox was also demonstrated to have desirable scavenging ability to protect the tissues against LPO (61). In order to examine the effectiveness of combined concentration of antioxidants on lipid peroxidation, the combined concentration of glutathione and trolox has proved to produce the best effect in lowering the spontaneous lipid peroxidation (72.6%) of untreated unsupplemented (control) sample, whereas other combinations, ascorbate + trolox and ascorbate + glutathione, were able to reduce the MDA levels by about 67.8 and 67.5%, respectively (Tables 16.1 and 16.2). On the other hand, in nicotine-treated samples the combination of ascorbate + trolox and in caffeine-treated samples the combination of glutathione +

trolox were substantiated to produce the best results. As cited earlier, the antioxidant defense system works in an integrated fashion in sperm cells to minimize the oxidative damage. Besides the activity of antioxidant enzymes, such as superoxide dismutase and catalase, α-tocopherol is present as a chain-breaking antioxidant in membranes and available to eliminate the generated ROS. Oxidation of α-tocopherol produces the tocopheryl radicals, which can be reduced by ascorbate molecules. The oxidation of ascorbate, in turn, gives rise to ascorbyl radical, which can be reduced and quenched by glutathione, producing the thyl ($GS^{\bullet}$) radicals (which are not as rapid as the oxidative attack of PUFA in membranes and therefore are not very harmful to cells) and oxidized GSH, which can be regenerated by glutathione reductase activity. As a consequence, the whole system has to work simultaneously and an alteration of one of the components, for example, inhibition of antioxidant enzymes and/or the presence of excessive amounts of each antioxidant or their interactions with metal ions, can lead to potentially damaging accumulation of ROS (62). Combinations of antioxidants can therefore be used to treat the sperm abnormality cases, as they can restore the physiological constitution of PUFA in the cell membrane (63). It is recommended that spermatozoa samples can be treated with antioxidants prior to *in vitro* fertilization; this procedure can also prove to be beneficial after cryopreservation, a condition in which an increase in peroxidative damage has been cited (64). The results came from a report indicating that glutathione can be used to maintain vitamin E concentration, thereby lowering the microsomal lipoperoxidation process in experimental conditions (65). Coantioxidant activity or synergism between vitamin E and C has also been observed to delay the MDA production during ferrous-catalyzed peroxidation of rat liver microsomal and phospholipid liposomes (62).

The sperm samples were subjected to 0.2 mM ferrous sulphate ($FeSO_4$), and it was proven that addition of ferrous (Fe^{2+}) to the untreated samples (control) caused a very sharp elevation in the extent of spontaneous LPO production by about 59.4% (P < 0.001). The resultant iron-catalyzed LPO was found to be extended upon addition of different concentrations of nicotine and caffeine to media (data not shown). Elevation in the level of MDA in treatment with the highest concentration of nicotine was 115.7%, and in the case of caffeine it was even raised by about 125.6% (P < 0.001). It can be suggested that the emerged complexes of Fe^{2+} with nicotine and/or caffeine may act as more potent oxidants, which is the reason behind the propagation of LPO throughout the membrane framework. At least for nicotine, a very plausible mechanism of action may be the ability of this compound to bind directly to Fe^{2+}, probably via its pyridine nitrogen (66). It can be speculated that complexes of Fe^{2+} and nicotine and/or caffeine could release more amounts of alkoxyl and peroxyl radicals (as LPO midproducts) from the preexisting lipid hydroperoxides (primary oxidized lipids) in the cell plasma and organelle membranes and finally give rise to MDA (as an endproduct of LPO) release in medium.

Our results showed that antioxidant supplementation caused a sharp decline in the levels of MDA (data not shown) except in the case of ascorbate (alone), which resulted in a further elevation in the rate of MDA formation in all the cases, *e.g.*, 89.2% (P

< 0.001), in untreated-Fe^{2+} supplemented (control) series. It may be suggested that a synergistic effect was established between ascorbate and ferrous as iron-ascorbate complex, which functioned as a LPO promoter.

Total Phospholipid Content

Mammalian cell membranes consist of a lipid bilayer composed primarily of phospholipids and cholesterol. Lateral diffusion of lipids in the membrane environment may allow proteins to undergo conformational changes necessary for receptor and transport functions. A report from Karnovsky and his co-workers indicated that most of the altered cellular functions are probably caused by direct modifications of the membrane lipid composition. Changes in lipid framework may thus lead to altered lateral mobility of proteins resulting in functional changes (67). Current theories of membrane fusion suggest that membrane fluidity is a prerequisite for normal cell function and that the fluidity and flexibility of cell membranes are mainly dependent on their lipid constitution, particularly phospholipid composition (68). Therefore, it can be suggested that any alteration in these membrane components will lead to a failure in the sperm-oocyte communication. It has been substantiated that the phospholipid sphingomyelin in human sperm cells can influence the rate of capacitation by slowing loss of sterols, particularly cholesterol, and that exogenous sphingomyelinase accelerates capacitation by speeding the loss of sterols and by generating ceramide (69).

The results from our laboratory substantiated that upon addition of nicotine (1 mM) and caffeine (7 mM) to the spermatozoa homogenates, a decline in the total phospholipid content was registered by about 40.3 and 16.3% ($P < 0.01$ and $P < 0.05$), respectively (Fig. 16.1 and 16.2). It is substantiated that nicotine has the ability to cross the membranes and reach the cytoplasm of ovarian cells, leading to perturbations in meiotic spindles (70). It is at the time of membrane crossing that nicotine can introduce some alterations into the lipid structure of plasma membranes. Caffeine is easily soluble in most organic solvents and is lipophilic enough to traverse through the cell membranes (71). The interaction and presence of caffeine in the lipid bilayer might bring about a change in the lipid fraction as judged by the induction of lipid peroxidation in the membrane elements. The total phospholipid and fatty acid content of phospholipid fractions of membrane can be altered under certain conditions, such as cryopreservation and aging. The total phospholipid content of spermatozoa decreased during liquid storage, whereas no quantitative decline in seminal plasma was observed. The decrease was significant in phosphatidylcholine content (72).

It was registered that antioxidants fail to lessen the drug-induced alterations in most of the sperm membrane lipid fractions when used in single concentrations (Fig. 16.1). On the other hand, combined concentrations of the antioxidants functioned satisfactory in mopping up the free radicals from the lipid media of sperm samples (Fig. 16.2). Trolox alone and also in combination with GSH exerted an effective scavenging role in lessening the peroxidative damages in media.

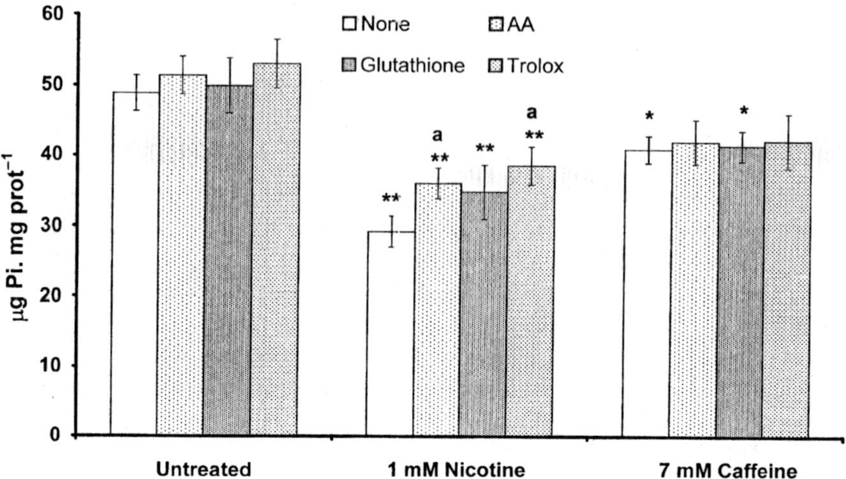

Fig. 16.1. Changes in total phospholipid content upon nicotine and caffeine additions plus antioxidants. *P* values as compared to the control are * *P* < 0.05 and ** *P* < 0.01. *P* value as compared to the respective drug-treated group is [a] *P* < 0.05.

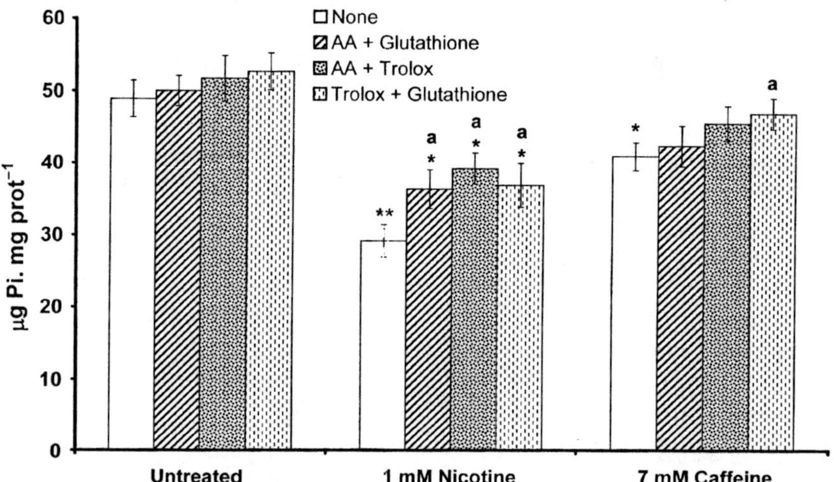

Fig. 16.2. Changes in total phospholipid content upon nicotine and caffeine additions plus antioxidants. *P* values as compared to the control are * *P* < 0.05 anf ** *P* < 0.01. *P* value as compared to the respective drug-treated group is [a] *P* < 0.05.

It can be taken into account that any decline in the extension of LPO by the function of antioxidants may be translated into an early improvement in peroxidation of lipid components of sperm membranes.

Glutathione Redox Ratio

One of the most prevalent nonenzymatic antioxidant defense systems against free radical insult in the cells is reduced glutathione, GSH, which is restrictedly related to the gamma-glutamyl compounds (68,73). The GSH redox ratio (GSH/GSSG) of a cell may be expressed as the ratio of the concentration of oxidizing equivalents to the concentration of reducing equivalents. In different biological systems, this status plays an important role in protecting the cells against oxidative damage. A high GSH/GSSG ratio will help spermatozoa to combat oxidative insult (74). The redox ratio has an inverse proportion to the oxidative stress. The level of the pro-oxidant molecules and antioxidant fluxes thus govern the fine redox balance within a cell. Therefore, an appreciation of the different sources of oxidants and the counteracting antioxidant (or reducing) system is necessary to understand what factors are involved in achieving a particular intracellular redox status (75). We showed that the GSH redox ratio was depressed upon drug treatments (Fig. 16.3) to the sperm samples by about 49.2 and 60.3% in nicotine-treated series and 20.7, 31.4, and 37.9% in caffeine-treated series. Reduction in the redox ratio in drug-treated groups is equal to the utilization of GSH molecules and formation of GSSG units. Antioxidant supplementations showed an elevation in the amount of redox ratio. The combined dosage of trolox + ascorbate was the best antioxidant result in sperm samples and showed an increase in redox ratio of 2.2-fold as compared to the controls (Fig. 16.3). Other increases were 1.2- and 1.3-fold in nicotine-treated samples and 1.3-, 1.2-, and 2.5-fold in caffeine-treated samples as compared to the respective drug treatments (Fig. 16.3). In human erythrocytes, it is also confirmed that oxidative stress causes GSH depletion with an increase in the

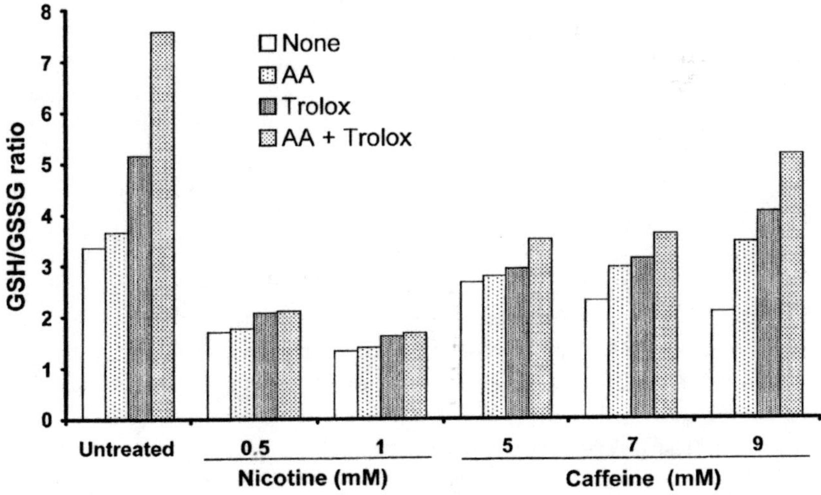

Fig. 16.3. Changes in glutathione redox ratio upon nicotine and caffeine additions plus antioxidants.

GSSG, which results in an elevated GSSG/GSH (or a decreased GSH/GSSG) ratio (76). An appreciation of the different sources of oxidants and the counteracting antioxidant system is necessary to understand what factors are involved in achieving a particular intracellular GSH redox status.

Sperm DNA Integrity

ROS may attack DNA integrity of human sperm cells. Generation of ROS induced by NADPH and the xanthine/xanthine oxidase system or by direct addition of H_2O_2 to the sperm samples was shown to cause a significant increase in DNA fragmentation (77). Furthermore, fragmentation of sperm DNA was shown to be inversely correlated with semen quality, particularly sperm morphology and motility and fertilization rate after *in vitro* fertilization (IVF) and intracytoplasmic sperm injection (ICSI) (77,78). Baseline DNA integrity in spermatozoa is lower than that of somatic cell types, possibly a reflection of its physiological role in fertilization (45,79). On the other hand, spermatozoa produced by infertile men were shown to have DNA that was more susceptible to damage by irradiation than that from fertile men. DNA damage may not prevent fertilization from occurring but may lead to fetal abnormalities that will be apparent later (80).

The comet assay proved to be a very sensitive test to examine the DNA strand breaks in the sperm chromatin. Single-stranded lesions in the sperm DNA should be repaired in the oocyte upon fertilization and should not be lethal. However, if a fertilizing spermatozoon possesses single-stranded DNA breaks of significant size, they may prove to be difficult for the oocyte to repair and may lead to failure in either the fertilization process or later in the development. Double-stranded breaks are considered to be more lethal lesions to the sperm DNA than single-stranded ones (81). In the present study, acridine orange stain was used to distinguish the single-stranded from double-stranded DNA breaks. When acridine orange binds to double-stranded DNA, it fluoresces green, but when it binds to single-stranded DNA breaks, it fluoresces red (82). Our results indicate that almost all the comet tails were double-stranded, and some single-stranded DNA breaks were also observed in both nicotine and caffeine-treated samples. Lopez and his coworkers demonstrated that men with a sperm population containing more than 25% DNA damage are more likely to experience a fertilization rate less than 20% after ICSI technique (77).

Both ROS generation and oxidative DNA base damage are elevated in the spermatozoa of infertile men. It may be suggested that ROS production and subsequent lipoperoxidation can be selected as predictors of the DNA damage in the spermatozoa samples (83). In our results nicotine (as a potent oxidative agent) could induce DNA damage with a percentage greater than that of caffeine (as a mild oxidant) in the spermatozoa samples as judged by the presence of more detected sperm comets in the treated samples (Fig. 16.4). It was also substantiated that human sperm chromatin becomes cross-linked under oxidative stress and exhibits increased DNA strand breaks (84). Smoking is associated with an increase in strand breaks in the sperm DNA structure as a result of oxidative stress (85). A sharp increase in the superoxide anion formation and

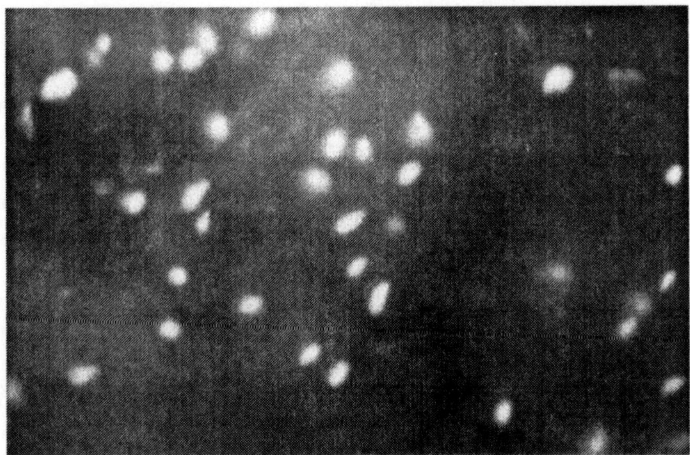

Fig. 16.4. Photomicrograph shows the effect of 1 mM nicotine on human sperm cells; bright spots are sperm DNA and comets are elongated cells.

DNA degradation and breaks following addition of 5 to 20 mM concentrations of caffeine to the culture medium of rat lung macrophages has been reported (51). Our data reveal that antioxidant supplementations can improve DNA integrity and protect sperm DNA from nicotine- and caffeine-induced free radical formation as judged by the lower percentage of sperm cells having the comet appearance. This effect was more prominent in caffeine-treated spermatozoa samples than in the nicotine-treated ones, which reversed the DNA damage to the control level when antioxidant combinations were added (data not shown). The combination of trolox and glutathione was found to produce better results in lowering the amount of DNA breaks. Addition of ascorbate and/or alpha tocopherol (trolox) to the sperm preparation did not affect the baseline DNA integrity but could provide sperm with complete protection against H_2O_2-induced DNA breaks (19). Addition of seminal plasma as a rich source of natural antioxidants to the sperm preparation resulted in a significant decrease in the DNA strand breaks and TBARS production (86). In disagreement with Hughes and his coworkers (79,80), who found that the addition of a combination of ascorbate and trolox to the spermatozoa samples could result in more DNA strand breaks, we observed that this combination can afford satisfactory protection to the sperm DNA against ROS. It may be suggested that there is a narrow physiological range in which antioxidants can work synergistically to act against the oxidative conditions.

Summary

Human spermatozoa have been found to be extremely vulnerable to the attack of ROS due to presence of unsaturated fatty acids in their membranes. It has been confirmed that oxidation of membrane elements results in a dramatic loss of spermatozoa function, impairing the fertilizing capacity of the sperm cells. The present investigation was designed to work out the antioxidative potential of ascorbate (1mM), glutathione (5 mM), and trolox (0.02 mM) (a water-soluble analogue of Vitamin E) singly and/or in combination in human ejaculated spermatozoa following treatment with nicotine (0.5, and 1 mM) and caffeine (5, 7, and 9 mM) in the different experimental conditions. The spontaneous LPO in the control group, measured as TBARS/MDA increased markedly with the addition of nicotine by 51.5 and 78%. On the other hand, caffeine caused an elevated level of MDA by about 14, 20, and 30% in the incubation mixture. It was speculated that nicotine and caffeine functioned as potent and mild oxidants, respectively, in promoting the rate of LPO in the spermatozoa samples. Using ferrous ions (Fe^{2+}) resulted in a further elevation in the TBARS level in the drug-treated samples as well as in the control. Trolox was observed to be a more effective antioxidant than glutathione and ascorbate, when used in single form, in lowering the rate of LPO generation. It has been established that in ferrous-treated samples antioxidant supplementation caused a sharp decline in the level of MDA, except in the case of ascorbate addition, which resulted in a further elevation in the rate of LPO. It may be suggested that a synergistic effect was established between Fe^{2+} and ascorbate functioning as an LPO promoter system.

The nicotine- (1 mM) and caffeine- (7 mM) induced lipid modifications in human spermatozoa homogenate with antioxidant modulations has been investigated. Nicotine and caffeine treatments caused a significant reduction in the content of total phospholipids, 40.3 and 16.3%, respectively. During the present investigation it was demonstrated that antioxidants used in a combined concentration were more efficient in mopping up the drug-induced free radicals than when used in single form.

The metabolism of glutathione as a most prevalent nonenzymatic antioxidant defense system in sperm cells is linked with the gamma-glutamyl cycle. The glutathione redox ratio (GSH/GSSG), which has an inverse proportion to oxidative stress, was found to be lowered following treatment with nicotine about 49.2 and 60.3%, and with caffeine by about 20.7, 31.4, and 37.9%, suggesting nicotine and caffeine as potent and mild oxidants, respectively.

The effect of drugs was evaluated on the sperm DNA integrity using the single cell gel electrophoresis (Comet) assay to detect the presence of DNA strand breaks in spermatozoa samples with antioxidant supplementation. It was observed that nicotine could induce severe DNA breaks in human spermatozoa samples as judged by the presence of different shapes of sperm comets in the samples. Caffeine functioned as a very mild oxidant agent in altering the sperm DNA integrity, which presented a lower percentage of comets than that of nicotine-treated samples. Antioxidant supplementation could improve and/or reverse the detrimental impact of the drugs in the spermatozoa samples.

Acknowledgements

This work was financed by the Ministry of Science, Research, and Technology (MSRT) of Iran and the Indian Council for Cultural Relations (ICCR) with the department of Zoology, Panjab University, Chandigarh, India. We also thank Dr. (Mrs.) Noha Eftekhari for her endless help.

References

1. Menkveld, R., Van Zylt, J.A., Kotze, T.J.W., and Joubert, G. (1986) Possible Changes in Male Fertility Over a 15-Year Period, *Arch. Androl. 17*, 143–144.

2. Menchini-Fabris, F., Rossi, P., Palego, P., Simi, S., and Turch, P. (1996) Declining Sperm Counts in Italy during the Past 20 Years, *Andrologia. 28*, 304–306.

3. Baird, D.D., and Wilcox, A.J. (1986) Future Fertility after Prenatal Exposure to Cigarette Smoke, *Fertil. Steril. 46*, 3–7.

4. Fleming, S., Green, S., and Hall, J. (1995) Analysis and Alleviation of Male Infertility, *Microsc. Anal. 35*, 37–39.

5. Rolf, C., Cooper, T.G., Yeung, C.H., and Nieschlag, E. (1999) Antioxidant Treatment of Patients with Asthenozoospermia or Moderate Oligoasthenozoospermia with High-Dose Vitamin C and Vitamin E: A Randomized, Placebo-Controlled, Double-Blind Study, *Reprod. 14*, 1028–1033.

6. Halliwell, B., and Gutteridge, J.M.C. (1989) *Free Radicals in Biology and Medicine,* 2nd edn., pp. 372–390, Clarendon Press, Oxford.

7. Aitken, R.J., Buckingham, D., West, K., Wu, F.C., Jikopouios, K., and Richardson, D.W. (1992) Differential Contribution of Leucocytes and Spermatozoa to High Levels of Reactive Oxygen Species on Human Spermatozoa, *J. Reprod. Fertil. 98*, 257–265.

8. Gomez, E., Buckingham, D.W., Brindle, J., Lanzafame, F., Irvine, D. S., and Aitken, R.J. 1996) Development of an Image-Analysis System to Monitor the Retention of Residual Cytoplasm by Human Spermatozoa-Correlation with Biochemical Markers of the Cytoplasmic Space, Oxidative Stress, and Sperm Function, *J. Androl. 17*, 276–287.

9. Jones, R., Mann, T., and Sherrins, R.J. (1973) Adverse Effects of Peroxidized Lipid on Human Spermatozoa, *Proc. R. Soc. Lond. (Biol.) 201*, 413–417.

10. Sharma, R.K., and Agarwal, A. (1996) Role of Reactive Oxygen Species in Male Infertility, *Urology. 48*, 835–850.

11. Gandini, L., Lenzi, A., Lombardo, F., Pacifici, R., and Dondero, F. (1999) Immature Germ Cell Separation Using a Modified Discontinuous Percoll Gradient Technique in Human Semen, *Hum. Reprod. 14*, 1022–1027.

12. Pakrashi, A., and Chatterjee, S. (1995) Effect of Tobacco Consumption on the Function of Male Accessory Sex Glands, *Int. J. Androl. 18*, 232–236.

13. Depuydt, C.E., Bosmans, E., Zalata, A., Schoonjans, F., and Comhaire, F.H. (1996) The Relation between Reactive Oxygen Species and Cytokines in Andrological Patients with or without Male Accessory Gland Infection, *J. Androl. 17*, 699–707.

14. Klinefelter, G.R., and Hess, R.A. (1998) Toxicology of the Male External Ducts and Accessory Sex Glands, in *Reproductive and Developmental Toxicology*, Korach, K.S., Marcel Dekker, New York, pp. 232–591.

15. Doba, T., Burton, G.E., and Ingold, K.U. (1985) Antioxidant and Co–Antioxidant Activity of Vitamin C. The Effect of Vitamin C Either Alone or in the Presence of Vitamin E or a Water Soluble Vitamin E Analogue, upon the Peroxidation of Multilamellar Phospholipid Liposomes, *Biohemica. Et. Biophysica. Acta. 835*, 298–303.

16. Chow, C.K. (1991) Vitamin E and Oxidative Stress, Free Radic. Biol. Med. 11, 215–232.

17. Dawson, E.B., Harris, W.A., Teter, M.C., and Powell, L.C. (1992) Effect of Ascorbic Acid Supplementation on the Sperm Quality of Smokers, *Fertil. Steril. 58*, 1034 –1039.

18. Surai, P., Cerolini, S., Wishart, G., Speake, B., Noble, R., and Sparks, N. (1998) Lipid and Antioxidant Composition of Chicken Semen and Its Susceptibility to Peroxidation, *Poult. Av. Biol. Rev. 9*, 11–23.

19. Donnelly, E.T., Neil, M., and Lwis, E. M. (1999) Antioxidant Supplementation *in Vitro* Does Improve Human Sperm Motility, *Fertil. Steril. 72*, 484–495.

20. Lewis, S.E.M., Boyle, P.M., McKinney, K.A., Young, I.S., and Thompson, W. (1995) Total Antioxidant Capacity of Seminal Plasma Is Different in Fertile and Infertile Men, *Fertil. Steril. 64*, 868–870.

21. Tarin, J.J., Brines, J., and Cano, A. (1998) Antioxidants May Protect Against Infertility, *Hum. Reprod. 13*, 1415 –1416.

22. Lenzi, A., Gandini, L., and Picardo, M. (1998) A Rationale for Glutathione Therapy, *Hum. Reprod. 13*, 1419–1421.

23. Aitken, R.J., and Clarkson, J.S. (1988) Significance of Reactive Oxygen Species and Antioxidants in Defining the Efficacy of Sperm Preparation Techniques, *J. Androl. 9*, 367–376.

24. *WHO* (World Health Organization) *Laboratory Manual: For the Examination of Human Semen and Sperm-Cervical Mucus Interaction* (1992), 3rd edn, Cambridge University Press, New York.

25. Stillman, R.J., Rosenberg, M.J., and Sachs, B.P. (1986) Smoking and Reproduction, *Fertil. Steril. 46*, 545–566.

26. Zenzes, M.T. (2000) Smoking and Reproduction: Gene Damage to Human Gametes and Embryos, *Hum. Reprod. Update 6*, 122–131.

27. Gorrod, J.W., and Wahren, J. (1993) *Nicotine and Related Alkaloids: Absorption, Distribution, Metabolism, and Excretion*, Chapman and Hall, London, Glasgow, New York, Tokyo, Madras.

28. Calzada, L., Wens, M.A., and Salazar, E.L. (1992) Action of Cholinergic Drugs on Accumulation of TPMP+ on Human Spermatozoa, *Arch. Androl. 28*, 19–23.

29. Pekarsky, A., Varn, E., Mathur, R.S., and Mathur, S. (1995) Effects of Nicotine on Sperm Attachment and Penetration of Zona-Free Hamster Eggs, *Arch. Androl. 34*, 77–82.

30. Gandini, L., Lombardo, F., Lenzi, A., Culasso, F., Pacifici, R., Zuccaro, P., and Dondero, F. (1997) The *in Vitro* Effects of Nicotine and Cotinine on Sperm Motility, *Hum. Reprod. 12*, 727–733.

31. Merino, G., Lira, S.C., and Martinez – Chequer, J.C. (1998) Effects of Cigarette Smoking on Semen Characteristics of a Population in Mexico, *Arch. Androl. 41*, 11–15.

32. Wong, W.Y., Thomas, C.M., Merkus, H.M., Zielhuis, G.A., and Doesburg, W.H. (2000) Cigarette Smoking and the Risk of Male Factor Subfertility: Major Association between Cotinine in Seminal Plasma and Semen Morphology, *Fertil. Steril. 74*, 930–935.

33. Wetscher, G.J., Bagchi, M., Bagchi, D., Perdikis, G., Hinder, P.R., Glaser, K., and Hinder, R. (1995a) Free Radical Production in Nicotine Treated Pancreatic Tissue, *Free Radic. Biol. Med. 18*, 877–882.

34. Wetscher, G.J., Bagchi, D., perdikis, G., Baghci, M., Redmond, E.J., Hinder, P.R., Glaser, K., and Hinder, R.A. (1995b) *In Vitro* Free Radical Production in Rat Esophaeal Mucosn Induced by Nicotine, *Dig. Dis. Sci. 40*, 853–858.

35. Cope, G.F. (1998) The *in Vitro* Effects of Nicotine and Continine on Sperm Motility, *Hum. Reprod. 13*, 777–778.

36. Blandchard, J., and Sawers, S.J.A. (1983) Comparative Pharmacokinetics of Caffeine in Young and Elderly Men, *J. Pharmacokinet Biopharm. 11*, 109–112.

37. Aitken, R.J., Best, F., Richardson, D.W., Schats, R., and Simm, G. (1983) Influence of Caffeine on Movement Characteristics, Fertilizing Capacity, and Ability to Penetrate Cervical Mucus of Human Spermatozoa, *J. Reprod. Ferti. 67*, 19–27.

38. Tesarik, J., Mendoza, C., and Carreras, A. (1992) Effects of Phosphodiesterase Inhibitors Caffeine and Pentoxifylline on Spontaneous and Stimulus-Induced Acrosome Reactions in Human Sperm, *Fertil. Steril. 58*, 1185–1190.

39. Hammit, D.G., Bedia, E., Rogers, P.R., Syrop, S.H., Donovan, J. F., and Williamson, R.A. (1989) Comparison of Motility Stimulants for Cryopreserved Human Semen, *Fertil. Steril. 52*, 495–502.

40. Mbizvo, M.T., Johnston, R.C., and Baker, G.H.W. (1993) The Effect of the Motility Stimulants, Caffeine, Pentoxifylline, and 2-Deoxyadenosine, on Hyperactivation of Cryopreserved Human Sperm, *Fertil. Steril. 59*, 1112–1117.

41. Levin, R.M., Greenberg, S.H., and Wein, A.J. (1981) Quantitative Analysis of the Effects of Caffeine on Sperm Motility and Cyclic Adenosine 3',5'-Monophosphate (AMP) Phosphodiesterase, *Fertil. Steril. 36*, 798–802.

42. Moussa, M.M. (1983) Caffeine and Sperm Motility, *Fertil, Steril. 39*, 845–848.

43. Buege, J.A., and Steven, A.D. (1978) in *Methods in Enzymology*, Colowick, S.P., and Kalpan, N.O., Academic Press, vol. 52, pp. 302–310.

44. Sedlak, J., and Lindsay, R.H. (1968) Estimation of Total, Protein Bound, and Non-Protein Bond Sulphydryl Groups in Tissues with Ellman's Reagent, *Anal, Biochem. 25*, 192–205.

45. Singh, N.P., McCoy, M.T., Tice, R.R., and Schneider, E.L. (1988) A Simple Technique for Quantitiation of Low Levels of DNA Damage in Individual Cells, *Exp. Cell Res. 175*, 184–191.

46. Pasqualotto, F.F., Sharma, R.K., Nelson, D.R., Thomas, A.J., Jr., and Agarwal, A. (2000) Relationship between Oxidative Stress, Semen Characteristics, and Clinical Diagnosis in Men Undergoing Infertility Investigation, *Fertil. Steril. 73*, 459–464.

47. Griveau, J.F., Grizard, G., Boucher, D., and Le Lannou, D. (1998) Influence of Oxygen Tension on Function of Isolated Spermatozoa from Ejaculates of Oligospermic Patients and Normospermic Donors, *Hum. Reprod. 13*, 3108–3113.

48. Kobayashi, H., Gil–Guzman, E., Mahran A.M., Sharma, R.K., Nelson, D.R., Thomas, A.J., Jr., and Agarwal, A. (2001) Quality Control of Reactive Oxygen Species Measurement by Luminal-Dependent Chemilumine-Scene Assay, *J. Androl. 22*, 568–574.

49. Alvarez, J.G., Touchstone, J.C., Blasco, L., and Storey, B.T. (1987) Spontaneous Lipid Peroxidation and Production of Hydrogen Peroxide and Superoxide in Human Spermatozoa. Superoxide Dismutase as Major Enzyme Protectant Oxygen Toxicity, *J. Androl. 8*, 338–348.

50. Ernster, L. (1993) Lipid Peroxidation in Biological Membranes: Mechanisms and Implications, in *Active Oxygen, Lipid Peroxides, and Antioxidants*, Yagi, K., CRC Press, Boca Raton, pp. 1–38.

51. Jafari, M., and Rabbani, A. (2000) Dose and Time Dependent Effects of Caffeine on Superoxide Release, Cell Survival and DNA Fragmentation of Alveolar Macrophages from Rat Lung, *Toxicology 149*, 101–108.

52. Rao, B., Soufir, J.C., Martin, M., and David, G. (1989) Lipid Peroxidation in Human Spermatozoa as Related to Midpiece Abnormalities and Motility, *Gamete Res. 24*, 531–537.

53. Oheninger, S., Blackmore, P., Mahony, M., and Hodgen, G. (1995) Effects of Hydrogen Peroxide on Human Spermatozoa, *J. Assist. Reprod. Genet. 12*, 41–47.

54. Rhemrev, J.P.T., Vermeiden, J.P., Haenen, G.R., De Bruijne, J.J., Rekers–Mombarg, L.T., and Bast, A. (2001) Progressively Motile Human Spermatozoa Are Well Protected

Against *in Vitro* Lipid Peroxidation Imposed by Induced Oxidative Stress, *Andrologia. 33*, 151–158.

55. Aitken, R.J., and Clarkson, J.S. (1987) Cellular Basis of Defective Sperm Function and Its Association with the Genesis of Reactive Oxygen Species by Human Spermatozoa, *J. Reprod. Fertil. 81*, 459–469.

56. Jain, S., Thomas, M., Kumar, G.P., and Laloraya, M. (1993) Programmed Lipid Peroxidation of Biomembranes Generating Kinked Phospholipids Permitting Local Molecular Mobility, *Biochem. Biophys. Res. Commun. 195*, 574–580.

57. Lewis, S.E.M., Sterling, E.S., Young, I.S., and Thompson, W. (1997) Comparison of Individual Antioxidants of Sperm and Seminal Plasma in Fertile and Infertile Men, *Fertil. Steril. 67*, 142–147.

58. Meister, A., and Anderson, M.E. (1983) Glutathione, *Ann. Rev. Biochem. 52*, 711–760.

59. Barclay, L.R.C., and Vinqvist, M.R. (1994) Membrane Peroxidation: Inhibiting Effects of Water–Soluble Antioxidants on Phospholipids of Different Charge Types, *Free Radic. Biol. Med. 16*, 779–788.

60. Lee, C. (2000) Antioxidant Ability of Caffeine and Its Metabolites Based on the Study of Oxygen Radical Absorbing Capacity and Inhibition of LDL Peroxidation, *Clinica. Chimia. Acta. 295*, 141–154.

61. Salvi, A., Carrupt, P., Tillement, J., and Testa, B. (2001) Structural Damage to Proteins Caused by Free Radicals: Assessment, Protection by Antioxidants, and Influence of Protein Binding, *Biochem. Pharmacol. 61*, 1237–1242.

62. Doba, T., Burton, G.E., and Ingold, K.U. (1985) Antioxidant and Co–Antioxidant Activity of Vitamin C. The Effect of Vitamin C Either Alone or in the Presence of Vitamin E or a Water Soluble Vitamin E Analogue, upon the Peroxidation of Multilamellar Phospholipid Liposomes, *Biohemica. et Biophysica. Acta. 835*, 298–303.

63. Hsu, P.C., Liu, M.Y., Hsu, C.C., Chen, L.Y., and Guo, Y.L. (1998) Effects of Vitamin E and/or C on Reactive Oxygen Species Related Lead Toxicity in the Rat Sperm, *Toxicology 128*, 169-179.

64. Royere, D., Barthelemy, C., Hamamah, S., and Lansac, J. (1996) Cryopreservation of Spermatozoa: A 1996 Review, *Hum. Reprod. Update 2*, 553–559.

65. Leedle, R.A., and Aust, S.D. (1990) The Effect of Glutathione on the Vitamin E Requirement for Inhibition of Liver Microsomal Lipid Peroxidation, *Lipids 5*, 241–245.

66. Linert, W., Bridge, M.H., Huber, M., Bjugstad, K.B., Grossman, S., and Arendash, G.W. (1999) *In Vitro* and *in Vivo* Investigating Possible Antioxidant Actions of Nicotine: Relevance to Parkinson's and Alzheimer's Disease, *Biochem. Biophys. Acta 1454*, 143–152.

67. Karnovsky, M.J., Kleinfeld, A.M., Hoover, R.L., and Klausner, R.D. (1982) The Concept of Lipid in Membranes, *J. Cell Biol. 94*, 1–6.

68. Lenzi, A., Gandini, L., Picardo, M., Tramer, F., Sandri, G., and Panfili, E. (2000) Lipoperoxidation Damage of Spermatozoa Polyunsaturated Fatty Acids (PUFA): Scavenger Mechanisms and Possible Scavenger Therapies, *Front. Biosci. 5*, E1–E15.

69. Cross, N.L. (2000) Sphingomyelin Modulates Capacitation of Human Sperm *in Vitro*, *Biol. Reprod. 63*, 1129–1134.

70. Racowsky, C., and Kaufman, M.L. (1992) Nuclear Degeneration and Meiotic Aberrations Observed in Human Oocytes Matured *in Vitro*: Analysis by Light Microscopy, *Fertil. Steril. 58*, 750–755.

71. Blandchard, J., and Sawers, S.J.A. (1983) Comparative Pharmacokinetics of Caffeine in Young and Elderly Men, *J. Pharmacokinet. Biopharm. 11*, 109–112.

72. Douard, V., Hermier, D., and Blesbois, E. (2000) Changes in Turkey Semen Lipids during Liquid *in Vitro* Storage, *Biol. Reprod. 63*, 1450–1456.
73. Meister, A., and Anderson, M.E. (1983) Glutathione, *Ann. Rev. Biochem. 52*, 711–760.
74. Irvine, D.S. (1996) Glutathione as a Treatment for Male Infertility, Rev. Reprod. 1, 6–12.
75. Gabbita, S.P., Robinson, K.A., Stewart, C.A., Floyd, R.A., and Hensley, K. (2000) Minireview: Redox Regulatory Mechanisms of Cellular Signal Transduction, *Arch. Biochem. Biophys. 376*, 1–13.
76. Nemeth, I., Orvos, H., and Boda, D. (2001) Blood Glutathione Redox Status in Gestational Hypertension, *Free Radic. Biol. Med. 30*, 715–721.
77. Lopez, S., Jurisicova, A., Sun, J.G., and Casper, R.F. (1998) Reactive Oxygen Species: Potential Cause for DNA Fragmentation in Human Spermatozoa, *Hum. Reprod. 13*, 896–900.
78. Host, E., Lindenberg, S., and Smidt-Jensen, S. (2000) The Role of DNA Strand Breaks in Human Spermatozoa Used for IVF and ICSI, *Acta. Obs. Gyn. Scandinavia. 79*, 559–563.
79. Hughes, C.M., Lewis, S.E.M., McKelvey-Martin, V.J., and Thompson, W. (1997) Reproducibility of Human Sperm DNA Measurements Using the Single Cell Gel Electrophoresis Assay, *Mut. Res. 347*, 261–268.
80. Hughes, C.M., Lewis, S.E.M., McKelvey-Martin, V.J., and Thompson, W. (1996) A Comparison of Baseline and Induced DNA Damage in Human Sperm from Fertile and Infertile Men, Using a Modified Comet Assay, *Mol. Hum. Reprod. 2*, 613–619.
81. Kizilian, N., Wilkins, R.C., Reinhardt, P., Ferrarotto, C., McLean, J.R.N., and McNamee, J. P. (1999) Silver-Stained Comet Assay for Detection of Apoptosis, *Biotechniques 27*, 926–930.
82. Zini, A., Bielecki, R., Phang, D., and Zenzes, M.T. (2001) Correlations between Two Markers of Sperm DNA Integrity, DNA Denaturation and DNA Fragmentation, in Fertile and Infertile Men, *Fertil. Steril. 75*, 674–677.
83. Barroso, G., Morshedi, M., and Oehninger, S. (2000) Analysis of DNA Fragmentation, Plasma Membrane Translocation of Phosphatidylserine and Oxidative Stress in Human Spermatozoa, *Hum. Reprod. 15*, 1338–1344.
84. Twigg, J.P., Irvine, D.S., and Aitken, R.J. (1998) Oxidative Damage to DNA in Human Spermatozoa Does Not Preclude Pronucleus Formation at Intracytoplasmic Sperm Injection, *Hum. Reprod. 13*, 1864–1871.
85. Potts, R.J., Newbury, C.J., Smith, G., Notarianni, L.J., and Jefferies, T.M. (1999) Sperm Chromatin Damage Associated with Male Smoking, *Mut. Res. 423*, 103–111.
86. Potts, R.J., Notarianni, L.J., and Jefferies, T.M. (2000) Seminal Plasma Reduces Exogenous Oxidative Damage to Human Sperm, Determined by the Measurement of DNA Strand Breaks and Lipid Peroxidation, *Mut. Res. 447*, 249–256.

Index

and GSH, 198, 199, 201, 234
hyperactivated, 136, 197
α-linoleic acid supplementation, 44
and linolenic acid, 154
and lipid peroxidation, 26, 188
and lipids components, 87
MDA production and, 217
n-3 fatty acid supplementation studies,
   44–45
PUFA, 186
and ROS, 163
and selenium levels, 222
and smoking, 252
and storage, 68
swim-up method, 33
Sperm plasma membrane
   biochemical constitution, 185
   fluidity, 69
   lipid composition, 24
   oxidative damage of, 6
   remodeling of, 24
   stabilizing, 230–231
   and vitamin E, 230–231
Sperm quality
   dietary supplementation, 109
   factors affecting, 3
   in last decades, 250
Sulfogalactosylglycerolipid. *See* SGG
Superoxidase dismutase (SOD), 219–221
Swim-up, 33, 166

T

TAC, 171
Tamoxifen, 5
Testicular cells, elongation of, 15
Testicular lipids
   incorporation of PUFA into, 18
   unsaturated fatty acids, 11
Testicular maturation, 24
Testis
   and aging, 192
   22-carbon PUFA, 17
   dietary supplementation in birds, 109
   enzyme activity in, 192

fatty acid composition in, 11
PHGPx activity in, 191–192
selenium concentration in, 222
undescended, 102
Testosterone, 102
α-tocopherol, 161, 194, 195, 230, 256
Topoisomerase II (topo II), 164
Toxic agents, 3
Trolox
   capability of, 255
   DNA strand breaks, 261
   effectiveness of, 255–256
Tuna orbita oil, 80
22:5n-6, 11
22:6n-3, 11, 12. *See also* Docosahexaenoic
   acid

U

Unsaturated fatty acids, 17
Utero-vaginal glands (UVG), 75

V

Varicocele, 3
Varicocelectomy, 173
Vitamic C. *See* Ascorbic acid
Vitamin D, 122
Vitamin E, 7, 65, 109, 161, 196
   in avian semen, 229–230
   concentration, 229
   as a dietary supplement, 229, 230
   and lipid peroxidation, 231–232
   recycling, 229
   and semen storage, 69

Z

ZP binding
   decrease in, 134
   inhibiting, 130–131
   initial, 131
   SGG role in, 131
   site, 129, 131
Zymosterol, 122